Handbook of Home Nutrition Support

Carol S. Ireton-Jones, PhD, RD, LD, CNSD, FACN

Nutrition Therapy Specialist
Carrollton, TX

Mark H. DeLegge, MD, FACG, AGAF, FASGE

Director of Nutrition
Digestive Disease Center
Medical University of South Carolina
Charleston, SC

JONES AND BARTLETT PUBLISHERS
Sudbury, Massachusetts
BOSTON   TORONTO   LONDON   SINGAPORE

World Headquarters
Jones and Bartlett Publishers
40 Tall Pine Drive
Sudbury, MA 01776
978-443-5000
info@jbpub.com
www.jbpub.com

Jones and Bartlett Publishers Canada
6339 Ormindale Way
Mississauga, Ontario
L5V 1J2
CANADA

Jones and Bartlett Publishers International
Barb House, Barb Mews
London W6 7PA
UK

Jones and Bartlett's books and products are available through most bookstores and online booksellers. To contact Jones and Bartlett Publishers directly, call 800-832-0034, fax 978-443-8000, or visit our website www.jbpub.com.

Substantial discounts on bulk quantities of Jones and Bartlett's publications are available to corporations, professional associations, and other qualified organizations. For details and specific discount information, contact the special sales department at Jones and Bartlett via the above contact information or send an email to specialsales@jbpub.com.

The editors and the publisher have made every effort to ensure that contributors to the *Home Nutrition Support* materials are knowledgeable authorities in their fields. Readers are nevertheless advised that the statements and opinions are provided as guidelines and should not be construed as official policy. The recommendations in this publication or the accompanying resource manual do not indicate an exclusive course of treatment. Variations taking into account the individual circumstances, nature of medical oversight, and local protocols may be appropriate. The editors and the publisher disclaim any liability or responsibility for the consequences of any action taken in reliance on these statements or opinions.

Library of Congress Cataloging-in-Publication Data
Handbook of home nutrition support / [edited by] Carol S. Ireton-Jones, Mark H. DeLegge.
p. ; cm.

Includes bibliographical references.
ISBN-13: 978-0-7637-4769-5 (alk. paper)
ISBN-10: 0-7637-4769-6 (alk. paper)
1. Parenteral feeding--Handbooks, manuals, etc. 2. Home nursing--Handbooks, manuals, etc. 3. Home care services--Handbooks, manuals, etc. 4. Nutrition counseling--Handbooks, manuals, etc. I. Ireton-Jones, Carol S. II. DeLegge, Mark H.
[DNLM: 1. Nutritional Support. 2. Home Care Services. WB 410 H2355 2007]
RM224.H3644 2007
615.8'54--dc22
2006034286

Production Credits
Publisher: Michael Brown
Production Director: Amy Rose
Associate Production Editor: Rachel Rossi
Associate Editor: Katey Birtcher
Marketing Manager: Wendy Thayer

Manufacturing Buyer: Therese Connell
Composition: ATLIS
Cover Design: Kristin E. Ohlin
Printing and Binding: Malloy Inc.
Cover Printing: Malloy Inc.

Printed in the United States of America
10 09 08 07 06   10 9 8 7 6 5 4 3 2 1

CPSIA information can be obtained
at www.ICGtesting.com
Printed in the USA
LVHW090117230521
688250LV00004B/207

9 798735 547839

Table of Contents

Preface

Nutrition support spans the spectrum of medical intervention from nutrition counseling to the provision of enteral and parenteral nutrition. At one time, the delivery of aggressive nutritional support could only occur in the hospital setting. Thanks to the pioneering efforts of a number of individuals, the provision of enteral and parenteral nutrition and other related infusion therapies (chemotherapy, antibiotics, biological agents) can now be delivered in the home environment. Experience with home nutrition therapies over the past 25 years has allowed patients to receive safe, effective nutrition therapy in the home setting. This has resulted in better patient quality of life, more involvement of patients in their medical nutrition therapy, and significant healthcare resource savings. A multidisciplinary team approach (physician, dietitian, pharmacist, nurse) to the care of these complex patients has become the standard of care. National organizations, such as the American Society for Parenteral and Enteral Nutrition have dedicated resources to establishing national guidelines for the delivery of enteral and parenteral nutrition at home and serve as an ongoing continuing education forum for clinicians practicing home nutrition support. The Oley Foundation, in Albany, NY, has evolved as a support organization for patients receiving enteral and parenteral nutrition at home. This book serves as a comprehensive review of the many aspects of the delivery of parenteral and enteral nutrition support at home.

Carol S. Ireton-Jones
Mark H. DeLegge

v

Dedication

This book is dedicated to Michael, Bill, Megan, Robbyn, Robin, and Colyn W. who taught me about real life on home nutrition support. They are living life to the fullest!

This book is also dedicated to pharmacists Amberley, Suzi, and Mindy and nurses Deborah and LeaAnn, the home care clinicians I learned from as they provided top notch care to their patients;

To Dr. Charles Baxter and Dr. William W. Turner, my mentors extraordinaire in nutrition support;

To Dr. Mark DeLegge, a wealth of knowledge in nutrition, nutrition support, and medicine, who is also always a pleasure to work with;

Finally, to my family Jim, Lauren, and Krissy, and Mom who provide support for me at home daily!

CIJ

This book is dedicated to Carol, Melinda, Alyce, Trisha, Karen, Mary, English, Chris, Ali, Amy, Addy, Emily, Kristen, Kristin, Jennifer, Carrie, Laura, Debbie, Kiely, and Kelley, an outstanding group of dietitians. It is also dedicated to Kathy, a world class doctor of pharmacy and Greg, a physician's assistant with compassion and extraordinary nutrition knowledge.

I would also like to thank my family Becky, Garrett, Madison, and Taylor who have always been there when I needed them.

MD

CHAPTER 1

Introduction to Home Infusion Therapy

Marc Stranz, Pharm D; Mark H. DeLegge, MD,
FACG, AGAF, FASGE; Carol S. Ireton-Jones,
PhD, RD, LD, CNSD, FACN; Betsy Rothley, RN,
NP; and Rafael Barrera, MD

INTRODUCTION

As many as 30 million adults and children in the United States will require medical treatment or supportive services during any particular time period. A large number of these will require home health care, including home infusion therapy. The National Home Infusion Association describes home infusion as the administration of medications, nutrients, or other solutions intravenously, subcutaneously, enterally, or epidurally to patients outside of the hospital. Like inpatient treatment, home infusion therapy encompasses a wide range of products and services and has frequently been described as a "hospital without walls."[1] Home infusion therapy for stable, non-life threatening conditions is considered a standard of practice in the United States. Provision of infusion therapy services at home is a continuum of the therapy that was provided to the patient in the hospital setting.

There are a variety of services and therapies that can be provided in the home setting in addition to home infusion therapy. These services include respiratory therapies, occupational and physical therapy, speech therapy, nursing services, home health aides, and companions and sit-

1

ters. In general, these services may be provided through a hospital-based home healthcare company or as a separate home healthcare commercial entity. These commercial entities may have a local, regional, or national presence.

Infusion therapies provided in the home setting are generally the most complex home services provided. This includes anti-infective therapies, inotropic therapies, pain management, chemotherapy, blood transfusions, and home parenteral or enteral nutrition (HPEN).[2,3] Virtually any medication that can be provided in the hospital or clinic can also be provided in the home setting. Yet because of the circumstances, home infusion therapy can be one of the most complex health care situations, with multiple professionals working in a highly coordinated manner without ever seeing each other or sharing a medical record. The structure and organization of the care team, which may consist of the physician, the patient, the pharmacist, the nurse, and the dietitian, is essential to achieving anticipated outcomes.

The major reason for providing these services in the home is cost savings coupled with patient convenience and an improved patient quality of life. Dalovisio and associates demonstrated that the costs of providing intravenous antibiotics in the home were 15% of the cost of providing the same therapy in the hospital and 22% of the cost of providing the same therapy in a skilled nursing facility.[1] A separate study by Esmond and associates compared antibiotic treatment at home or in the hospital for upper respiratory tract infections in patients with cystic fibrosis.[4] Quality of life parameters were better in patients treated in the home setting. The provision of home parenteral nutrition (HPN) has been shown to be cost effective, saving up to 70% of the cost of providing the same parenteral therapy for patients in the hospital setting.[5]

HOME NUTRITION SUPPORT AND HOME NUTRITION SUPPORT TEAMS

Parenteral nutrition and enteral nutrition support in a hospital environment is often delivered through a fragmented system. A dietitian, a pharmacist, a nurse, or a physician may take responsibility for advising clinicians on their patient's nutritional status and for suggesting and monitoring nutritional therapy. In some facilities, comprehensive nutrition support teams (NSTs) have evolved. These teams consist of a nurse, a dietitian, a pharmacist, and often a physician working together to provide a cohesive approach to nutritional therapy. Multidisciplinary NSTs have been shown to improve patient care and patient outcomes by creating treatment protocols and controlling overall costs. With the recent trend for shorter hospital stays, often only the sickest patients are hospitalized. This results in more complex patients who experience nutrition-related problems being treated outside of the hospital setting. The Home Nutrition Support Team (HNST) transfers the successful multidisciplinary inpatient nutrition management concept to the outpatient setting. The HNST is responsible for not only monitoring a patient on HPN or home enteral nutrition (HEN), but also determining the goals of nutrition therapy including wound healing, weight maintenance, muscle mass maintenance, and improvement of a patient's quality of life.[6,7]

OTHER COMMON HOME INFUSION THERAPIES

In addition to HPEN, many patients at home also require one or more additional infusion therapies. Most commonly prescribed additional therapies are anti-infective therapies and pain management therapies. The patients may be discharged with these therapies or the therapies may be initiated in the home while the patient is receiving HPEN. Patients who are receiving intravenous anti-infectives, pain management, or other infusion therapies at home may also have parenteral or enteral nutrition initiated in the home. Any therapy initiated for a patient in the home setting must begin with a careful evaluation of the patient's clinical status in order to ensure success.

Anti-Infectives

Careful consideration needs to be given to many drug and patient factors before taking the steps to administer or initiate intravenous antibiotics or antifungals in the home environment. These considerations include:

- Safety profile of the agent
- Previous patient history of agent tolerance
- Ability to achieve adequate penetration into the target tissues and fluids
- Profile of the agent as to either a long half-life or a half-life convenient for home dosing

- Specificity of the infection as demonstrated through appropriate cultures
- Stability of the agent after mixing or preparation in a manner to retain needed stability prior to dosing

A randomized study compared the use of antibiotics at home for infectious processes compared to similar regimens provided in the hospital.[8] Total treatment time duration averaged 11 days. Quality of life of the home antibiotic infused group was maintained. The cost of home infusion was 50% less than that of hospital-based infusion.

The Infectious Disease Society of America has published guidelines for the delivery of antimicrobial therapy in the home setting.[9] Their guidelines state that the literature supports the use of outpatient parenteral antimicrobial therapy (OPAT). They stress the need for communication between the physician, the patient, and the members of the home infusion therapy team. They also stress the importance of continuing clinical outcome measures of OPAT to ensure therapy effectiveness and quality of care.

Pain and Symptom Management

Pain and pain-related symptoms that are not well controlled become the primary impetus for hospital readmissions and emergency room visitations for patients with varying disease processes. Home management of pain issues provides a proactive solution for the prevention of hospital visitation and creates an environment to augment a patient's quality of life.

The least invasive route of pain management therapy administration is preferred, including oral, rectal, and topical alternatives. When concurrent disease processes impede these routes from being used, or when the pain or related symptoms remain unstable, invasive pain management therapies, such as intravenous, subcutaneous, or intrathecal delivery, is optimal. Once these routes are maximized for pain and symptom control, and as the disease exacerbation is declining, these invasive pain management modalities can be weaned and transitioned back to a less invasive therapy. The arena of postoperative regional nerve block anesthesia with continuous infusion at home has become a therapy that now can be delivered, which offers yet another alternative to the pain management regimen.[10,11]

Home pain management requires proper assessment and development of a plan of care. Changes or adjustments in pain management therapy require assessment for patient tolerance and continued pain therapy adjustment until patient comfort is achieved. In order to obtain these goals, the patient's primary disease process, previous pain management history, psychological profile, social situation, home environment and concurrent medical regimen must also be thoroughly assessed. Controlling pain often has a very positive effect on the medical management of the patient's overall disease process and co-morbidities.

Inotropic Therapy

Outpatient positive inotropic support and implantation of an automatic implantable cardiac defibrillator (AICD) may be used as a successful bridge to cardiac transplantation in patients with end-stage heart failure.[12] Upadya reported on a $70,000–120,000 per patient cost savings for patients awaiting heart transplantation for heart failure when treated with a home inotropic therapy/AICD regimen as compared to in-hospital treatment. Outpatient inotropic therapy is not only cost-effective and efficacious, but also safe to deliver in the home setting.[13]

CONCLUSION

The multidisciplinary team allows complex medical patients to be treated in the home setting safely and effectively. Medical technology has assisted in this movement of therapies from the hospital to the home setting. Portable, small ambulatory infusion pumps allow continuous low volume delivery of nutrition, medication, or chemotherapy.[14] Pre-filled syringes can accommodate for decreased strength or fine motor skills of patients or their families, disabilities which could otherwise impact therapy delivery. Elastomeric pumping devices can be pre-filled and can allow the delivery of a medication without electricity, pump programming, or alarm difficulties.[15] Attention to all components of the home infusion therapy model including the patient, clinician personnel, physician oversight, home environment, office delivery capabilities, psychosocial patient issues, therapy risks and benefits, and desired outcomes will ensure positive patient experiences.

REFERENCES

1. Available at http://www.nhianet.org/ppopresources/index.html#overview. Accessed June 13, 2006.
2. Szterling LN. Home blood transfusion, a four-year experience. *Transfus Apher Sci.* 2005;33:253–256.
3. Ramsey KM, Vande Waa JAA. Outpatient parenteral antibiotic therapy; not so crazy after all these years. *South Med J.* 2005;98:590–595.
4. Esmond G, Butler M, Mccormack AM. Comparison of hospital and home intravenous antibiotic therapy in adults with cystic fibrosis. *J Clin Nurs.* 2006;15:52–60.
5. Wesley JR. Nutrition support teams: past, present and future. *Nutr Clin Pract.* 1995;10(6):219–228.
6. Schattner M, Barrera R, Nygard S, Scott F, Quesada O, Brown P, Shike M. Outcome of long term home enteral nutrition in patients with malignant dysphagia. *Nutr Clin Pract.* 2001;16:292–295.
7. Barrera R, Schattner M, Nygard S, Ahdoot M, Ahdoot A, Adeyeye S, Groeger J, Shike M. Outcome of direct percutaneous endoscopic jejunostomy tube placement for nutritional support in critically ill, mechanically ventilated patients. *J Crit Care.* 2001;16(4):178–181.
8. Wolter JM, Cagney RA, McCormack JG. A randomized trial of home vs hospital intravenous antibiotic therapy in adults with infectious diseases. *J Infect.* 2004;48(3):263–268.
9. Tice AD, Rehm SJ, Dalvovisio JR, et al. Practice guidelines for outpatient parenteral antimicrobial therapy. *Clin Infect Dis.* 2004;38:1651–1672.
10. Ilfeld BM, Enneking FK. Continuous peripheral nerve blocks at home: a review. *Anesth Analg.* 2005;100(6):1822–1833.
11. Greengrass RA, Nielsen KC. Management of peripheral nerve block catheters at home. *Int Anesthesiol Clin.* 2005 Summer; 43(3):79–87.
12. Upadya SP, Sedrakyan A, Saldarriaga C, et al. Comparative costs of home inotropic infusion versus in-hospital care in patients awaiting cardiac transplantation. *J Card Fail.* 2004;10(5):384–389.
13. Gorski LA. Positive inotropic drug infusions for the patient with heart failure. *Home Care Provid.* 2001;6(3):78–80.
14. Bean CA. High-tech homecare infusion therapies. *Crit Care Nurs Clin North Am.* 1998;10(3):287–303.
15. Oseland SA, Querciagrossa AJ. Collaboration of nursing and pharmacy in home infusion therapy. *Home Healthc Nurse.* 2003;21(12):818–826.

CHAPTER 2

What is Home Nutrition Support?

Theresa Han-Markey, MS, RD, CNSD

WHAT IS HOMECARE?

Health care services provided in the home setting have evolved over the past 20 years. "homecare" is a general term describing a wide range of health and social services.[1] As the delivery of health care increasingly moves from the hospital to the home environment, some researchers have fashioned the phrase "dehospitalization."[2] Table 2–1 lists potential services available in the homecare setting.

Clinicians have successfully "dehospitalized" both enteral nutrition (EN) support and parenteral nutrition (PN) support. Home nutrition support (EN or PN) improves patients' or clients' quality of life and can be cost effective when compared to hospitalized nutrition support delivery in certain patient populations. Researchers today debate the cost-effectiveness of homecare services to frail, elderly individuals as compared to nursing home care.[3] However, this chapter will be limited in its scope to nutrition support in appropriate home candidates.

MALNUTRITION IN THE HOME CARE SETTING

Estimates of the incidence of malnutrition in the home care setting range from 5% to upwards of 50%.[3,4] In 1998, home care agencies in the United States documented an increase in health care costs associated

---

TABLE 2–1   Spectrum of Available Home Health Care Services

Skilled care (Under the direction of a physician):

1. Services provided by health care professionals, such as nurses and therapists

2. Activities, such as home dialysis, medical social work and physical therapy

Home support services:

1. Activities of Daily Living assistance, such as getting in and out of bed, walking, bathing, toileting, and dressing

2. Light housecleaning

3. Running errands

4. Meal preparation

5. Laundry

6. Companionship

Reference: http://www.mayoclinic.com

---

with malnutrition.[5] Recent work utilizing the Mini Nutritional Assessment tool in a South Australian population identified approximately 42% of 250 homecare clients aged 67–99 years old who were either at risk of malnutrition or malnourished.[6] Though over-nutrition or obesity has now become a global threat, clinicians must remain vigilant and be adept at nutrition screening for under-nutrition in the homecare population. Nutrition screening and assessment are integral components of home care. As of 1999–2000, the Joint Commission on Accreditation of Healthcare Organizations (JCAHO) standards require homecare providers to perform nutrition screening of all homecare patients at moderate to high risk.[7] A 2003 publication confirms the association of moderate and large weight loss and risk of nursing facility admission.[8] This study utilized a large cohort of data available longitudinally and included 6,746 white subjects. The moderate and large weight loss groups had 1.60 and 2.41 hazard ratios, respectively, as compared to weight maintenance groups for nursing care facility admission.

Malnutrition in homecare patients results in adverse clinical complications such as poor wound healing, increased infection rate, and increased falls.[9] Malnourished patients also utilize more health care resources, which is measured by hospital length of stay, homecare agency visits, physician visits, and drug utilization. In addition, malnourished patients, once hospitalized, have an increased risk of developing other complications such as pneumonia, increasing their morbidity and mortality. Homecare clinicians strive to keep clients well nourished, replete the malnourished, and thereby prevent hospitalization. Most general homecare patients do not require specialized home nutrition support services such as EN or PN support. If malnutrition is suspected or a patient has a disease process such as diabetes, renal disease, or cancer, then the patient can benefit from one or several visits with a dietitian employed by the homecare provider or the hospital where the patient is seen for his or her disease management. Patients who are discharged while on PN or EN support need specialized services to ensure successful therapy outcomes. General homecare services such as durable medical equipment supplies, nursing aides, or home health aides often provide adjunct services and supplies to many home nutrition support patients.

HOME NUTRITION SUPPORT MODALITIES

Home nutrition support, via EN or PN, is a specialized aspect of homecare. Clinicians deliver both modalities of nutrition support to clients in a home setting. The enteral route is the delivery of nutrition therapy by way of the gastrointestinal tract. Enteral access devices such as gastrostomy (stomach) or jejunostomy (small intestine) tubes are placed in a clinical setting. Patients receive training on enteral formula administration and enteral access device maintenance either in the hospital prior to discharge or in the home prior to initiation of therapy. Patient and/or caregiver independence with nutrition therapy is the overall goal of home nutrition support services. Depending on the enteral feeding provider, patients may receive little or no clinical monitoring in the home, such as with a Durable Medical Company provider (DME) or regular clinical monitoring and assessment of the enteral nutrition (EN) therapy by nutrition support clinicians such as with a home infusion provider.[10]

Parenteral nutrition (PN) support is the delivery of nutrition therapy intravenously. Clients receive intravenous macro- and micronutrients through peripheral, or more commonly, central venous access. Parenteral nutrition delivery requires close clinical monitoring because of its complexity and associated potential complications. Regular assessment of a patient's fluid and electrolytes, nutritional status, vitamin and mineral status, disease status, and quality of life are imperative. Central venous catheter (CVC) maintenance care and complication prevention education by the HNS team improves overall patient outcomes. A provider of home PN support should have experienced clinicians and support personnel to work with the patient and caregiver to obtain the best health care outcomes. Most often home PN is provided by a home infusion company specialized in providing high tech home infusion therapy such as PN.

INDICATIONS FOR HOME NUTRITION SUPPORT

A patient's medical condition and overall nutrition assessment determines their clinical need for PN or EN support. Whether the patient resides in an acute care facility or is being transitioned to their home, these medical indications for therapy do not differ.[11] Patients requiring EN support cannot voluntarily meet their nutrition requirements by mouth. These patients have a functioning gastrointestinal tract. Home enteral nutrition is commonly used in patients with stroke induced dysphagia, head and neck cancers, gastroparesis and other neurological disorders affecting the ability to swallow (see Chapter 9). Parenteral nutrition supports patients who have a nonfunctioning gastrointestinal tract to maintain a well-nourished nutritional status. Utilizing a nutrition registry, a 2005 publication identified the top five CPT codes for patient receiving home parenteral nutrition as malabsorption, pancreatic disease, regional enteritis (Crohn's disease), intestinal obstruction, and nutritional deficiency.[12] The need for PN may be temporary or permanent (see Chapter 8).

Home care standards for nutrition support exist and are updated on a routine basis.[13] The homecare company delivering these nutrition services should have written policies and procedures addressing the management of home EN or PN. In addition to patient's nutritional medical suitability for these therapies, other equally important factors must be evaluated in order for HNS to be successful. These assessments include home environment evaluation, social and economic constraints, educational abilities, and psychosocial factors.[6]

THE BENEFITS OF HOME NUTRITION SUPPORT

The quality of the patient or client's life can be improved with home EN or PN. Home EN caregivers for children with cerebral palsy report significant improvement in physical, social, and emotional functioning six months after gastrostomy tube placement.[14] Caregivers also play a large role in developing an acceptable feeding schedule and improved medication delivery techniques in their children, giving them a sense of control over their child's nutritional and medical issues. A study published in 2004 documented that care time for children requiring gastrostomy tube feeding is significantly greater than those without a tube; however, both maternal caregiver groups did not differ in depressive mood measures.[15] Maternal caregivers of tube fed children were no less satisfied with their lives compared to maternal caregivers of children without tube feeding. In adult patients requiring home EN, quality of life, measured by functional and symptom scales, improved in both neurologically intact and modestly impaired individuals.[16] Malnutrition impacted these patients' quality of life. Once nutritional status improved, patients experienced improved physical functioning and decreased fatigue.

Patients receiving home PN often improve their nutritional status and subsequently improve physical and functional progress. However, lifelong PN dependency results in depressive tendencies, chronic disease complications, and other psychosocial problems.[17] homecare providers should assess psychosocial coping issues and suggest patient referrals to appropriate ancillary medical personnel for treatment. A 2004 nursing study documented the impact on health insurance changes on the quality of life in 29 home PN patients.[18] As the increase in health care costs shift toward employees, the financial and psychological impact on home PN patients must be considered. This study documented that changes in insurance providers was associated with an increase in home PN patient depression.

Numerous studies have documented the cost-effectiveness of HNS services as compared to hospital-based care. A retrospective study in Brazil reported an average $3100 per patient savings when nutrition care was administered in the home versus the hospital.[2] The hospital also had a higher bed rotation and decreased length of hospital stay. These authors reference a number of other publications supporting the overall health care savings in home-based delivery of nutrition support. Costs between homecare and residential care have also been studied.[19] Costs for community clients were significantly less than residential clients, even when informal caregivers' time was assigned an associated wage.

Residential care was more expensive because of facility related expenses such as room and board.

A.S.P.E.N. GUIDELINES AND STANDARDS FOR HOME NUTRITION SUPPORT

The American Society for Parenteral and Enteral Nutrition (A.S.P.E.N.) is an organization contsisting of health care professionals representing medicine, nursing, pharmacy, dietetics, and nutrition science.[11] The mission of A.S.P.E.N. is to serve as a preeminent, interdisciplinary, research-based patient-centered clinical nutrition society throughout the world. The A.S.P.E.N. organization promulgates safe and effective patient care by nutrition support practitioners, and clinical guidelines assist in this mission. The guidelines were created in accordance with the Institute of Medicine recommendations as "systematically developed statements to assist practitioner and patient decisions about appropriate health care for specific clinical circumstances." The following A.S.P.E.N. practice guidelines are specific to home specialized nutrition support (HSNS):

1. HSNS should be used in patients who cannot meet their nutrient requirements by oral intake and who are able to receive therapy outside of an acute care setting.
2. When HSNS is required, home enteral nutrition is the preferred route of administration when feasible.
3. When HSNS is indicated, home parenteral nutrition should be used when the gastrointestinal tract is not functional and in patients who cannot be adequately supported with home enteral nutrition.

These guidelines are supported by strength of evidence "B" (Table 2–2). This grading is a modified version of the Agency for Health Care Research and Quality, US Department of Health and Human Services method of assessing the strength of clinical evidence. "B" strength states there is fair research-based evidence to support the guideline (well-designed studies without randomization). In addition to these guidelines, A.S.P.E.N. also publishes standards for home nutrition support.[13] These standards aim to ensure sound and efficient home nutrition support care. They represent a fair consensus of A.S.P.E.N.'s membership of the

---

TABLE 2–2   A.S.P.E.N. Clinical Evidence Rating System[12]

Level A: There is good research-based evidence to support the guideline (prospective, randomized trials).

Level B: There is fair research-based evidence to support the guideline (well-designed studies without randomization).

Level C: The guideline is based on expert opinion and editorial consensus.

TABLE 2–3   Competent Care Required of homecare Delivery Companies

1. Definitions of Terms

2. Organization

3. Nutrition Screening

4. Nutrition Assessment

5. Patient Selection

6. Development of a Nutrition Care Plan

7. Implementation and Education

8. Patient Monitoring

9. Review and Revision of the Nutrition Care Plan

10. Termination of Therapy

---

range of performance of competent care that should be subscribed to by any homecare organization providing these services (Table 2–3).

HOW TO CHOOSE A HOMECARE COMPANY

Patients often receive an introduction to home health care services upon discharge from a hospital or another health care setting. Discharge coordinators and social workers provide information on homecare providers to patients and families. Patients and families should ask for a list of community providers. The decision of which homecare agency or home infusion provider to choose should be as important as choosing a physician. In addition, there are "checklist" questions that patients and families can use to assist in choosing their home nutrition support provider.[20,21] Table 2–4 lists questions which should assist in the selection of a provider.

TABLE 2–4   Patient Questions for Choosing a Home Health Care
Provider

1. Does the agency serve my community? How long has the company been serving
   my community?
2. Does the provider supply literature explaining its services, eligibility requirements,
   fees, and funding sources?
3. Does the provider furnish patients with a detailed "Patient Bill of Rights?"
4. What kind of training does the agency require for caregivers? Will the same
   caregiver be sent to my home for each visit?
5. What are the procedures to handle emergencies? Are caregivers available 24
   hours a day, seven days a week?
6. Is there a written plan of care for each patient? Does the agency involve the
   patient and caregivers in designing the plan and educate them about the care
   provided?
7. Can the provider supply a list of references, such as doctors, discharge planners,
   patients or their family members who are familiar with the provider's quality of
   service?

SUMMARY

Homecare and HNS has rapidly evolved over the past 25 years. The intensity of care of today's homecare patient requires a home health care team that can deliver a wide range of clinically competent and socially sensitive medical interventions. The quality of care provided to home patients has a direct impact on hospital readmissions and on patient quality of life.

REFERENCES

1. How to Choose a homecare Provider. 1996. Available at: http://www.nahc.
   org/consumer/wihc.html. Accessed February 18, 2005.
2. Baxter YC, Dias MC, Maculevicius J, et al. Economic study in surgical patients of a new model of nutrition therapy integrating hospital and home vs the conventional hospital model. *JPEN*. 2005;29(suppl 1):S96–S105.
3. Posner BM, Jette A, Smigelski C, et al. Nutritional risk in New England elders. *J Gerontol*. 1994;49(3):M123–M124.
4. http://www.aafp.org/x16093.xml. Accessed March 1, 2005.
5. Gallagher-Allred CR, Vott AC, Koop KL. The effect of medical nutrition therapy on malnutrition and clinical outcomes. *Nutrition*. 1999;15(6): 512–514.

6. Visvanathan R, Macintosh C, Callary M, et al. The nutritional status of 250 older Australian recipients of domiciliary care services and its association with outcomes at 12 months. *J Am Geriatr Soc.* 2003;51(7):1007–1011.

7. Joint Commission: 1999–2000 Comprehensive Accreditation Manual for homecare. Oakbrook Terrace, Ill: Joint Commission on Accreditation of Health Care Organization; 1998.

8. Zizza C, Herring A, Domino M, et al. The effect of weight change on nursing care facility admission in the NHANES I Epidemiologic Followup Survey. *J Clin Epidemiol.* 2003;56(9):906–913.

9. Arnaud-Battandier F, Malvy D, Jeandel C, et al. Use of oral supplements in malnourished elderly patients living in the community: a pharmacoeconomic study. *Clin Nutr.* 2004;23(5):1096–1103.

10. Ireton-Jones C. Home enteral nutrition from the provider's perspective. *JPEN.* 2002 Sep-Oct;26(suppl 5):S8–S9.

11. August D, Teitelbaum DH, Albina J, et al. Guidelines for the use of parenteral and enteral nutrition in adult and pediatric patients. *JPEN.* 2002;26(1): 14SA–21SA.

12. Ireton-Jones C, DeLegge M. Home parenteral nutrition registry: a five-year retrospective evaluation of outcomes of patients receiving home parenteral nutrition support. *Nutrition.* 2005;21(2):156–160.

13. ASPEN Board of Directors. Standards for home nutrition support. *Nutr Clin Pract.* 1999;14(3);151–162.

14. Sullivan PB, Juszczak E, Bachlet AM, et al. Impact of gastrostomy tube feeding on the quality of life of carers of children with cerebral palsy. *Dev Med Child Neurol.* 2004;46(12):796–800.

15. Heyman MB, Harmatz P, Acree M, et al. Economic and psychologic costs for maternal caregivers of gastrostomy-dependent children. *J Pediatr.* 2004;145(4):511–516.

16. Loeser C, von Herz U, Kuchler T, et al. Quality of life and nutritional State in Patients on Home Enteral Tube Feeding. *Nutrition.* 2003;19(7–8): 605–611.

17. Persoon A, Huisman-de Waal G, Naber TA, et al. Impact of long-term HPN on daily life in adults. *Clin Nutr.* 2005;24(2):304–313.

18. Gaskamp CD. Quality of life and changes in health insurance in long-term homecare. *Nurs Econ.* 2004;22(3):135–139.

19. Chappell NL, Dlitt HB, Hollander MJ, et al. Comparative costs of homecare and Residential Care. *Gerontologist.* 2004;44(3):389–400.

20. Home health checklist [American Association for Homecare Web site]. Available at: http://www.aahomecare.org/displaycommon.cfm?an=1&sub articlenbr=85. Accessed March 28, 2005.

21. How to choose a homecare provider. Available at: http://www.nahc.org/Consumer/hdistrhcp.html. Accessed March 28, 2005.

CHAPTER 3

Preparing the Patient for Discharge on Home Nutrition Support

M. Patricia Fuhrman, MS, RD, LD, FADA, CNSD

INTRODUCTION

Although on the surface it appears relatively simple to send a patient home on nutrition support, there are nuances about home nutrition support that when understood can facilitate the patient's discharge. Table 3–1 delineates some of the management and philosophical differences between acute care and home care. The patient is now a consumer who can choose his/her home infusion provider. The patient and care partner are most often the individuals responsible for infusing the therapy. Overall, home nutrition support focuses on incorporation of the therapy into the patient's lifestyle.

The American Society for Parenteral and Enteral Nutrition (A.S.P.E.N.) has published practice guidelines for home nutrition support.[1] Home nutrition support is indicated when patients cannot meet nutrient requirements with oral diet and it is possible to provide nutrition therapy outside the acute care setting. As always, enteral nutrition, when feasible, is preferred over parenteral. Parenteral nutrition (PN) is indicated when the patient cannot meet nutritional needs via the gastrointestinal (GI) tract or when the GI tract is not functional. The American Society for Parenteral and Enteral Nutrition practice guide-

TABLE 3–1   Differences in Nutrition Support in Acute Care and at Home

	Acute Care	Home Care
Terminology	Patient	Consumer
Nutritional regimen	Provided by nurse and healthcare providers	Provided by consumer and care partner(s)
Management	Crisis management	Life management
Goals of therapy	Sustain patient during critical illness Survival	Optimize health and well-being Improving quality of life
Nutrient requirements	Permissive underfeeding with high protein	Meet needs for weight loss, gain or maintenance with modest protein
Complications	Hyperglycemia Acute fluid/electrolyte management Sepsis Diarrhea Aspiration Immune compromise	Hyper/hypoglycemia Long-term fluid and electrolyte management Infection/sepsis Constipation/diarrhea Dehydration Hepatic steatosis/cholestasis Metabolic bone disease Micronutrient inadequacies and excesses Feeding access malfunction and breakage
Frustrations	Inconsistent delivery of nutrition Residual volumes	Consumer compliance with regimen Therapy reimbursement—meeting Medicare and commercial insurance guidelines
Nutrients	Antioxidants Specialty formulas Conditionally essential amino acids	Justification for specialty enteral formulations Provision of specialty PN formulas

Reprinted with permission from Fuhrman MP, Newton A. Transitioning the Patient from Acute Care to Home Care [DNS Home & Alternate Site Home Page]. Available at: http://www.dnsdpg.org. Accessed 11/06/06.

lines and standards also recommend discharge planning and follow-up be performed by an interdisciplinary team consisting of a dietitian, pharmacist, physician, and nurse.[1,2]

SELECTING A HOME INFUSION PROVIDER

The first step to discharging a patient on home nutrition support is to determine who will manage the patient at home. This needs to be the initial step because the home infusion provider is an active participant in the decision of whether the patient is a candidate for home nutrition support and proactively determines the patient's reimbursement for the therapies needed.

Essential components and attributes of a home infusion provider are given in Table 3–2. Policies and procedures should be in place that delineate clinician roles and competencies, describe processes and criteria for care, and address patient admission, management, education, and discharge-from-service.[2] There should also be an emergency preparedness plan for the home infusion provider and for their patients.

A home infusion provider should also be selected based on reported quantitative and qualitative outcomes.[2,3] A list of questions to ask about the experience and outcomes of a home infusion provider is given in Table 3–3. One of the most important questions is what are the outcomes concerning complications and quality of life for the patients.[4] Very little is reported in the literature on home nutrition support outcomes. This is primarily because of the complexities of collecting and interpreting the data as well as the fragmentation of home care.[5]

PATIENT SELECTION

Not all patients who require nutrition support beyond the finite period of hospitalization are candidates for home nutrition support. The patient must be clinically and medically stable for discharge.[6,7] This means that the patient is clearly on the road to recovery with laboratory indices and a physical examination that are relatively predictable versus the labile status during critical illness. The feeding access whether for tube feeding or PN should be a permanent device appropriate for the home. The patient should be tolerating the nutrition support modality. However, it is not necessary for the patient to be at full formula volume or infusion rate prior to discharge. Progression of feeding as well as initiation of a cycled regimen can safely and effectively be provided in the home environment by a home nutrition support team.

TABLE 3–2   Essential Components of a Home Nutrition Support Provider

- 24-hour accessibility to clinicians, 7 days per week
- Experienced dietitians, pharmacists, and nurses on staff
- Close contact between the consumer and the home nutrition support provider, regarding deliveries, tolerance, and response to therapy
- An open invitation by the provider to the consumer, physician, case manager, or hospital clinicians to visit the home infusion office and meet the employees
- Adherence to A.S.P.E.N's *Safe Practices for Parenteral Nutrition*
- Willingness to assist with reimbursement questions
- Accurate, timely, and courteous home deliveries
- Routine home visits to monitor response to therapy and access site by the nurse and dietitian
- Nutrition assessments and summaries regularly provided to the physician, case manager, and relevant clinicians

Reprinted with permission from Fuhrman MP, Newton A. Transitioning the Patient from Acute Care to Home Care [DNS Home & Alternate Site Home Page]. Available at: http://www.dnsdpg.org. Accessed 11/06/06.

TABLE 3–3   Questions to Ask Potential Providers of Home Infusion Therapy[3]

1. How many home nutrition support patients do you service per year?
2. How many patients per year do you service with this particular diagnosis?
3. Who manages your home nutrition support patients?
4. Do you perform in-home nutrition assessments?
5. Do you have policies and procedures for managing patients on home nutrition support?
6. What is your rate of complications, particularly catheter-related infections?
7. Can you quantify cost savings that you achieve with effective clinical management?
8. What outcome parameters do you measure? What are your outcomes in these areas? Do you report these outcomes?

The A.S.P.E.N. practice guidelines state that home nutrition support should only be provided if patients have a safe home environment.[1] The home environment should be clean, and have electricity, a safe source of water, storage space for supplies, and refrigeration. A.S.P.E.N. guidelines also state that pediatric patients must have care partners who are able and willing to provide care.[1] Ideally, adults will have a care partner initially, but as the long-term therapy becomes more routine, the patient

TABLE 3–4   Home Nutrition Support Patient Selection Criteria[6,7]

Patient's route of feeding is appropriate for clinical condition

Patient is clinically stable

Patient has permanent feeding access

Patient and care partner consent to therapy at home

Patient and care partner are able and willing to provide therapy

Patient's home environment is safe and adequate

Refrigeration	Water supply
Electricity	Telephone
Storage space	General cleanliness
Work space	Evaluation of safety issues

Supplies and clinical/technical support and follow-up are available

Patient has source of reimbursement for the therapy at home

generally performs the tasks independently with care partners becoming involved only as needed.[6] Table 3–4 lists the criteria for selection of patients for home enteral and parenteral nutrition. If the patient does not fit the criteria for discharge home on nutrition support, then the social worker at the hospital can assist in finding a facility that can take the patient. However, many patients are able to go home on very complex therapies with adequate teaching and support from their home infusion provider.

It is imperative to confirm the patient's reimbursement benefits for nutrition support before sending him or her home. Insurance may dictate the home infusion provider as well as the therapy that the patient can receive at home. If no reimbursement is available, the patient may be willing and able to self-pay for the therapy, but this must be confirmed before discharge. Refer to Chapter 15 on reimbursement.

EDUCATION OF PATIENT AND/OR CARE PARTNER

The goal of educating and training the patient and his or her care partner on the preparation and infusion of home parenteral and enteral therapy is to enable them to independently provide effective and safe therapy in the home. The A.S.P.E.N. practice guidelines recommend that education of patients and care partners is started in the hospital and continued in the home following discharge.[1] Starting the education and training process early in the discharge planning phase enables the home infusion clinician to determine the patient and care partner willingness to perform the tasks needed and to determine the best teaching style to facilitate learning with each patient. Pumps and equipment used at home are smaller and more portable than the equipment used in the hospital. It can be comforting for patients to see what they will actually use at home before they leave the hospital. Teaching should continue after discharge because the home is often a more relaxed, comfortable environment that is more conducive to learning than the hospital. Teaching in the home also gives the home infusion clinician the opportunity to observe the conditions under which the nutrition therapy will be prepared and infused. If it is not feasible to initiate training and education in the hospital, then teaching can begin as soon as the patient gets home.

Education includes hands-on practice of techniques, written materials, and technical and clinical support following discharge. The teaching manual for the patient should have illustrations and step-by-step instructions for tasks. Education should involve demonstration by the patient and care partner of ability to perform all the tasks required for the home enteral or parenteral therapy. The teaching techniques and materials should be based on the patient and care partner's assessed learning needs, capabilities, and readiness to learn.[2] Ideally, the patient's competency is verified yearly because techniques can become less precise over time.

A study in complex inflammatory bowel disease patients found anxiety about managing PN at home decreased from 60% of patients being quite or a little anxious to 13% of patients being a little anxious after one week at home.[8] The greatest contributors to anxiety were concerns about community nursing care (33%), about who to call with problems (33%), and about the safety of the peripherally-inserted central catheter (13%). Education and communication can alleviate the concerns and increase the patient and care partner comfort with home infusion therapy.

COMMUNICATION

The transition of a patient from in-patient management to home nutrition support requires communication between the in-patient management team and the home nutrition support team. Another important aspect of a successful transition of nutrition support from acute care to home is timely referral. It can take time to determine reimbursement status, clarify the most appropriate enteral or parenteral formulation and feeding method for home, and set-up teaching and delivery schedules. Pharmacist to pharmacist communication and documentation is required when patients transfer from one healthcare facility to another or to home to ensure accuracy of the parenteral nutrition prescription.[9]

Experienced home infusion pharmacists, dietitians, and nurses work with the responsible physician to assist in the management of home nutrition support. The PN prescription and enteral orders from the hospital should be carefully reviewed with the physician and modified, if necessary, in order to best meet the patient's nutrition needs in the home care setting. For example, nocturnal feedings may be disruptive to sleep patterns and the patient may prefer daytime infusions. Many patients discharged home on nutrition support may also require additional therapies, such as anti-infectives, pain management, wound care, catheter care, hydration, and blood products. Coordination of these therapies requires competent clinicians and effective communication among all those involved with care. Table 3–5 provides the steps to successful transition from hospital to home for patients on nutrition support.

PATIENT SUPPORT

The focus on clinical management can overlook the personal struggles of the patient and family on home nutrition support. An article by Robbyn Kindle brought to the forefront the challenges and isolation felt by patients on long-term home parenteral nutrition.[10] Winkler and Wetle reported long-term home parenteral nutrition patients using nurturing terms such as "baby" to refer to parenteral nutrition and "umbilical cord" to refer to intravenous tubing.[4] Kindle called her parenteral nutrition "Fred."[10] This emotional connection to a life-saving therapy demonstrates the depth of dependence and familiarity that long-term patients have with their home parenteral nutrition. A study in 30 elderly home enteral patients reported that the patients experienced weight loss, consumed inadequate fluid, and had GI complications following discharge.[11] This study also demonstrated that elderly home enteral nutrition patients require frequent monitoring, reassessment, and intervention from a multidisciplinary team. The 24/7 availability of the home

---

TABLE 3–5   Steps to Successful Discharge Home on Nutrition Support

1. Identify home infusion provider

2. Determine patient's appropriateness for discharge home
   a. Clinical and medical stability
   b. Willingness to perform therapy
   c. Appropriate home environment
   d. Reimbursement

3. Education on preparation and infusion of therapy
   a. Initiate teaching in hospital and continue after discharge
   b. Teach with equipment and supplies to be used in the home
   c. Written, verbal, and demonstration teaching techniques
   d. Have patient demonstrate competency

4. Identify who will write nutrition prescription and monitor outcomes of patient following discharge
   a. Determine timing and method of communication preferred
   b. Distribute contact information to patient, home infusion provider, and physician

5. Finalize nutrition prescription prior to discharge
   a. Determine appropriateness of nutrition formula for home
   b. Specify infusion schedule
   c. Determine schedule for labs and re-ordering nutrition prescription
   d. List nutrition goals and anticipated outcomes

6. Day of discharge
   a. Supplies and formula are delivered to the home if not already done
   b. Home infusion clinician meets patient at the home to begin therapy

---

nutrition support team clinicians provides a connection for the patient for troubleshooting clinical problems as well as for sharing personal challenges and triumphs. The Oley Foundation is a national support group and advocate for patients on long-term enteral and PN therapy.[12]

SUB-ACUTE CARE AND ALTERNATE SITE DISCHARGE

If a patient is being prepared for discharge on home nutrition support from a community hospital, skilled nursing facility, nursing home, or clinic, there may be fewer resources available for in-house management as well as for facilitation of discharge. In this case it is even more important to involve the home infusion provider as soon as possible to assist with the teaching and discharge process. Many smaller facilities do not have nutrition support teams or nutrition support experts to manage the patients. Nutrition care is often contracted with limited monitoring and evaluation. The home infusion provider will provide nutrition support expertise to optimize the discharge prescription and facilitate the education process for the patient and their care partner. Routine use of the same home infusion provider can create a predictable transition of patient care for all those involved.

SUMMARY

The transition of nutrition support from the acute care or sub-acute care setting to the home can and should be a smooth and natural progression of the recovery process. Although sometimes there are long-term health issues and challenges in the home setting, the consumers and care partners are enthusiastic to be with their families and friends after days, weeks, or months spent away from home. Involving the home infusion provider early in the discharge process improves communication and collaboration among those involved in the transfer of care. The A.S.P.E.N. practice guidelines and standards can provide the necessary tools to identify the aspects of care that should be provided.[1,2]

REFERENCES

1. A.S.P.E.N. Board of Directors and The Clinical Guidelines Task Force. Guidelines for the use of parenteral and enteral nutrition in adult and pediatric patients. *J Parenter Enteral Nutr.* 2002;26(suppl 1):20SA–21SA, 137SA–138SA.
2. American Society for Parenteral and Enteral Nutrition Board of Directors and the Standards for Specialized Nutrition Support Task Force. Standards for specialized nutrition support: home care patients. *Nutr Clin Pract.* 2005;20(5):579–590.
3. Ireton-Jones C. Outcomes of home nutrition support: fact or fiction? *Support Line.* 2006;28(1):25–28.
4. Winker MF, Wetle T. A pilot study of qualitative interview guide for quality of life in home parenteral nutrition patients. *Support Line.* 2006;28(1): 19–25.

5. Ireton-Jones CS, DeLegge MH. Home parenteral nutrition registry: a five-year retrospective evaluation of outcomes of patients receiving home parenteral nutrition support. *Nutrition.* 2005;21(2):156–160.

6. Ireton-Jones CS, DeLegge MH, Epperson LA, Alexander J. Management of the home parenteral nutrition patient. *Nutr Clin Pract.* 2003;18(4):310–317.

7. Ireton-Jones CS. Home care. In Matarese LE, Gottsclich MM, eds. *Contemporary Nutrition Support Practice: A Clinical Guide.* 2nd ed. Philadelphia, Pa: Saunders; 2003:301–314.

8. Evans JP, Steinhart AH, Cohen Z, McLeod RS. Home total parenteral nutrition: an alternative to early surgery for complicated inflammatory bowel disease. *J Gastrointest Surg.* 2003;7(4):562–566.

9. Task Force for the Revision of Safe Practices for Parenteral Nutrition. Safe practices for parenteral nutrition. *J Parenter Enteral Nutr.* 2004;28(6):S39–S70.

10. Kindle R. Life with fred: 12 years of home parenteral nutrition. *Nutr Clin Pract.* 2003;18(3):235–237.

11. Silver HJ, Wellman NS, Arnold DJ, et al. Older adults receiving home enteral nutrition: enteral regimen, provider involvement, and health care outcomes. *J Parenter Enteral Nutr.* 2004;28(2):92–98.

12. Oley Foundation. Available at http://www.oley.org. Accessed April 18, 2006.

CHAPTER 4

Nutrition Screening and Assessment in Home Nutrition Support

M. Patricia Fuhrman, MS, RD, LD, FADA, CNSD

INTRODUCTION

Nutrition screening and assessment are interrelated but separate processes for determining nutritional risk and for developing a nutrition care plan to prevent or reverse nutritional risk. A nutrition screening process enables clinicians to use pre-selected criteria to identify patients who require an in-depth nutrition assessment. The goal of a nutrition assessment is not only to determine the degree of nutritional risk and existence of a nutritionally deficient or excessive state, but also to develop a nutrition care plan that focuses on a nutrition intervention and the desired versus actual outcomes of the implemented interventions. Figure 4–1 is an algorithm that provides a general overview of the nutrition screening and assessment process.

Nutrition Screening

According to the American Society of Parenteral and Enteral Nutrition (A.S.P.E.N.) Clinical Guidelines, "screening is a dynamic process" designed to identify patients at nutritional risk.[1] The screening process examines risk factors and determines whether the patient is or is not at risk. If a patient is deemed to be at nutritional risk, then the patient is

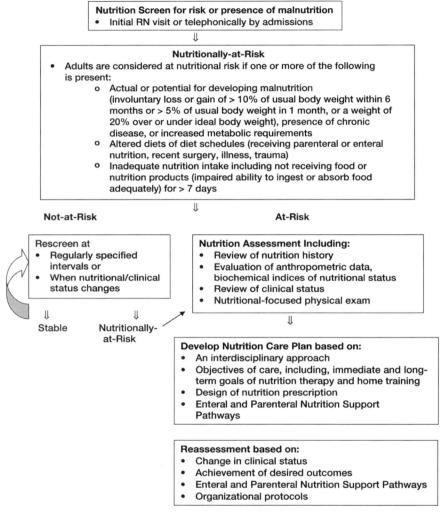

Adapted with permission from the A.S.P.E.N. Board of Directors. *Clinical pathways and algorithms for delivery of parenteral and enteral nutrition support in adults.* Silver Spring, Md: A.S.P.E.N.; 1998.

FIGURE 4–1   Screening and Assessment Algorithm for Adults on Home Nutrition Support

referred to a registered dietitian (RD) for an in-depth nutrition assessment that determines the degree of risk and the nutrition interventions required to reduce or eliminate the risk.

Every homecare provider should have a process in place to screen patients for nutritional risk.[1,2] Patients on enteral or parenteral nutrition support should be automatically referred for a nutrition assessment by an

RD. All other patients should undergo a nutrition assessment if the patient is at nutritional risk.

The nutrition screening process must identify the following:[1]

- who will perform the screen,
- what criteria will be used to determine who is at nutritional risk,
- when rescreening will be done, and
- how the information on at-risk patients will be communicated to the RD.

Often an RD is not a part of the homecare provider's team; therefore, a qualified clinician should evaluate the results of the nutrition screen to determine nutritional risk. It is not unusual to identify a patient referred for hydration therapy, chemotherapy, or antibiotics at nutritional risk.

A screening process should be quick and easy to perform. The parameters used to identify risk should be reliable as indicators of nutritional status and inexpensive to obtain.[3]

The screening criteria for nutritional risk can include:

- history of weight loss,
- gastrointestinal (GI) symptoms (chronic vomiting, fistula or ostomy losses, and diarrhea),
- appetite changes,
- chewing and swallowing impairments,
- food allergies and intolerances, and
- chronic and recent dietary intake.

According to the A.S.P.E.N. Clinical Guidelines, a nutrition screen should include information on height, weight, weight change, primary diagnosis, and co-morbidities.[1] Laboratory values are often not readily available and current and should not be relied upon. For efficiency, the screening tool should be a checklist or a series of questions that are part of the routine admission process. Most screening tools are scored to determine if the patient should be referred to an RD or other qualified clinician for a nutrition assessment. If the patient is not at nutritional risk according to the pre-determined criteria, then the patient should be rescreened according to a pre-determined schedule as set in the company's policies and procedures for the type of home infusion therapy being provided.[1,2] The length of time before rescreening should not exceed two weeks.

Figure 4–2 provides a sample of a nutrition-screening tool. The tool used in each facility should be specific for its patient population. The effectiveness of the screening process and the screening tool should be routinely evaluated to ensure that the process is running smoothly and that the criteria used with the tool are sufficient to identify at-risk patients. Semi-annual chart audits should be performed to identify adherence to the screening policy as well as the effectiveness of the screening tool to identify patients at nutritional risk.

NUTRITION ASSESSMENT

Patients at nutritional risk should undergo a thorough nutrition assessment by an RD. If an RD is not available to perform the nutrition assessment, then a qualified clinician with specialized training in nutrition care can perform the assessment. Nutrition assessment is the on-going process of examining all the contributing factors (nutritional and metabolic) to the presence or potential of an impaired nutritional state and identifying nutrition interventions to sustain, improve, or control deterioration of the patient's nutritional status.[1] The American Dietetic Association has developed an intricate nutrition care process that incorporates nutrition assessment, nutrition diagnosis, nutrition intervention, and nutrition monitoring and evaluation.[4] This process is designed to promote quality care, standardize the nutrition assessment process and facilitate outcome management and reporting.

Table 4–1 lists parameters reviewed and monitored throughout the nutrition assessment process. One single factor cannot define a patient's nutritional risk. It is important to examine all clinical and metabolic factors in order to assess and monitor nutritional status.

According to the A.S.P.E.N. Clinical Guidelines,[1] the nutrition assessment should

- include objective and subjective data to specify the degree of nutritional risk,
- provide specific recommendations for micronutrient and macronutrient requirements, and
- delineate goals of providing nutrition support.

Referral Therapy (circle all that apply):   anti-infectives   pain management

IVF   parenteral nutrition*   enteral nutrition*   blood products

transplant   Other: _____

Diagnosis/Co-morbidities (circle all that apply):   GI disease*   cancer*

pancreatitis*   hyperemesis gravidarum*   transplant   diabetes

heart disease   Other: _____

Food Consumption (2 or more * = RD referral)

    Appetite: increased   no change   decreased (> 7 days or
                                                      > 1 meal/day)*

    Chewing difficulties: yes*   no

    Swallowing difficulties: yes*   no

    Gastrointestinal losses: no   ileostomy*   colostomy*

                                        fistula*   chronic diarrhea*   chronic vomiting*

Weight Change over past 6 months:

decreased (intentional/non-intentional*)   no change   increased

usual weight: _____   current weight: _____   percent weight change: _____ %
(if non-intentional weight loss > 10% usual body weight, refer to RD)*

*Immediate referral to RD for in-depth nutrition assessment

FIGURE 4–2   Example of a homecare Screening Form[1-3]

The subjective and objective data comes from the patient's medical record as well as from the patient interview and physical examination.

Subjective data is information told to the clinician without documentation of authenticity. Often the height of the patient is stated versus an actual measurement. Dietary recall, symptom complaints, and recent weight changes can be subjective in nature. Subjective data is as valuable as objective data, but it can be difficult to quantify and measure changes

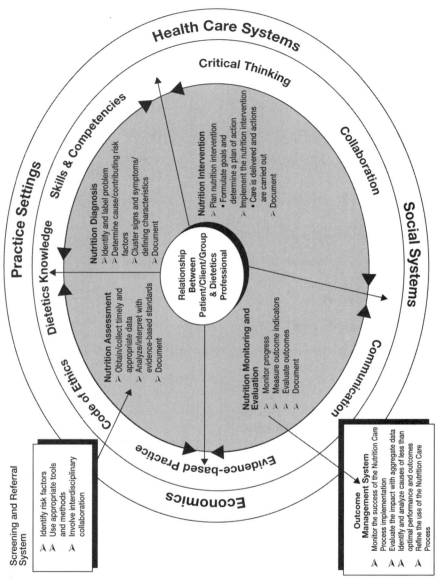

Reprinted with permission from Lacey K, Pritchett E. Nutrition care process and model: ADA adopts road map to quality care and outcomes management. *J Am Diet Assoc*. 2003;103:1062.

FIGURE 4–3   American Dietetic Association's Nutrition Care Process and Model

TABLE 4–1   Home Nutrition Assessment Parameters

Medical and Surgical History

Nutrient intake

Anthropometrics

Physical assessment

Functional status

Laboratory data

Safety and appropriateness of the home environment

Patient's willingness to change behaviors and learn new techniques

for outcome reporting. Objective data, on the other hand, is measurable. It has been quantified, and improvements are measured and compared to previous results. Examples of objective data are measured changes in weight or height, laboratory data, results of diagnostic tests and procedures, indirect calorimetry, and quality of life and functional status measurement tools. Table 4–2 lists some of the signs and symptoms derived from the nutrition assessment that can indicate a nutrient deficiency or toxicity.

COMPONENTS OF THE NUTRITION ASSESSMENT

Medical and Surgical History

The patient's medical and surgical history lays the foundation for existing and potential health issues of the patient.

- Co-morbidities, such as diabetes mellitus, chronic kidney and liver disease, Crohn's disease, and cardiovascular and pulmonary disease, impact nutrient absorption, utilization, and excretion.
- Surgical procedures can directly impact the capacity of the GI tract to assimilate nutrients. The section and length of the bowel removed will directly influence the digestion, absorption, and excretion of nutrients. The potential for nutrient deficiencies and toxicities as well as bowel adaptation depends on the disease process and length and the section of bowel remaining.[5]

TABLE 4–2   Signs and Symptoms of Nutrient Deficiency and Toxicity[28-30, 57-59]

Alopecia
Anemia
Anorexia
Confusion
Diarrhea
Hair color changes
Hematologic disorders
Impaired immunity
Nail abnormalities
Neurological defects
Neuropathy
Skeletal disorders
Skin abnormalities
Tissue inflammation (oral cavity, lips, eyes, skin, etc.)
Vision abnormalities
Vomiting
Weakness
Weight change

Adapted with permission from Fuhrman MP. Overview of micronutrients and parenteral nutrition. *Support Line*. 2002;24(3):7.

- Medications can impact nutrient availability and assimilation. Patients often take multiple medications further complicating the risk of interference with nutrient availability and utilization.
  - Clinicians do not always investigate the patient's use of herbal and dietary supplements. These over-the-counter therapies can be problematic or even dangerous depending on the patient's medical condition and other medications and therapies.[6,7]
  - It is also important to know the pharmacokinetics of the medication to be sure it is effective when given via the oral, enteral or parenteral route. For instance, a medication that requires gastric acid for dissolution will not be effective if given through a jejunal feeding tube.

Nutrient Intake

A thorough diet history is an invaluable key to determining nutrient inadequacies and excesses. Even if the patient is primarily dependent on nutrition support for nutrients and energy requirements, the type and amount of food consumed could impact GI losses as well as the potential for intestinal rehabilitation.[5] In many cases, patients on home nutrition support receive enteral or parenteral nutrition three to five days a week and therefore rely on their oral diet to provide a portion of their nutrient requirements. Maximizing the oral intake may help the patient decrease their reliance on nutrition support. A thorough diet history in conjunction with a comprehensive nutrition-focused physical examination can also enable the clinician to differentiate between signs and symptoms of nutrient deficiencies and toxicities versus physical manifestations of disease or medications (see Table 4–2).

It is important to ensure that the patient is receiving 100% of the Recommended Dietary Allowance for vitamins and minerals every day.[8–12] If the patient has undergone surgery that changed the anatomy of the small or large bowel, then it is important to know what nutrients will be affected and hence may require additional supplementation.

Anthropometrics

Anthropometrics are measurements of body size and generally focus on height and weight.[13,14] Height is often estimated or stated by the patient rather than measured, especially in the homecare setting. This can contribute to error in estimating energy requirements because most of the equations commonly used rely on height as one of the parameters within the equation.

- As a rule, individuals tend to over-estimate their height. Some patients may "shrink" with age because of compression of the spinal cord with metabolic bone disease.
- Height can be indirectly measured by arm span, summation of body parts, and knee height.[15]

Weight is reported in several ways: ideal body weight (IBW), usual body weight (UBW), but the most accurate weight is the patient's actual, measured body weight (ABW). Ideal body weight is a reference range based on height using either the Hamwi[16] method, life insurance actuarial tables,[17] or epidemiological data.[18–20] There are caveats with each

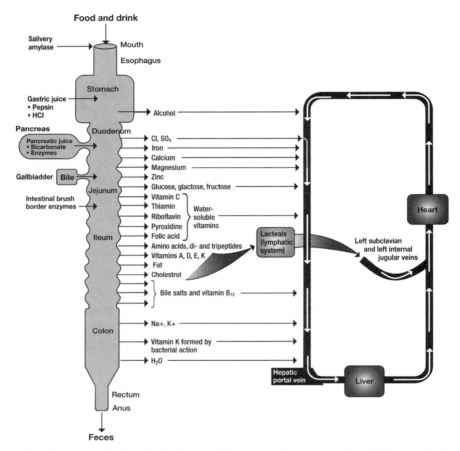

Reprinted with permission from Beyer PL. Digestion, absorption, transport and excretion of nutrients. In: Mahan LK, Escott-Stump S, eds. *Krause's Food, Nutrition, & Diet Therapy*. 11th ed. Philadelphia, Pa: Saunders; 2004:18.

FIGURE 4–4   Sites of Secretion and Absorption in the Gastrointestinal Tract

method, but the Hamwi method is the easiest for the homecare setting and provides a starting point.

- Men: 106 pounds for the first 5 feet of height and 6 pounds for each additional inch.[16]
- Women: 100 pounds for the first 5 feet of height and 5 pounds for each additional inch.[16]

TABLE 4–3   Methods for Estimating Height[15]

Method	Measurement
Arm span	Extend arms straight out to the sides at a 90-degree angle from the torso. Measure from longest fingertip on one hand to longest fingertip on the other hand.
Summation of body parts	Add together the measured length of each of the following: heel, leg, pelvis, spine, and skull.
Knee height	Bend the knee at 90-degree angle. Measure from the heel of the foot to the anterior surface of the thigh. Male: Height (cm) = 64.19 – [0.04 × age (yrs)] + [2.02 × knee height (cm)] Female: Height (cm) = 84.88 – [0.24 × age (yrs)] + [1.83 × knee height (cm)]

TABLE 4–4   Body Mass Index

BMI = weight (kg)/height (m²)	
BMI	**Interpretation**
14–15 kg/m²	associated with mortality
<18.5 kg/m²	underweight, health risks low
18.5–25 kg/m²	healthy weight
>25 kg/m²	overweight, health risk increased
>30 kg/m²	obese, health risk moderate
>35 kg/m²	severe obese, health risk severe
>40 kg/m²	morbid obesity, health risk very severe

Adapted from National Institutes of Health: Clinical guidelines on the identification and treatment of overweight and obesity in adults — the evidence report, *Obes Res*. 1998; 6:51S–209S.

Calculations of IBW should take into account amputations and spinal cord injury. Subtract 5–10% from the IBW with paraplegia and 10–15% with quadriplegia.[21]

The percentage of body weight provided by individual body parts has been estimated[22] to be

- 16% for an entire leg,
- 5.9% for lower leg and foot,
- 1.5% for a foot,
- 5% for an entire arm,
- 2.3% for forearm and hand, and

- 0.7% for a hand.

Actual body weight is the patient's actual weight at the time of assessment. Fluid status impacts measured weight and can result in a misleading assessment of body cell mass. Therefore, it is important to assess the presence of fluid deficit or overload, edema, and ascites. Usual body weight is most reliable for the ambulatory population who has a chronic disease process or who suddenly requires homecare or home infusion therapy.

A change from usual body weight is one of the most reliable measurements of energy excess or inadequacy. The following are suggestive of malnutrition and should be investigated:[1]

- Involuntary weight loss or gain of $\geq$ 10% of UBW within six months
- $\geq$ 5% UBW within one month is suggestive of malnutrition
- If UBW is unknown or unreliable, then a change of 20% above or below IBW.

It is then important to determine the factors contributing to the weight change. Weight changes can be related to fluid accumulation or losses. Patients with chronic diseases and increased metabolic requirements are more likely to be underweight; while obese patients are at greater risk of chronic diseases, such as cardiovascular disease, hypertension, and diabetes mellitus.[1]

Body mass index (BMI) uses the patient's height and weight to determine the health risk and degree of obesity.[2,3] [Body mass index eliminates the need to determine frame size in order to assess appropriateness of weight to height. As with any calculation, the accuracy of BMI is only as good as the accuracy of the measurements of height and weight used in the equation. Body mass index does not identify body composition and can be misleading in those who are overweight with a large proportion of lean body mass (weight lifters) and those who are underweight or normal weight who have a larger proportion of body fat.

Body composition measurements are most often restricted to research. Clinical tools available in the home setting include tricep skinfold and mid-arm circumference measurements. These allow the clinician to monitor changes in body composition rather than being limited to extrapolation from height and weight alone. If done serially on a patient by the same clinician, there is greater accuracy in the data.

Bioelectrical impedance assessment (BIA) measures electrical conductivity and impedance within the body. Lean tissue has a greater conductivity and lower impedance than fat tissue. Bioelectrical impedance assessment is a reliable, safe, noninvasive, and rapid method to determine body composition.[24] Portable BIA equipment make this more feasible in the home setting, but the clinician must be cognizant of factors that can impact the validity of the measurement as well as the equations used by the equipment.[25] Accuracy is better when the patient is well hydrated, has not exercised for 4–6 hours, and has not consumed alcohol within the past 24 hours.[26] Egger and associates compared BIA and subjective global assessment to anthropometry and laboratory measurement of hepatic proteins and lymphocyte count in 47 home parenteral nutrition patients.[27] Bioelectrical impedance assessment did not accurately reflect fat free mass possibly because of the effect of nocturnal parenteral nutrition infusion impacting fluid status. They found that the optimal method of assessing nutritional status was weighing combined with subjective global assessment. Application of BIA to the home setting is limited because of potential inaccuracy, the cost of the equipment, and the availability of skilled clinicians to perform the measurement.

Physical Examination

A nutrition-focused physical examination is a visual and tactile examination of the patient looking for signs and symptoms of nutrition-related complications.[28–30] The physical exam should be done in a head-to-toe approach so that no area is overlooked. The patient's overall appearance is examined as well as inspection and palpation of integumentary and musculoskeletal systems. Table 4–5 provides a list of physical findings with potential nutrient toxicities and deficiencies. However, physical manifestations are neither specific nor sensitive indicators of nutritional excess or depletion. Therefore, all components of the nutrition assessment must be incorporated into the determination of whether physical findings are nutritional in etiology. Physical examination allows the clinician to determine body mass distribution as with cachexia and adiposity.

TABLE 4-5 Clinical Interpretation of Physical Examination Findings

	Normal	Clinical Findings	Suspect Deficiency	Other Comments
Eyes	• Bright, clear, shiny, smooth cornea • Pink and moist membranes	• Pale conjunctiva	• Iron	• Non-nutritional anemia
		• Night blindness	• Vitamin A	• Heredity • Eye diseases
		• Bitot's spots	• Vitamin A	
		• Xerosis	• Vitamin A	• Aging • Allergies
		• Redness, fissuring in corners of eyes	• Riboflavin • Pyridoxine	
	• Normal eye movement to follow objects	• Opthalmoplegia	• Thiamin • Phosphorus	• Brain lesion
Hair	• Shiny, firm, not easily plucked	• Flag sign • Easily plucked with no pain	• Protein • Seen in kwashiorkor and occasionally marasmus	• Over processing hair as in excess bleaching
	• Normal appearing or thick	• Sparse	• Protein • Biotin • Zinc	• Alopecia from aging, chemotherapy or radiation to the head • Endocrine disorders
	• Normal appearing hair shaft and emergence from skin	• Corkscrew hair • Unemerged coiled hairs	• Vitamin C	

	Normal	Clinical Findings	Suspect Deficiency	Other Comments
Nails	• Uniform, rounded, smooth	• Transverse ridging	• Protein	
		• Koilonychia	• Iron	• Considered normal if seen on toenails only
Skin	• Uniform color	• Scaling	• Vitamin A	• Vitamin A excess
	• Smooth, healthy appearance	• Nasolabial seborrhea	• Zinc	• Nasal congestion
			• Riboflavin	
			• Essential fatty acids	
			• Pyridoxine	
		• Petechiae, especially perifollicular	• Vitamin C	• Abnormal blood clotting
				• Severe fever
				• Red spots from flea bite
		• Purpura	• Vitamin C	• Warfarin
			• Vitamin K	• Injury
				• Thrombocytopenia
				• Excessive vitamin E
		• Follicular hyperkeratosis	• Vitamin A	
			• Vitamin C	
		• Pigmentation	• Niacin	
		• Desquamation of sun-exposed areas		
		• Cellophane appearance	• Protein	• Aging process
		• Yellow pigmentation of palms of hands		• Excess beta-carotene

	Normal	Clinical Findings	Suspect Deficiency	Other Comments
	with normal white sclera	• Body edema • Round, swollen face (moon face)	• Protein • Thiamin	• Medications, esp steroids
		• Poor wound healing • Decubitus ulcers	• Protein • Vitamin C • Zinc • Kwashiorkor	• Poor skin care • Diabetes • Steroid use
		• Pallor • Fatigue	• Iron	• Blood loss
Oral	• Lips smooth without sores	• Cheilosis • Angular stomatitis	• Riboflavin • Pyridoxine • Niacin	• Excessive salivation due to ill-fitting dentures • Dry skin (winter) • Dehydration
	• Tongue, red without swelling • Normal surface	• Atrophic lingual papillae	• Riboflavin • Niacin • Folate • Vitamin B_{12} • Protein • Iron	
	• Normal taste and smell	• Hypoguesia • Hyposmia	• Zinc	• Medications such as antineoplastic agents or sulfonylureas • Nasal congestion

	Normal	Clinical Findings	Suspect Deficiency	Other Comments
	• Normal gums and teeth	• Mottled tooth enamel		• Excess fluoride
		• Eroded enamel		• Suspect bulimia
		• Cavities • Missing teeth		• Poor dental hygiene
		• Retracted gums		• Peridontal disease
		• Swollen, bleeding gums • Retracted gums with teeth	• Vitamin C	• Poor oral hygiene • Pregnancy
Neurologic	• Psychological stability	• Dementia	• Niacin • Vitamin B_{12}	• Disease or age related • Increased calcium • Medications • Aluminum toxicity
		• Confabulation • Disorientation	• Thiamin (Korsakoff's psychosis)	
	• Normal reflexes and sensations	• Foot and wrist drop	• Thiamin	
		• Peripheral neuropathy with weakness and parasethesias • Ataxia and decreased tendon reflexes, fine	• Thiamin • Pyridoxine • Vitamin B_{12}	

Normal	Clinical Findings	Suspect Deficiency	Other Comments
	tactile vibrator and position sense		
	• Tetany	• Calcium • Magnesium • Vitamin D	
Others	• Parotid enlargement • Hepatomegaly	• Protein • Bulimia	• Disease of the parotid or liver • Excess vitamin A
	• Rickets or osteomalacia	• Vitamin D	

Adapted with permission for Morrison SG. Clinical nutrition physical examination. *Support Line.* 1997;19(2):16–18.

TABLE 4–6 Functional Status

Activities of Daily Living (ADLs)	Instrumental Activities of Daily Living (IADLs)
Eating	Using the telephone
Moving into/out of beds and chairs	Traveling
Being mobile indoors/outdoors	Shopping
Dressing	Preparing meals
Bathing	Doing light housework
Toileting	Taking medication
Maintaining continence	Managing money

Reprinted with permission from Harris NG. Nutrition in aging. In: Mahan LK, Escott-Stump S, eds. *Krause's Food Nutrition, and Diet Therapy*. 11th ed. Philadelphia, Pa: Saunders; 2004:324.

Functional Status

Functional status evaluation determines what the patient is physically capable of performing. Tools used to quantify physical capabilities include hand-grip dynamometry and lung function testing. However, these may not be practical for use in the home setting. It may be more practical and useful to track the patient's ability to participate in the activities of daily living (ADLs) and the instrumental activities of daily living (IADLs).[31]

A component of functionality is psychosocial abilities and limitations. For long-term nutrition support patients, quality of life (QOL) is an important factor to consider. Several tools are available to measure a patient's QOL. A simple and useful tool in the homecare setting is Karnofsky's Performance Status Scale.[32] Karnofsky's scale incorporates the ADLs and IADLs into a scored classification of functional status and has been used in home patients receiving hospice care[33] and home enteral nutrition.[34] A study by Loeser and associates used Karnofsky's scale and found that malnutrition was associated with a decreased QOL and some aspects of QOL could be improved within 4 months of home enteral nutrition therapy.[34]

Laboratory Data

Laboratory data that can be tracked over time to monitor changes in organ function and metabolic losses and demands.[35–37] The results of laboratory studies must be evaluated in the context of the patient's disease, nutrition support modality, and ongoing losses and gains. Frequency of laboratory testing is generally less in the homecare setting because patients are more stable.

KARNOFSKY PERFORMANCE STATUS SCALE DEFINITIONS RATING (%) CRITERIA		
Able to carry on normal activity and to work; no special care needed.	100	Normal no complaints; no evidence of disease.
	90	Able to carry on normal activity; minor signs or symptoms of disease.
	80	Normal activity with effort; some signs or symptoms of disease.
Unable to work; able to live at home and care for most personal needs; varying amount of assistance needed.	70	Cares for self; unable to carry on normal activity or to do active work.
	60	Requires occasional assistance, but is able to care for most of his personal needs.
	50	Requires considerable assistance and frequent medical care.
Unable to care for self; requires equivalent of institutional or hospital care; disease may be progressing rapidly.	40	Disabled; requires special care and assistance.
	30	Severely disabled; hospital admission is indicated although death not imminent.
	20	Very sick; hospital admission necessary; active supportive treatment necessary.
	10	Moribund; fatal processes progressing rapidly.
	0	Dead

Source: http://www.hospicepatients.org/karnofsky.html. Accessed July 12, 2005.

FIGURE 4–5   Karnofsky's Performance Status Scale

There is a common misconception that hepatic proteins reflect nutritional status. However, hepatic proteins are more responsive to hydration and inflammation than nutrition.[38] Decreases in albumin, transferrin, and prealbumin (negative acute phase proteins) that occur during inflammation coincide with decreased intake induced by the inflammatory state. When the patient recovers from inflammation, these hepatic proteins increase, as does the appetite and nutrient intake. Hence a

TABLE 4–7 Laboratory Monitoring for Home Enteral Nutrition Support

Lab Test	Frequency of Monitoring
Sodium, potassium, chloride, glucose, BUN, creatinine, calcium, phosphorus, magnesium	Weekly 1st month or until stable. Then monthly for 3 months. Then quarterly.
Albumin, CBC	Quarterly

Adapted with permission from the American Society for Parenteral and Enteral Nutrition (ASPEN), from the following: Kovacevich DS, Canada T, Lown D. Monitoring home and other alternate site nutrition support. In: Gottsclich MM, ed. *The Science and Practice of Nutrition Support: A Case-Based Core Curriculum.* Dubuque, Iowa: Kendall/Hunt Publishing Company; 2001:734. ASPEN does not endorse the use of this material in any other form than in its entirety.

TABLE 4–8 Laboratory Monitoring for Home Parenteral Nutrition Support

Lab Test	Frequency of Monitoring
Sodium, potassium, chloride, bicarbonate, glucose, BUN, creatinine, calcium, phosphorus, magnesium	Weekly until stable. Then monthly for 3 months followed by every other month if stable.
CBC, triglycerides	Monthly for 3 months, then every other month.
Albumin, AST, ALT, ALP, total bilirubin*, PT, INR	Every 3–6 months.
Vitamins, minerals, trace elements**	Every 6–12 months based on facility policy.
Iron studies	Baseline with admission, at 3 months, and then every 6 months.

* ALT and AST may increase within 1–3 weeks of PN initiation and can be associated with hepatic steatosis. ALP and gamma-glutamyl transferase may also rise (usually later) and may be associated with cholestasis. An elevation in total bilirubin occurs less frequently and is typically observed last. ALP should be fractionated to determine if elevation is from liver or bone.

** Commonly seen lab changes with metabolic bone disease include increased alkaline phosphatase, decreased PTH and 1,25 dihydroxy vitamin D, normal 25 hydroxy vitamin D, hypercalciuria, and intermittent hypercalcemia.

Adapted with permission from the American Society for Parenteral and Enteral Nutrition (ASPEN), from the following: Kovacevich DS, Canada T, Lown D. Monitoring home and other alternate site nutrition support. In: Gottsclich MM, ed. *The Science and Practice of Nutrition Support: A Case-Based Core Curriculum.* Dubuque, Iowa: Kendall/Hunt Publishing Company; 2001:734. ASPEN does not endorse the use of this material in any other form than in its entirety.

cause-and-effect was believed to occur with decreased nutrient intake and decreased albumin, transferrin, and prealbumin levels when, in fact, changes in the hepatic protein levels and nutrient intake were both impacted by the inflammatory process. Albumin and prealbumin levels are prognostic indicators and help identify the sickest patients who, without aggressive nutrition support, have the greatest capacity to become malnourished or to worsen their nutritional state. Transferrin's role in identifying nutritional status has not been extensively studied and is directly impacted by iron status and inflammation.[1] Hepatic proteins should not be used to determine nutritional status and effectiveness of nutrition therapy, however, levels are used to qualify patients for Medicare reimbursement and as such should be monitored.

Safety and Appropriateness of the Home Environment

During the home visit for the nutrition assessment, the clinician must critically evaluate the home environment for safety and appropriateness for home nutrition support. The patient must have a clean environment with electricity, refrigeration, adequate storage space for supplies, and a space for preparing enteral or parenteral solutions for infusion.

Patient's Readiness to Learn and Change Behavior

Patient education is an integral component to management of nutrition support in the home environment.[39] It is the patient's/care partner's responsibility to adhere to sterile or clean technique, infuse the feeding according to the prescription, and monitor vital signs and weights per protocol. Adherence to the overall management requires the patient's and care partner's ability to understand and willingness to perform the procedures of the feeding modality. Without compliance to the established regimen, it is impossible for the clinician to know when and how to adapt the regimen when the actual outcome is not what was desired.

Subjective Global Assessment

The subjective global assessment (SGA)[40] is an assessment technique that combines the following to determine the degree of nutrition risk:

- nutrition-related history,
- physical examination, and
- functional capacity.

This technique does not incorporate laboratory values into the process because laboratory values are either not available or are skewed by disease process and fluid status. Variations of the SGA are used in cancer,[41] elderly,[42] and renal[43] patients.

ASSESSMENT OF NUTRIENT REQUIREMENTS

Energy Expenditure

The most commonly used equation for predicting energy expenditure and therefore calories requirements for most individuals is the Harris-Benedict equation (HBE), which was published in 1919 in a study involving 236 healthy subjects.[44–46] There is ongoing debate whether this is the most accurate equation to use in healthy and hospitalized patients.[47] An evidence-based analysis of predictive equations in healthy subjects (normal weight and obese) found that the Mifflin-St Jeor equation had better accuracy than the HBE.[48]

Energy requirements in the homecare population differ from the acute care population.

- Acute care patients have increased requirements from an exacerbation of a critical illness or the presence of trauma.[49,50]
- homecare patients can have an underlying inflammatory process, but it is not generally as full-blown as it is in the acute care setting.
- In addition, the homecare patient's activity can range from bedbound to triathlon training.

A study in Crohn's patients found that the energy expenditure was the same during a flare as without a flare of the disease.[51] When disease activity increased, physical activity decreased, and when disease activity abated, physical activity resumed. Therefore, the homecare clinician must balance disease activity and physical activity into the estimation of energy requirements.

Indirect calorimetry measures oxygen consumption and carbon dioxide production through pulmonary gas exchange to identify energy utilization at the cellular level.[52–54] Measured energy expenditure had not been practical in the outpatient setting because of the equipment requirements and technical expertise required to perform the measurements. However, development of a hand-held indirect calorimetry device enables the homecare clinician to measure and monitor changes in

TABLE 4–9   Commonly Used Predictive Equations[44-46, 57-59]

Harris Benedict Equation

Male: 66.5 + 13.8 (W) + 5 (H)–6.8 (A)

Female: 655 + 9.6 (W) + 1.9 (H)–4.7 (A)

Kcal per kg

Weight gain: 40 kcal/kg

Weight maintenance: 30 kcal/kg

Weight loss: 20 kcal/kg

Mifflin St Jeor Equation

Male: 10 (W) + 6.3 (H)–4.9 (A) + 5

Female: 10 (W) + 6.3 (H)–4.9 (A)–161

Ireton-Jones Equation

Spontaneously breathing: EEE = 629–11(A) + 25(W)–609 (O)

Ventilator-dependent: EEE = 1794–11 (A) + 5(W) + 244 (G) + 239(T) + 804 (B)

Abbreviated Version for Persons of Normal Weight and Height

Female: REE = kg × 0.95 kcal/kg × 24 hr

Male: REE = kg × 1 kcal/kg × 24 hr

A=age in years; W=actual body weight in kg; H=height in cm; O= obesity, >30% IBW (0=absent, 1=present); G=gender (1=male, 2=female); T=trauma (0=absent, 1=present); B=burn (0=absent, 1=present)

energy expenditure in the home nutrition support patient. The accuracy of this device has been validated[55] and it has been used in the homecare setting.[56]

Despite the availability and accuracy of the hand-held indirect calorimeter, many clinicians rely on energy estimation equations to identify the patient's energy requirements. There are more than 200 equations that estimate energy requirements, some of which are designed for specific patient populations—healthy, burn, pediatric, intensive care, and so on. Table 4–9 provides some of the more commonly used equations in healthy subjects.[44-46,57-59]

Protein Requirements

As stated earlier, serum albumin and other negative acute phase proteins are inappropriate to use to determine a patient's protein requirements. Collection of a 24-hour urine sample and measurement of nitrogen bal-

TABLE 4–10   Estimating Fluid Requirements[8,60]

Milliliter Per Kilogram Method

Adults: 35 mL/kg

Elderly: 30 mL/kg

Holliday-Segar Method

1000 mL for first 10 kg

500 mL for next 5 kg

20 mL/kg for all kg >15

Body Surface Area Method

1500 mL/m²

RDA Method

1 mL per kcal estimated needs

ance is impractical for the home setting. Protein needs are generally estimated according to the diagnosis and potential on-going losses. Protein requirements can range from 0.8 to 1.5 gm/kg per day depending on the patient's disease process.[60] Providing >1 gm protein/kg per day for the long-term parenteral nutrition patient can increase hypercalciuria and its associated risk for metabolic bone disease.

Fluid Requirements

Fluid requirements are usually based roughly on milliliters per kilogram of body weight. This amount is then adjusted according to changes in hydration status.

- Patients with renal, hepatic, and cardiac dysfunction may require less fluid volume.
- Patients with gastric decompression, ileostomies, chronic diarrhea, and fistulae may require additional fluid.
- Patients unable to respond to thirst because of inability to consume fluids volitionally by mouth will have to have all fluid needs met via the enteral or parenteral route.

Table 4–10 provides calculations to estimate fluid requirements.

Micronutrient Requirements

Regardless of whether the patient is receiving oral diet, tube feeding, parenteral nutrition, or a combination thereof, it is imperative to ensure that the patient receives 100% of estimated micronutrient requirements daily. Parenteral vitamin and mineral preparations should provide micronutrients according to the American Medical Association Nutrition Advisory Group.[12] However, there is debate as to whether these preparations are inadequate in some nutrients and excessive in others for the long-term patient. There are also some disease states where there may be an increased need for some nutrients while others should be given in smaller quantities. It is important to monitor serum levels of any micronutrient that is given above the American Medical Association Nutrition Advisory Group guidelines as well as those reduced or omitted from parenteral solutions because there is a risk of the patient developing toxicity or deficiency. The frequency of monitoring can range from monthly to yearly depending on the patient's medical condition, the presence of physical manifestations of adverse effects, and the amount of a specific nutrient given or omitted.

Home parenteral nutrition patients should be assessed every 6 months to a year for potential micronutrient deficiencies and toxicities.[61] Risk of deficiencies is greater in patients with ongoing GI losses or sustained inflammation. Toxicities can occur when excretion routes are impaired as they are in renal and hepatic failure. Elevated levels of manganese have been reported in patients with normal liver function receiving the standard trace element preparations.[62] Clinical manifestations of manganese toxicity were not seen despite elevated serum levels.

Absolute identification of micronutrient deficiencies and toxicities can be difficult. As shown in Tables 4–2 and 4–5, the clinical manifestations are often indistinguishable from disease-related, medication-induced, or environment-produced signs and symptoms. In addition biochemical confirmation is often elusive because of errors in collection and storage, blood tests that are not sensitive for tissue/storage amounts, and functional testing of the micronutrient is not available.[63]

SUMMARY

Nutrition screening is a process that identifies patients who require a comprehensive nutrition assessment. Nutrition assessment is the process of discovering why the patient is malnourished or at nutritional risk and developing a nutrition care plan to reduce, reverse, or eliminate the risk. A global nutrition assessment includes medical, surgical, and diet history, laboratory values, psychosocial evaluation, physical assessment, and functional status. A nutrition assessment for home nutrition support should include a home visit in order to perform the physical assessment and to assess the safety and appropriateness of the home environment. The patient's willingness to change behaviors and implement the feeding regimen should be assessed. An important key to the nutrition assessment process is to identify nutrition interventions and desired outcomes and to monitor the actual outcomes of the implemented interventions. When desired outcomes are not achieved, the clinician must reassess and identify an alternative intervention.

REFERENCES

1. A.S.P.E.N. Board of Directors and The Clinical Guidelines Task Force. Guidelines for the use of parenteral and enteral nutrition in adult and pediatric patients. *J Parenter Enteral Nutr.* 2002;26(suppl 1):9SA–12SA.
2. A.S.P.E.N. Board of Directors. *Clinical pathways and algorithms for delivery of parenteral and enteral nutrition support in adults.* Silver Spring, Md: ASPEN; 1998.
3. Charney P, Marian M. Nutrition screening and risk assessment. In: Charney P, Malone A, eds. *ADA Pocket Guide to Nutrition Assessment.* Chicago, Ill: American Dietetic Association; 2004:1–22.
4. Lacey K, Pritchett E. Nutrition care process and model: ADA adopts road map to quality care and outcomes management. *J Am Diet Assoc.* 2003;103(8):1061–1072.
5. Matarese LE, Seidner DL, Steiger E. Growth hormone, glutamine, and modified diet for intestinal adaptation. *J Am Diet Assoc.* 2004;104(8):1265–1272.
6. WHO Guidelines: Developing information on proper use of traditional, complementary, and alternative medicines. Geneva: World Health Organization. June 22, 2004. Available at http://www.who int. Accessed August 5, 2004.
7. Ernst E. The risk-benefit profile of commonly used herbal therapies: Ginkgo, St. John's Wort, Ginseng, Echinacea, Saw Palmetto, and Kava. *Ann Intern Med.* 2002;136(1):42–53.
8. Food and Nutrition Board, National Research Council, National Academy of Sciences. *Recommended Dietary Allowances*, 10th ed. Washington, DC: National Academy Press; 1989.
9. Standing Committee on the Scientific Evaluation of Dietary Reference Intakes of the Food and Nutrition Board, Institute of Medicine, The National

Academies in collaboration with Health Canada. *Dietary Reference Intakes for Energy, Carbohydrates, Fiber, Fat, Protein and Amino Acids (Macronutrients)*. Washington, DC: National Academy of Sciences; 2002.

10. Trumbo P, Yates AA, Schlicker S, Poos M. Dietary reference intakes: Vitamin A, vitamin K, arsenic, boron, chromium, copper, iodine, iron, manganese, molybdenum, nickel, silicon, vanadium, and zinc. *J Am Diet Assoc*. 2001;101(3):294–301.

11. WHO. *Energy and protein requirements*. Report of a Joint FAO/WHO/UNU Expert Consultation. (Technical Report Series 724). Geneva: World Health Organization; 1985.

12. Task Force for the Revision of Safe Practices for Parenteral Nutrition: Mirtallo J, et al. Safe practices for parenteral nutrition. *J Parenter Enteral Nutr*. 2004;28(6):S39–S70.

13. Howell WH. Anthropometry and body composition analysis. In: Matarese LE, Gottschlich MM, eds. *Contemporary Nutrition Support Practice*: A Clinical Guide. 2nd ed. Philadelphia, Pa: Saunders; 2003:31–44.

14. Malone A. Anthropometric assessment. In: Charney P, Malone A, eds. *ADA Pocket Guide to Nutrition Assessment*. Chicago, Ill: American Dietetic Association; 2004:142–152.

15. Shopell JM, Hopkins B, Shronts EP. Nutrition Screening and Assessment. In: Gottschlich MM, ed. *The Science and Practice of Nutrition Support: A Case-based Core Curriculum*. Dubuque, Iowa: Kendall/Hunt Publishing Company; 2001:107–140.

16. Hamwi GJ. Changing dietary concepts. In: Danowski TS, ed. *Diabetes Mellitus: Diagnosis and Treatment, Vol. 1*. New York: American Diabetes Association, Inc; 1964:73–78.

17. Metropolitan Life Insurance Company. Statistical Bulletin. January-June, 1983.

18. National Center for Health Statistics. Plan and Operation of the Health and Nutrition Examination Survey, United States, 1971–1973 (Part A-Development, Plan, and Operation) Vital and Health Statistics. Series 1, No. 10a. DHEW Publ. No. (PHS) 79–1310. Washington, DC: US Government Printing Office; 1977.

19. National Center for Health Statistics. Plan and Operation of the Health and Nutrition Examination Survey, United States, 1971–1973 (Part B-Data Collection Forms of the Survey) Vital and Health Statistics. Series 1, No. 10b. DHEW Publ. No. (PHS) 79–1310. Washington, DC: US Government Printing Office; 1977.

20. National Center for Health Statistics. Plan and Operation of the Health and Nutrition Examination Survey, United States, 1976–1980 (Part A-Development, Plan, and Operation) Vital and Health Statistics. Series 1, No. 15. DHEW Publ. No. (PHS) 81–1317. Washington, DC: US Government Printing Office; 1981.

21. Peiffer SC, Blust P, Leyson JF. Nutritional assessment of the spinal cord injured patient. *J Am Diet Assoc.* 1981;78(5):501–505.
22. Osterkamp LK. Current perspective on assessment of human body proportions of relevance to amputees. *J Am Diet Assoc.* 1995;95(2):215–218.
23. National Institutes of Health. Clinical guidelines on the identification and treatment of overweight and obesity in adults—the evidence report. *Obes Res.* 1998;6(suppl 2):51S–209S.
24. Barak N, Wall-Alonso E, Cheng A, Sitrin M. Use of bioelectrical impedance analysis to predict energy expenditure of hospitalized patients receiving nutrition support. *J Parenter Enteral Nutr.* 2003;27(1):43–46.
25. Frankenfield D. Energy dynamics. In: Matarese LE, Gottsclich MM, eds. *Contemporary Nutrition Support Practice: A Clinical Guide.* 2nd ed. Philadelphia, Pa: Saunders; 2003:77–93.
26. Hammond KA. Dietary and clinical assessment. In: Mahan LK, Escott-Stump S, eds. *Krause's Food, Nutrition, & Diet Therapy*, 11th ed. Philadelphia, Pa: Saunders; 2004:407–435.
27. Egger NG, Carlson GL, Shaffer JL. Nutritional status and assessment of patients on home parenteral nutrition: anthropometry, bioelectrical impedance, or clinical judgment? *Nutrition.* 1999;15(1):1–6.
28. Hammond K. History and physical examination. In: Matarese LE, Gottsclich MM, eds. *Contemporary Nutrition Support Practice: A Clinical Guide.* 2nd edition. Philadelphia, Pa: Saunders; 2003:14–30.
29. Bates B, Bickley L, Hoekelman RA, eds. *A Guide to Physical Exam and History Taking.* 6th edition. Philadelphia, Pa: JB Lippincott Company; 1995.
30. Fuhrman MP. Nutrition-focused physical exam. In: Charney P, Malone A, eds. *ADA Pocket Guide to Nutrition Assessment.* Chicago, Ill: American Dietetic Association; 2004:41–62.
31. Harris NG. Nutrition in aging. In: Mahan LK, Escott-Stump S, eds. *Krause's Food Nutrition, and Diet Therapy.* 11th ed. Philadelphia, Pa: Saunders; 2004: 318–337.
32. Karnofsky DA, Burchenal JH. The clinical evaluation of chemotherapeutic agents in cancer. In: *Evaluation of chemotherapeutic agents.* New York: Columbia University Press; 1949:191.
33. Dobratz M. A comparative study of variables that have an impact on non-cancer end-of-life diagnoses. *Clin Nurs Res.* 2004;13(4):309–325.
34. Loeser C, von Herz U, Kuchler T, Rzehak P, Muller MJ. Quality of life and nutritional state in patients on home enteral tube feeding. *Nutrition.* 2003;19(7–8):605–611.
35. Thompson C. Laboratory assessment. In: Charney P, Malone A, eds. *ADA Pocket Guide to Nutrition Assessment.* Chicago, Ill: American Dietetic Association; 2004:63–141.
36. Russell MK. Laboratory monitoring. In: Matarese LE, Gottsclich MM, eds. *Contemporary Nutrition Support Practice: A Clinical Guide.* 2nd edition. Philadelphia, Pa: Saunders; 2003:45–62.

37. Kovacevich DS, Canada T, Lown D. Monitoring home and other alternate site nutrition support. In: Gottslich MM, ed. *The Science and Practice of Nutrition Support: A Case-Based Core Curriculum.* ASPEN. 2001:731–756.

38. Fuhrman MP, Charney P, Mueller CM. Hepatic proteins and nutrition assessment. *J Am Diet Assoc.* 2004;104(8):1258–1264.

39. Rosal MC, Ebbeling CB, Lofgren I, et al. Facilitating dietary change: the patient-centered counseling model. *J Am Diet Assoc.* 2001;101(3):332–341.

40. Detsky AS, McLaughlin JR, Baker JP, et al. What is subjective global assessment of nutritional status? *J Parenter Enteral Nutr.* 1987;11(1):8–13.

41. Ottery FD. Cancer cachexia prevention, early diagnosis, and management. *Cancer Pract.* 1994;2(2):123–131.

42. Davidson J, Getz M. Nutritional risk and body composition in free-living elderly participating in congregate meal-site programs. *J Nutr Elder.* 2004;24(1):53–68.

43. National Kidney Foundation. K/DOQI clinical practice guidelines for nutrition in chronic renal failure. *Am J Kidney Dis.* 2000;35(6 suppl 2):S1–S140.

44. Harris JA, Benedict FG. *A biometric study of basal metabolism in man.* Publication No. 279, Washington, DC, 1919, Carnegie Institute.

45. Benedict GF. Basal metabolism data on normal men and women (series II) with some considerations on the use of prediction standards. *Am J Physiol.* 1928;85(3):607–620.

46. Benedict GF. Old age and basal metabolism. *N Engl J Med.* 1935;212(24):1111–1122.

47. Frankenfield DC, Muth ER, Rowe WA. The Harris-Benedict studies of human basal metabolism: history and limitations. *J Am Diet Assoc.* 1998;98(4):439–445.

48. Frankenfield D, Rowe WA, Smith JS, Cooney RN. Validation of several established equations for resting metabolic rate in obese and nonobese people. *J Am Diet Assoc.* 2003;103(9):1152–1159.

49. Daly JM, Heymsfield SB, Head CA, et al. Human energy requirements: overestimation by widely used prediction equation. *Am J Clin Nutr.* 1985;42(6):1170–1174.

50. Long CL, Schaffel N, Geiger JW, et al. Metabolic response to injury and illness: estimation of energy and protein needs from indirect calorimetry and nitrogen balance. *J Parenter Enteral Nutr.* 1979;3(6):452–456.

51. Stokes MA, Hill GL. Total energy expenditure in patients with Crohn's disease: measurement by the combined body scan technique. *J Parenter Enteral Nutr.* 1993;17(1):3–7.

52. Matarese LE. Indirect Calorimetry: technical aspects. *Support Line.* 1997;14(1):6–12.

53. Headley JM. Indirect calorimetry: a trend toward continuous metabolic assessment. *AACN Clin Issues.* 2003;14(2):155–167.

54. Weir JB. New methods for calculating metabolic rate with special reference to protein metabolism. *J Physiol.* 1949;109(1):1–9.

55. Nieman DC, Trone GA, Austin MD. A new handheld device for measuring resting metabolic rate and oxygen consumption. *J Am Diet Assoc.* 2003;103(5):588–593.

56. Ireton-Jones CS. Kearney JT. Measuring resting metabolic rate of patients receiving home parenteral nutrition: a useful adjunctive therapy? Poster presentation at A.S.P.E.N. Clinical Nutrition Week in Orlando, Fla, 2005.

57. Johnson RK. Energy. In: Mahan LK, Escott-Stump S, eds. *Krause's Food, Nutrition, and Diet Therapy.* 10th ed. Philadelphia, Pa: WB Saunders; 2000:26.

58. Mifflin MD, St. Jeor ST, Hill LA, et al. A new predictive equation for resting energy expenditure in healthy individuals. *Am J Clin Nutr.* 1990;51(2):241–247.

59. Ireton-Jones CS, Turner WW, Liepa GW, Baxter CR. Equations for estimating energy expenditures in patients with burns with special reference to ventilatory status. *J Burn Care Rehabil.* 1992;13(3):330–333.

60. Russell MK, Malone A. Nutrient requirements. In: Charney P, Malone A, eds. *ADA Pocket Guide to Nutrition Assessment.* Chicago, Ill: American Dietetic Association; 2004:153–188.

61. Fuhrman MP. Identifying your patient's risk for a vitamin deficiency. *Nutr Clin Pract.* 2001;16:S8–S11.

62. Siepler JK, Nishikawa RA, Diamantidis T, Okamoto R. Asymptomatic hypermanganesemia in long-term home parenteral nutrition patients. *Nutr Clin Pract.* 2003;18(5):370–373.

63. Fuhrman MP, Parker M. Micronutrient assessment. *Support Line.* 2004;26(1):17–24.

CHAPTER 5

Access for Home Enteral Nutrition

Mark H. DeLegge, MD, FACG, AGAF, FASGE

INTRODUCTION

Enteral nutrition is the act of receiving nutrients through the gut, either orally or through an enteral access device. The use of enteral access devices for enteral nutrition delivery has long been practiced in the hospital and the nursing home setting. Recently, the number of patients receiving home enteral nutrition (HEN) through enteral access devices in the United States has progressively increased. The absolute numbers of HEN patients in the United States remains difficult to determine.

Home enteral nutrition has become a growing segment of the home care arena. In 1992 Medicare estimates noted that there were approximately 73,000 HEN patients with an average yearly expenditure of $136 million.[1] Today's expenditure estimates are very difficult to obtain, not only from the Medicare population, but also for the Medicaid and private insurer populations. General consensus is that the HEN population continues to grow at a rapid rate both in numbers and in dollars spent.

There are many common patient disease groups that make up the majority of the HEN population. This includes patients with neurological dysfunction, upper GI cancers, anorexia and failure to thrive. These patients, by in large, have difficulty with transfer of food from the oral cavity to the stomach. A review of the available data from 1987 to 1991 gives an excellent sample of the types of patients that were sent home on enteral nutrition.[2] The majority of these patients had a primary cancer as the cause of their poor oral intake. The second most common group was patients with swallowing disorders, such as patients with cerebral vascular accident, or with a neuromuscular dysfunction.

The management of home enteral nutrition requires decisions that are made early on by physicians regarding enteral access, enteral formula, route of formula delivery, monitoring, complication management, and appropriateness for therapy. Careful attention must be given to each of these decisions in order to prevent complications and to ensure good patient outcomes.

Enteral access devices are the foundation for providing enteral feeding. Knowledge of these devices is imperative in order for patients to receive safe, effective enteral nutrition. In general enteral access devices can be broken down into two categories: short-term access (nasal or orally placed feeding tubes) and long-term access (percutaneous or surgically placed feeding tubes).

ENTERAL ACCESS HISTORY

The history of enteral access can be difficult to trace. In 1598, Capiccaveus is reported to have used a hollow tube to put liquid down a patient's esophagus.[3] In the 1600's, Von Helmont manufactured a flexible leather tube for esophageal tube feeding. In the 1700's, Boerhave suggested that tubes be passed into the stomach for feeding.[4] Often these tubes had a funnel or syringe attached to their ends for feeding. Hunter, in 1790, was reported to have used an orogastric tube made of whale bone covered with eel skin to feed a mixture of jellies, eggs, sugar, wine and milk.[5] Pap boats, boat-shaped vessels with a lip or a spout on one end, were used for the oral delivery of bread soaked in wine with sugar or other "nutrients."

In the 1800's, rectal feeding was considered as good as if not better than gastric feedings. Long pieces of rubber tubing were attached to funnels or wooden syringes.[6] It was widely believed that it was necessary to use ground pancreatic gland in the rectal feeding solutions. Other components of the rectal feedings could be milk, wine, beef broth, tobacco or meats.

In 1910, Einhorn first developed duodenal feeding for patients with gastric intolerance.[4] In 1916, Jones introduced the drip method for delivering enteral feedings. In 1918, Anderson passed a tube into the jejunum and fed a combination of milk, dextrose and whiskey.[7] In 1939, Abbot and Rawson developed a double lumen feeding tube with one opening in the stomach for decompression and a separate opening in the small bowel for feeding.[8]

One of the most prolific papers in enteral access was published by Michael Gauderer and Jeff Ponsky in 1980.[9] They described a new technique for obtaining gastric access percutaneously, without the need for laparotomy, by using an endoscope. This information was presented at the American Society of Gastrointestinal Endoscopy Annual Meeting in 1980 and was embraced immediately by the gastroenterologists. This was the birth of percutaneous endoscopic gastrostomy, better known as PEG. The development of PEG has led to new innovations in the science of gastric and small bowel access.

NASOENTERIC TUBE ACCESS

Nasoenteric tube placement techniques have been developed for the bedside, for use with endoscopy, for use with fluoroscopy, or to be placed during surgery. These techniques all have their indications, benefits, and risks. The final position of an enteral access tube is either the stomach, for gastric feedings, or the jejunum, for small bowel feedings. A patient who is intolerant of gastric feedings, such as a patient with gastroparesis, or a patient who has had their stomach surgically removed, will receive small bowel feedings.

Bedside nasoenteric tube placement is the most common enteral access technique used in the hospital. However, it is the least common enteral access technique for use in the home or long-term care environment. There is very limited use of nasojejunal (NJ) tubes in the home setting and therefore it will not be discussed further.

Nasoenteric Tube Placement

There are many techniques available for passing bedside nasogastric (NG) tubes. Typically, an 8–12 fr NG tube is passed into the stomach after the tube has been lubricated, the head is flexed, and the patient ingests sips of water to assist in passing the tube into the stomach.[10] Many clinicians promote bedside abdominal auscultation with a stethoscope for confirmation of an adequate position of the NG tube. However, this can be misleading as inappropriate tube locations such as in the lung, in the pleural cavity after perforation, or coiled in the esophagus may be misinterpreted as in proper position by bedside abdominal auscultatory techniques. For this reason, every patient should have an abdominal radiograph to confirm proper position of a nasogastric or nasojejunal tube before initiating feedings.[11]

Nasoenteric Tube Maintenance

The decision to use a nasogastric tube also should warrant some very specific instructions regarding its care. The lumen of these tubes is much smaller (10 fr – 12 fr) than a percutaneous endoscopic gastrostomy (PEG) tube (20 fr – 24 fr) and therefore they are prone to occlusion and clogging. These tubes should be flushed after every tube feeding and medication instillation. Only liquid medications, or completely dissolved medications, should be placed through an NG tube in order to reduce the chances of tube occlusion. Care should be taken to stop tube feedings during infusion of medication such as theophylline or potassium chloride, products that are known to coagulate tube feedings and obstruct the NG tube. In general, NG tube size does not limit the type of tube feeding formula ordered. Collier et al. has shown that the use of a fiber containing formula is quite safe, even through a 5 fr feeding tube.[12] However, the addition of a protein powder supplement to tube feeding formulas does promote clogging in smaller diameter NG tubes (<10 fr).

Fixation of the NG tube to the patient's head is important for preventing NG tube migration and dislodgement. Many of these fixation devices contain an adhesive bandage which is placed across the nose. The NG tube is connected to the bandage with either an attached clip or additional adhesive. Some clinicians prefer to tape the tube to the patient's forehead. There are no randomized trials comparing different methods of NG tube fixation. Bridling or suturing the tube to the patient's nose is discouraged because of the high risk for nasal mucosal ulceration and tissue damage.

Nasoenteric Tube Complications

Complications of nasogastric tube placement have been reported in up to 12% of patients[13] (Table 5–1). Early identification of these complications is important in preventing interruptions in tube feeding administration.

TABLE 5–1   Complications of Nasogastric Tube Placement

Nasal mucosal ulceration

Otitis media

Pharyngitis

Pneumothorax

Sinsusitis

Tracheoesophageal fistula

Tube migration

Aspiration pneumonia

Tube obstruction

PERCUTANEOUS ENDOSCOPIC ENTERAL ACCESS

If a patient will require enteral access for greater than 1 month, endoscopic percutaneous procedures are preferred as compared to nasoenteric access. These procedures include PEG, percutaneous endoscopic gastrojejunostomy (PEG/J), and direct percutaneous jejunostomy (DPEJ). All of these procedures require the use of conscious sedation or deep anesthesia and can be performed in the endoscopy suite, in the operating room, or at the bedside in the hospital. In comparison to nasogastric access, PEG has been shown to be a more reliable enteral access tube allowing patients to receive more calories per day because of a reduction in tube dysfunction.[14]

PERCUTANEOUS ENDOSCOPIC GASTROSTOMY

Percutaneous endoscopic gastrostomy was developed by Ponsky and Gauderer in the early 1980s.[15] This procedure has become the standard of care for gastric access. Compared to surgical gastrostomy, PEG insertion is associated with reduced procedure related costs and morbidity. Prospective evaluations of PEG placement have found this procedure to be associated with few procedure-related complications.[16] However, PEG is usually performed in patients with numerous co-morbid diseases. Because of this, the survival of patients after PEG tube placement at 1 month is often close to 40%. In one study there was a reported 48% mortality at 7 days after PEG placement if the patient had prior aspiration episodes, had a concurrent urinary tract infection, or were older than 75 years. This was compared to a reported 4% mortality at 7 days if none of the aforementioned risk factors were present.[17]

Percutaneous Endoscopic Gastrostomy Outcome Data

Percutaneous endoscopic gastrostomy may be used successfully in many disease states, but most commonly for diseases associated with dysphagia. Outcome data for PEG placement for some of the more common processes are:

Cancer Patients

One area of oncology in which PEG tubes are of proven benefit is in patients with head and neck cancer. The benefit of PEG tubes in this setting was illustrated in a retrospective study that had 40% (32/88) of patients receiving a PEG tube prior to chemotherapy and radiotherapy. The majority of these patients received home enteral feedings. Those who received a PEG lost an average of 3.1 kg compared to 7 kg of weight loss for those without a PEG. The same PEG group had significantly fewer hospitalizations for dehydration and malnutrition and had no interruption in treatment of their cancer as compared to the group which did not receive PEG.[18]

Cerebral Vascular Accident

Data supports the use of PEG tubes in those with dysphagia-associated central nervous system disorders. In one study, the authors reported a 1-, 8-, and 48-month survival of 78%, 35%, and 27% respectively after PEG placement, when the most common indication was a hemispheric cerebral vascular accident (CVA).[19] Approximately 50% of those patients discharged from the hospital with a PEG tube post-CVA will receive HEN. Most of the remaining patients will be managed in a long-term, step-down or rehabilitation center setting.

Dementia

Dementia is a frequent disorder of the elderly and a common patient population referred for PEG. Approximately 36,000 elderly patients with dementia receive a PEG each year.[20] However, the benefit of providing enteral nutrition in these patients is less clear.[21] No large, randomized trials have demonstrated a difference in survival in dementia patients with or without a PEG, although these trials are very difficult to construct ethically. A recent, retrospective analysis suggested there was no difference in mortality among dementia patients who did or did not receive a PEG tube.[22] However, this study did not address whether the use of PEG tubes in this population for hydration and medication delivery would be appropriate. The use of PEG tube feedings for dementia patients at home or in the long-term care facility remains common.

Percutaneous Endoscopic Gastrostomy Design

Percutaneous endoscopic gastrostomy kits are commercially available from multiple manufacturers. The most common sizes for adult patients are from 16 fr to 24 fr. Most tubes are made of silicone or polyurethane.

The PEG tube itself consists of an internal bolster, the tube lumen, an external bolster and a feeding adaptor (Figure 5–1). The internal bolster prevents the PEG tube from being accidentally dislodged or "falling out" of the patient. Most internal bolsters made today are flexible and designed to fold-up such that these tubes can be removed with external traction (externally removeable). It generally will take 8–10 lbs of external pull pressure to remove the tubes. Combative patients may also remove their own PEG tubes. In some cases, these combative patients will need to wear protective mittens or have an abdominal binder placed over the PEG tube site to prevent them from removing their own PEG tubes.

Percutaneous Endoscopic Gastrostomy Post-procedure Care

After initial placement, the external bolster of the PEG tube is maintained 1–2cm from the anterior abdominal wall to avoid tissue compression and wound breakdown (Figure 5–2). The wound should be cleaned daily with hydrogen peroxide. A notched sponge or "tracheostomy" sponge is placed over the external bolster, around the tube. Dressings should not be placed under the external bolster. This will lead to extra pressure on the PEG tube wound promoting the development of wound leakage and wound infection.

Percutaneous Endoscopic Gastrostomy Dysfunction

Percutaneous endoscopic gastrostomy tubes usually start to degrade or malfunction after 1–2 years, often from yeast implantation in and degra-

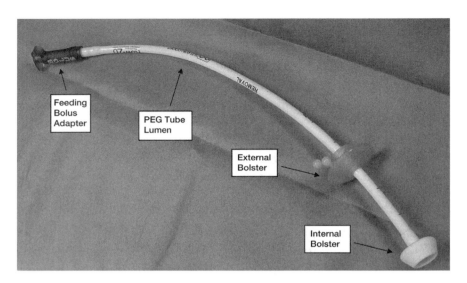

FIGURE 5–1   PEG Tube Design.

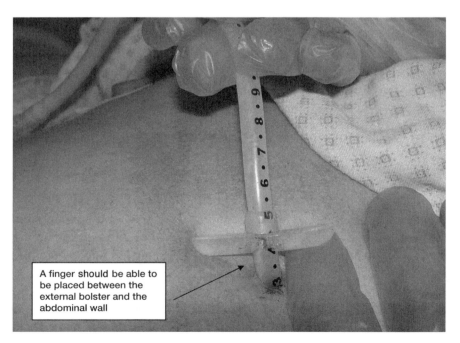

FIGURE 5–2   Proper Placement of the External Bolster of a PEG on the Abdominal Wall.

dation of the PEG tube wall.[23] Once a PEG tube malfunctions, degrades, or is no longer needed it can be removed at the bedside by external traction[24] Some PEG tubes have a rigid internal bolster and can be removed only with an endoscope. They are labeled as "endoscopic removal." Although there is an associated increase in cost with the use of endoscopic removal PEG tubes because of the need for a repeat upper endoscopy to accomplish the removal, they may be safer in patients who are confused or combative and at risk for pulling their PEG tube out after initial placement.

Percutaneous Endoscopic Gastrostomy Tube Replacement

Replacement PEG tubes are broadly divided into two categories, replacement gastrostomy tubes or low profile devices. Replacement gastrostomy tubes usually have a balloon-type internal bolster (Figure 5–3). These balloon tubes can be inserted blindly through the gastrostomy site into the gastric lumen. The balloon is inflated to serve as the internal bolster. An external bolster is slid down the PEG tube against the abdominal wall to keep the PEG tube from migrating. There are also PEG tubes with a distensible internal bolster (Figure 5–4). The internal bolster is stretched with a stylet and pushed blindly through the gastrostomy site into the gastric lumen. The stylet is removed and the internal bolster assumes its previous shape.

PEG tubes may also be replaced with low profile gastrostomy devices (Figure 5–5). These devices provide a skin level access to the gastric lumen. The internal bolster may be a balloon inflatable design or a distensible internal bolster that requires a stylet for placement. These devices come in predetermined lengths. The gastrostomy tract length must be measured in order to choose the correct length low profile device. In order to access the device for feeding or gastric decompression, an access tube must be used to engage a valve in the top of the low profile device. Although these tubes are cosmetically appealing, the small internal diameter of the access tubing and the valve make them more prone to valve and access tube occlusion. They are also more costly than standard balloon gastrostomy replacement tubes.

After a bedside replacement PEG device has been placed, appropriate position of the PEG tube tip within the gastric lumen must be confirmed. This can be done by a combination of ausultation of the stomach for air rapidly infused by a syringe through the PEG tube and visual-

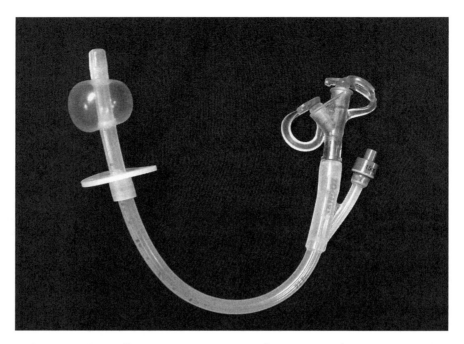

FIGURE 5-3   Balloon Gastrostomy Replacement Tube.

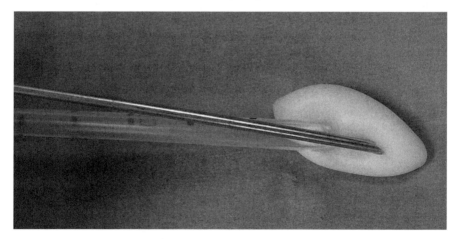

FIGURE 5-4   Stylet Drive Gastrostomy Replacement Tube.

ization of gastric contents aspirated by an attached syringe. In the event of a question regarding the PEG tube tip position, a contrast fluoroscopic study through the PEG tube should be obtained. This is especially important when the originally placed PEG tube has been in position for 1

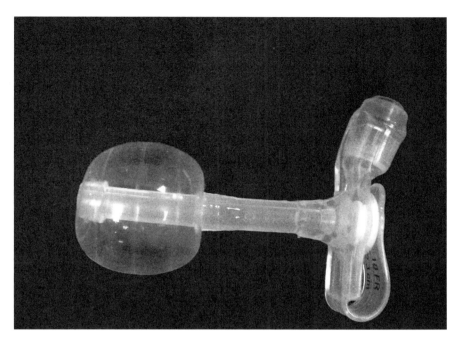

FIGURE 5–5   Low Profile Gastrostomy Tube.

month or less. Early PEG tube removal may result in the stomach separating from the abdominal wall because the PEG tube tract has not completely formed. In these cases, blind, bedside PEG tube replacement may result in the replacement PEG tube being inadvertently positioned into the peritoneal cavity.

Percutaneous Endoscopic Gastrostomy Complications

Complications of PEG arise more frequently in patients with co-morbidities such as poor wound-healing, aspiration, or coagulopathy.[25–27] The most common complication is peristomal wound infection.[25,28] Excessive tightening of the external bolster against the abdominal wall can cause tissue ischemia, wound leakage, and necrotizing fasciitis.[29] Peristomal wound infections are often treated for seven days with an oral antibiotic such as cephalexin® in order to cover skin-related microorganisms. The infected area should also have twice daily topical cleansing with or without the application of an antibiotic ointment. The PEG tube should be removed in cases of worsening infection.

Major reported complications are rare and include hematoma, peritonitis, necrotizing fasciitis, gastric or colonic perforation, hepatogastric, gastrocolic or colocutaneous fistulas.[26–28,30] A colocutaneous fistula is the inadvertent placement of a percutaneous feeding tube through the colon before it enters the stomach. Often this does not become evident until the patient has their original PEG tube exchanged for a replacement PEG tube. The replacement tube tip is pushed through the abdominal wall and into the colon, but does not find its way from the colon into the stomach. If the enteral feedings are restarted, the patient will develop diarrhea as the tube feeding is now being infused directly into the colon. In cases of a colocutaneous fistula, the PEG tube should be removed and the patient's condition should be monitored for appropriate closure of the fistulous tract. If the tract does not heal, surgery is warranted to repair the fistula.

Minor reported complications include peristomal leakage, pneumoperitoneum, fever, ileus, cutaneous or gastric ulceration, and tube extrusion or migration.[26,28,30–32] Peristomal leakage may be resolved by holding tube feedings for a few days to reduce gastric drainage, making sure that the external bolster is not tight against the abdominal wall and protecting the patient's abdominal wall surface from the effects of acid and bile by using a skin barrier cream. Persistent, worsening peristomal wound leakage may require PEG tube removal.

There is little data concerning PEG tube complications in the HEN population. A recent retrospective study by Silver et al. focused on the experiences of older patients receiving HEN.[33] The majority of these patients had gastrostomies. Most of these patients relied upon their families for help and had little other nursing or dietitian intervention. One third of the patients reported tube clogging or leaking and one third reported G-tube displacement. More input from the clinician regarding home enteral access care would be important in order to prevent these frequent tube-related complications.

Percutaneous Endoscopic Gastrostomy Tube Obstruction

Percutaneous endoscopic gastrostomy tubes may occlude from medications, feeding formula or blenderized foods placed through the PEG. Obstructed PEG tubes may be cleared with the use of warm water and a syringe. In some cases, pancreatic enzymes mixed in a bicarbonate solution can also be effective.[34] There is no data to support the use of juices, soft drinks or meat tenderizers to unclog a PEG tube. Commercially available PEG tube cleaning brushes are also available. Flushing the PEG tube between feedings and also with medication instillation will reduce the possibility of PEG tube occlusion.

New Technologies in Percutaneous Endoscopic Gastrostomy

One of the more challenging patients receiving PEG is the patient who is unable to open their mouth for passage of the endoscope or patients in whom any sedation for endoscopy is dangerous because of their severe underlying comorbid diseases. Dumortier et al recently reported on transnasal PEG placement using a 5.9 mm endoscope pass through the nare into the stomach.[35] This procedure was performed in unsedated patients. A 20 fr PEG with a flexible internal bolster was passed through the nare into position on the abdominal wall by the pull technique. This is exactly the same pull technique used for PEG placement through the oral cavity. Twenty-three patients received a transnasal PEG without any sedation. The procedure was successful in 91% of patients with 2 failures secondary to inability to transilluminate the abdominal wall. There was 1 episode of transient epistaxis, 1 subsequent PEG wound infection and one episode of peritubular leakage. None of these complications resulted in PEG tube removal. Transnasal endoscopy appears to be safe and well tolerated for PEG placement and may be an option for some patients.

PERCUTANEOUS ENDOSCOPIC GASTROJEJUNOSTOMY

In those patients in whom small bowel feedings are required endoscopic, percutaneous, small bowel access may be obtained by two methods. The first method, percutaneous endoscopic gastrojejunostomy (PEG/J), places a jejunal feeding tube through an existing PEG into the small bowel using an over-the-guidewire endoscopy method. After PEG placement, the patient is re-endoscoped and a 9 or 12 fr J-tube is passed over a guidewire, through the existing PEG and into position in the small bowel (Figure 5–6).[36] This PEG/J system allows for gastric decompression and small bowel feeding concurrently. The PEG tubes are 20–24 fr and the J-tubes are 9–12 fr in size. The average longevity of the J-tube within the PEG/J system is 3–6 months. [36,37]

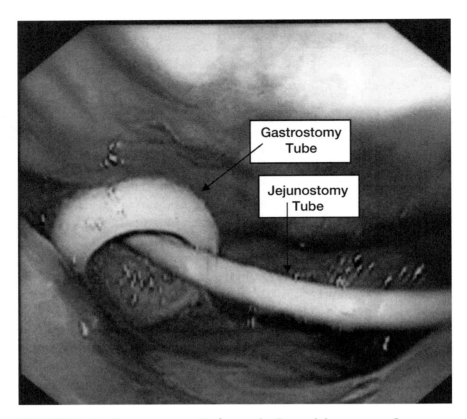

FIGURE 5–6   Percutaneous Endoscopic Gastrojejunostomy System.

Percutaneous Endoscopic Gastrojejunostomy Management

The management of PEG/J tubes is similar to that of PEG tubes. Jejunal tubes need to be flushed aggressively as to avoid clogging. Reported clogging rates of J-tubes have ranged from 3.5% to 35%.[38,39] Pushing poorly dissolved medications or bulking medications such as Metamucil® through the J-tube or checking for tube feeding residuals through the J-tube all lead to an increased incidence of J-tube occlusion.[40] Medication may be administered through the gastrostomy tube, the larger diameter tube. The gastrostomy tube may also be used for decompression in those with gastroparesis or gastric outlet obstruction. There is little literature regarding the use of a PEG/J systems in the home environment although it is not an uncommon practice.

Percutaneous Endoscopic Gastro/Jejunostomy Complications

Complications of PEG/J tubes include those already discussed for a PEG. In addition, the J-tube may experience retrograde migration or luminal dysfunction secondary to kinking or clogging. Tube migration occurs most commonly in those patients who have persistent vomiting or in instances where the J-tube was not originally positioned properly through the PEG tube. In instances of J-tube dysfunction, a new J-tube may be placed through the PEG into the small bowel with the use of endoscopy or fluoroscopy.

DIRECT PERCUTANEOUS JEJUNOSTOMY

The second method of endoscopic jejunal access, direct percutaneous jejunostomy (DPEJ), directly places a J-tube into the small bowel using an endoscope, similar to the PEG technique. Good success with this procedure has been reported by Shike.[41,42] There were some minor complications reported, including local site infection, but no reported cases of peritonitis nor bowel infarction. Because of the larger diameter of DPEJ tubes (18–24 fr), they are less likely to occlude than the jejunal tubes in PEG/J systems (9–12 fr). In addition, because the DPEJ tube is placed directly into the small intestine, the J-tube does not migrate back into the stomach as seen with the PEG/J system. There is little literature regarding the use of a DPEJ in the home environment although it is not an uncommon practice.

Direct Percutaneous Endoscopic Jejunostomy Tube Management

Immediately after DPEJ placement, it may be helpful to leave the J-tube unclamped for 1–2 hours so as to decompress the small bowel from the substantial amount of air that is insufflated during the procedure. Otherwise, the management is similar to that of PEG and PEG/J tubes.

Direct Percutaneous Endoscopic Jejunostomy Complications

Complications and technical failures have been reported in three retrospective series on DPEJ outcomes. Technical failure rates ranged for placement from 12–28 %. Complications included bleeding, abdominal wall abscesses, colonic perforations, peristomal infections, enteric ulcers, and enteric leakage. Tube-related malfunctions similar to PEG tubes have also occurred.[42–44]

SURGICAL ENTERAL ACCESS

Surgical enteral access was the standard of care for many years. These procedures included gastrostomy, gastrojejunostomy, and jejunostomy. These procedures may be performed via a standard, open surgical technique or with laparoscopic guidance. In recent years, the advent of PEG, PEG/J and DPEJ have relegated surgical enteral access placement to patients who are in the operating room for another surgical procedure or in patients where endoscopic or radiologic enteral access is technically impossible. In a review by Meyers et al, patients received surgical jejunostomies as an additional technique during other major abdominal surgery in 95% of cases and as the sole surgical technique in 5% of cases.[45] Multiple studies have compared surgical gastrostomy to PEG. These studies have either shown a cost-savings or a reduction in morbidity with PEG.[46,47]

Surgical Jejunostomy

Surgical jejunostomy is a procedure in which a tube is placed into the lumen of the proximal jejunum. In 1891, Witzel first described the most well known technique for jejunostomy which has subsequently undergone a number of modifications.[48] In the standard feeding jejunostomy, a transverse laparotomy is performed and a jejunal loop is identified. An 8–12 fr silicone or rubber catheter is inserted through the abdominal wall and into the jejunum. The tube itself is sutured to the abdominal wall to keep it from migrating. These tubes usually do not have an internal or an external bolster as do PEG and DPEJ tubes. Therefore, they are dependent on the use of sutures or tape to fix them to the abdominal wall to prevent inadvertent tube dislodgement. The decision to place a surgical J-tube follows the same decision analysis as the decision to place any jejunal feeding tube. Typically, patients who are intolerant to gastric feedings, patients at high risk for aspiration of tube feedings or patients in whom the stomach is either diseased or surgically absent, will receive a surgical J-tube. Surgical jejunostomy is a common procedure used to obtain feeding access in trauma patients. Surgical J-tubes are used for HEN although there is little reportable outcome data.

Surgical Jejunostomy Complications

Complications associated with surgical J-tube placement include wound infection, wound breakdown, tube occlusion, and tube dislodgment. Holmes et al reported a complication rate of 10% and a mortality rate of 1.4% in trauma patients receiving a surgical jejunostomy directly related to the procedure.[49] There is limited published information regarding the outcome of surgical jejunostomy in HEN patients.

Needle Catheter Jejunostomy

Needle catheter jejunostomy (NCJ) is an alternative tube system which can be placed surgically within the small intestine. This involves the placement of a 5 or 7 fr catheter into the jejunum, via a submucosal tunnel. It was hypothesized that this technique would have fewer complications compared with standard jejunostomy as the entrance to the jejunum was much smaller in comparison. However, the small size of the needle catheter jejunostomy makes it prone to early occlusion and dislodgement. These catheters must be flushed aggressively. Medications, other than those available in liquid form, should not be infused via a NCJ because of its small diameter. In general, NCJ are not used for HEN.

Laparoscopic Enteral Access

Laparoscopic placement of J-tubes and G-tubes was developed in the early 1990s. Initially it was proposed that these procedures were associated with less morbidity and operative stress than standard surgical jejunostomy and gastrostomy. However, it was later determined that these laparoscopic techniques did not significantly add any advantage compared with standard surgical gastrostomy or jejunostomy with relation to operative time nor associated procedure morbidity.[50]

FLUOROSCOPIC PERCUTANEOUS ENTERAL ACCESS

Placement of percutaneous gastrostomy and gastrojejunostomies with fluoroscopic guidance has continued to gain acceptance since their introduction in the early 1980s.[51,52] These procedures are usually performed by radiologists in the fluoroscopy suite. After topical anesthesia of the abdominal wall, and occasional conscious sedation, the inferior margin of the liver is identified by ultrasound and marked on the patient's abdominal wall skin surface. A nasogastric tube is passed into the stomach for insufflation. After gastric insufflation, the stomach is punctured with an introducer catheter that is pushed through the abdominal wall into the gastric lumen. A guidewire is placed into the stomach through the introducer. The puncture site is serially dilated over a guidewire to a size of 10 to 14 fr. A gastrostomy tube is passed over the guidewire into the stomach or into the small intestine if a gastrojejunostomy tube is desired. Some radiologist will attach the stomach to the anterior abdominal wall with T-fasteners, whereas others will not. These T-fasteners are placed through the abdominal wall by the use of a small cutting catheter and advanced into the gastric lumen. Usually, 3–4 T-fasteners are placed in a circle around the feeding tube. This allows the stomach to be pulled up and sutured to the abdominal wall.

Fluoroscopic Enteral Access Complications

The major criticism of fluoroscopic enteral tube placement focuses on procedure-related and tube-related complications. The majority of the procedure-related complications involve either inadvertent puncture of contiguous abdominal organs or separation of the abdominal and gastric wall during gastrostomy tract dilation. This separation of the abdominal and gastric wall may lead to gastric leakage peritonitis. Other tube-related complications include both tube occlusion, because of the small tube size, or inadvertent tube dislodgement.

ENTERAL ACCESS OUTCOMES IN HOME ENTERAL NUTRITION

Outcome studies of enteral access outcomes in HEN patients are small in number. A study by Wilcock et al focused on HEN complications in 19 patients over one year, a very small number.[53] Enteral stomal infections frequently resulted in a visit to the physician or the healthcare worker. The same was true for the onset of diarrhea. Flatulence, although a common complaint, rarely resulted in a physician visit. They reported 14 incidents where patients couldn't obtain their tube feeding from their home provider, 2 cases of equipment failure and 10 cases where the feeding tube became obstructed. Only one of those problems resulted in a visit to a healthcare provider.

Shatner, et al reported on home enteral nutrition use in patients with dysphagia.[54] This was a retrospective review over the course of eight years. The patient's nutrition therapy was followed by a nutrition support team, who also monitored their outcomes. There were 82 patients with a mean age of 61. Most of them had head and neck cancer. Most of the patients were at home on gastric feedings, the minority of them were home on small-bowel feedings. Diarrhea occurred in approximately 20% of the whole group. Tube site stomal infection or stomal irritation and leakage occurred in 6% to 7% of the total patient group.

In a preoperative head and neck cancer study, preoperative enteral nutrition support was given to a group of patients with weight loss.[55] Forty-six patients received an NG-tube and 43 patients received a PEG. All received at-home enteral nutrition training. Their pre-treatment weight loss was approximately 12%. On follow-up, there were no significant HEN complications. The NG-tube fed patients only had a 15% compliance rate with NG-feedings. Those who were fed with a PEG had a 68% compliance with their home tube feeding regime. Because of nutrition compliance issues, the PEG-fed patients had a 30% reduction in their hospital stay as compared to the NG fed patients.

SUMMARY

Home enteral nutrition has become a commonly prescribed home therapy. In order to provide this therapy, enteral access needs to be established. Enteral access placement techniques may involve the nurse, the radiologist, the endoscopist, or the surgeon. The patient's current disease state, co-morbidities, medical therapy, life expectancy, expected time of need of their enteral access device and home environment will help determine the appropriate enteral access technique for tube placement (Table 5–2). Knowledge of all enteral access devices and techniques for placement is imperative in order to provide the safest and most effective route for enteral nutrition.

TABLE 5-2   Endoscopic Enteral Access Methods

Type of access	Used for	Length of need
Surgical or percutaneous access Gastrostomy	Gastric feeding Gastric decompression	>1 month
Gastrojejunostomy	Gastric decompression Jejunal feeding	1–6 months
Jejunostomy	Jejunal feeding	>1 month
Nasal/Oral access Nasal/Oral Gastric Tube	Gastric feeding Gastric decompression	<1 month
Nasal/Oral Gastrojejunal Tube	Gastric feeding Gastric decompression Jejunal feeding	<1 month
Nasal/Oral Small Bowel Tube	Jejunal feeding	<1 month

REFERENCES

1. North American home enteral and parenteral patient registry; Annual Reports 1985–1990. Albany, NY: The Oley Foundation; 1987–1992.
2. Howard L, Heaphey L, Fleming CR, et al. Four years of North American registry home parenteral nutrition outcome data and their implications for patient management. *JPEN*. 1991;15(4):384–393.
3. Randall HT. The history of enteral nutrition. In: Rombeau JL, Caldwell MD, eds. *Enteral and Parenteral Nutrition*. Philadelphia, Pa: WB Saunders; 1984:1–10.
4. Harkness L. The history of enteral nutrition therapy: from raw eggs and nasal tubes to purified amino acids and early postoperative jejunal delivery. *J Am Diet Assoc*. 2002;102(3):399–404.
5. Kravetz RE. Pap boat. *Am J Gastroenterol*. 2000;95(1):271.
6. Jones-Humphreys RM. An easy method of feeding per rectum. *Lancet*. 1891;1:366–367.
7. Anderson AFR. Immediate jejunal feeding after gastro-enterostomy. *Ann Surg*. 1918;67:565–566.
8. Abbott WO. Fluid and nutritional maintenance by the use of the intestinal tract. *Ann Surg*. 1940;112:584–593.
9. Gauderer MW, Ponsky JL, Izant RJ Jr. Gastrostomy without laparotomy: a percutaneous endoscopic technique. *J Pediatr Surg*. 1980;15(6):872–875.
10. Caulfield KA, Page CP, Pestana C. Technique for intraduodenal placement of transnasal enteral feeding catheters. *Nutr Clin Pract*. 1991;6(1):23–26.
11. McWrey RE, Curry NS, Schabel SI, Reines HD. Complications of nasoenteric feeding tubes. *Am J Surg*. 1988;155(2):253–257.

12. Collier P, Kudsk KA, Glezer J, Brown RO. Fiber–containing formula and needle catheter jejunostomies: a clinical evaluation. *Nutr Clin Pract.* 1994; 9(3):101–103.

13. Cataldi–Betcher EL, Seltzer MH, Slocum BA, Jones KW. Complications occurring during enteral nutrition support: a prospective study. *JPEN.* 1983;7(6):546–552.

14. Park RHR, Allison MC, Long J, et al. Randomized comparison of percutaneous endoscopic gastrostomy vs nasogastric feedings in patients with persistent neurological dysphagia. *Br Med J.* 1992;304:1406–1409.

15. Ponsky JL, Gauderer MW. Percutaneous endoscopic gastrostomy: a nonoperative technique for feeding gastrostomy. *Gastrointest Endosc.* 1981;27(1): 9–1

16. Steigman GV, Goff JS, Silas D, et al. Endoscopic versus operative gastrostomy: Final results of a prospective, randomized trial. *Gastrointest Endosc* 1990; 36:1–5.

17. Light VL, Slezak FA, Porter JA, et al. Predictive factors for early mortality after percutaneous endoscopic gastrostomy. *Gastrointest Endosc.* 1995;42(4): 330–335.

18. Lee JH, Machtay M, Unger LD, et al. Prophylactic gastrostomy tubes in patients undergoing intensive irradiation for cancer of the head and neck. *Arch Otolaryngol Head Neck Surg.* 1998;124(8):871–875.

19. DeLegge MH. PEG placement: Justifying the intervention. UpToDate 2001;9(1).

20. Gillick MR. Rethinking the role of tube feeding in patients with advanced dementia. *New Engl J Med.* 2000;342(3):206–210.

21. Sanders DS, Carter MJ, D'Silva J, et al. Survival analysis in percutaneous endoscopic gastrostomy feeding: a worse outcome in patients with dementia. *Am J Gastroenterol.* 2000;95(6):1472–1475.

22. Murphy LM, Lipman TO. Percutaneous endoscopic gastrostomy does not prolong survival in patients with dementia. *Arch Intern Med.* 2003;163(11): 1351–1353.

23. Marcuard SP, Finley JL, MacDonald KG. Large-bore feeding tube occlusion by yeast colonies. *JPEN.* 1993;17(2):187–190.

24. DeLegge MH, Kirby DF. Enteral nutrition overview. Part 1: Enteral Access Devices. Pract Gastro 1992;XV:21–6.

25. Steiner M, Bourges HR, Freedman LS, Gray SJ. Effect of starvation on the tissue composition of the small intestine in the rat. *Am J Physiol.* 1968; 215(1):75–77.

26. Alverdy J, Chi HS, Sheldon GF. The effect of parenteral nutrition on gastrointestinal immunity. The importance of enteral stimulation. *Ann Surg.* 1985;202(6):681–684.

27. Adams S, Dellinger EP, Wertz MF, et al. Enteral versus parenteral nutritional support following laparotomy for trauma: a randomized prospective trial. *J Trauma.* 1986;26(10):882–991.

28. Jain NK, Larson DE, Schroeder KW, et al. Antibiotic prophylaxis for percutaneous, endoscopic gastrostomy. A prospective, randomized, double-blind clinical trial. *Ann Intern Med.* 1987;107(6):824–828.

29. DeLegge MH, Lantz G, Kazacos E, et al. Effect of external bolster tension on PEG tube tract formation. *Gastrointest Endosc.* 1996;43:A349.

30. Foutch PG, Talbert GA, Waring JP, et al. Percutaneous endoscopic gastrostomy in patients with prior abdominal surgery: virtues of the safe tract. *Am J Gastroenterol.* 1988;83(2):147–150.

31. Wolfsen HC, Kozarek RA, Ball TJ, et al. Tube dysfunction following percutaneous endoscopic gastrostomy and jejunostomy. *Gastrointest Endosc.* 1990;36(3):261–263.

32. Kirby DF, DeLegge MH, Fleming CR. American Gastroenterological Association technical review on tube feeding for enteral nutrition. *Gastroenterology.* 1995;108(4):1282–1301.

33. Silver HJ, Wellman NS, Arnold DJ, et al. Older adults receiving home enteral nutrition: enteral regimen, provider involvement, and health care outcomes. *JPEN.* 2004;28(2):92–98.

34. Sriram K, Jayanthi V, Lakshmi RG, et al. Prophylactic locking of feeding tubes with pancreatic enzymes. *JPEN.* 1997;21(6):353–356.

35. Dumortier J, Lapalus MG, Pereira A, et al. Unsedated transnasal PEG placement. *Gastrointest Endosc.* 2004;59(1):54–57.

36. DeLegge MH, Patrick P, Gibbs R. Percutaneous endoscopic gastrojejunostomy with a tapered tip, nonweighted jejunal feeding tube: improved placement success. *Am J Gastroenterol.* 1996;91(6):1130–1134.

37. Gore DC, DeLegge MH, Gervin A, et al. Surgically placed gastro-jejunostomy tubes have fewer complications compared to feeding jejunostomy tubes. *J Am Coll Nutr.* 1996;15(2):144–146.

38. Meyers JG, Page CP, Stewart RM, et al: Complications of needle catheter jejunostomy. *Ann Surg.* 1985;55:466–469.

39. Holmes JH, Brundage SI, Yeun P, et al. Complications of surgical feeding jejunostomy in trauma patients. *J Trauma.* 1999;47(6):1009–1012.

40. DeWald CL, Heitte PO, Sewall LE, et al. Percutaneous gastrostomy and gastrojejunostomy with gastropexy: experience in 701 procedures. *Radiology.* 1999;211(3):651–656.

41. Shike M, Berner YN, Gerdes H, et al. Percutaneous endoscopic gastrostomy and jejunostomy for long-term feeding in patients with cancer of the head and neck. *Otolaryngol Head Neck Surg.* 1989;101(5):549–554.

42. Shike M, Latkany L, Gerdes H, et al. Direct percutaneous endoscopic jejunostomies for enteral feeding. *Gastrointest Endosc.* 1996;44(5):536–540.

43. Varadarajulu S, DeLegge MH. Use of a 19-gauge needle as a direct guide for percutaneous endoscopic jejunostomy tube placement. *Gastrointest Endosc.* 2003;57(7):942–945.

44. Fan AC, Baron TH, Rumalla A, et al. Comparison of direct percutaneous endoscopic jejunostomy and PEG with jejunal extension. *Gastrointest Endosc.* 2002;56(6):890–894.
45. Meyers JG, Page CP, Stewart RM, et al. Complications of needle catheter jejunostomy in 2,022 consecutive applications. *Am J Surg.* 1995;170(6): 547–550.
46. Steigmann GV, Goff JS, Silas D, et al. Endoscopic versus operative gastrostomy: final results of a prospective randomized trial. *Gastrointest Endosc.* 1990;36(1):1–5.
47. Scott JS, de la Torre RA, Unger SW. Comparison of operative versus percutaneous endoscopic gastrostomy tube placement in the elderly. *Am Surg.* 1991;57(5):338–340.
48. Rombeau JL, Caldwell MD, Forlaw L, et al. *Atlas of Nutrition Support Techniques.* Boston, MA: Little Brown; 1989:167–174.
49. Holmes JH, Brundage SI, Yeun P, et al. Complications of surgical feeding jejunostomy in trauma patients. *J Trauma.* 1999;47(6):1009–1012.
50. Edelman DS, Unger SW, Russin DR. Laparoscopic gastrostomy. *Surg Laparosc Endosc.* 1991;1(4):251–253.
51. Ho CS. Percutaneous gastrostomy for jejunal feeding. *Radiology.* 1983; 149(2):595–596.
52. Ho CS, Yeung EY. Percutaneous gastrostomy and transgastric jejunostomy. *AJR Am J Roentgenol.* 1992;158(2):251–257.
53. Wilcock H, Armstrong J, Cottee S, et al. Parenteral Nutrition support for the Cambridge Health District. Health Trends. *Am J Clin Nutr.* 1991;23:93–100.
54. Shattner M, Barrera R, Nygard S, et al. Outcome of Home Enteral Nutrition in patients with malignant dysphagia, NCP 2001;16:292–295.
55. Holden CE, Puntis JW, Charlton CP, et al. Nasogastric feeding at home: acceptability and safety. *Arch Dis Child.* 1991;66(1):148–151.

CHAPTER 6

Home Enteral Nutrition Support in Adults

Carol S. Ireton-Jones, PhD, RD, LD, CNSD, FACN

Home enteral nutrition is the most common home nutrition therapy provided with more than 344,000 people of all ages in the United States receiving enteral nutrition at home.[1] Enteral nutrition is defined as nutrients provided via the gastrointestinal tract.[2] Therefore, enteral nutrition can mean oral nutrition (diet) as well as nutrition is provided through a tube, catheter, or stoma that delivers nutrients distal to the oral cavity.[2] Sometimes people who require enteral nutrition support at home are able to consume some nutrients orally, but many rely on the enteral tube feeding to provide the bulk of their nutritional needs. This chapter will focus specifically on enteral (tube) nutrition in adults. Chapter 9 reviews home enteral nutrition in pediatrics.

INDICATIONS FOR ENTERAL NUTRITION

The major considerations for selecting the feeding route and nutrition support formula include gastrointestinal (GI) function, expected duration of nutrition therapy, aspiration risk, and the potential for or the actual development of organ dysfunction.[3] The American Society of Parenteral and Enteral Nutrition has developed practice guidelines for both enteral and parenteral nutrition support which deal with hospitalized and home care patients.[3] These guidelines are useful to practitioners who provide nutrition therapies often as well as those who are infrequently faced with patients requiring nutrition support.

Enteral nutrition support can be accomplished in a wide variety of patients with many disease processes. Often quoted is the phrase, "if the gut works, use it." In order to utilize the GI tract, a minimum of 100 cm jejunal and 150 cm ileal length of functioning small bowel with the ileocecal valve intact is necessary for sufficient absorption of nutrients.[4] Enteral nutrition is most often used when there is a malfunction of the mechanism to pass food from the mouth to the stomach. Appropriate patients include those who cannot swallow such as after a stroke, due to a debilitating neurological disease or patients who have a disease process or therapy that interferes with swallowing such as head and neck cancer patients. Patients who have gastroparesis may have a tube placed distal to the stomach and those with pancreatitis may have a feeding tube placed into the jejunum, allowing them to meet their nutritional needs enterally. Patients with malabsorption, high output fistulas or severe enterocolitis, severe nausea, vomiting or diarrhea are not probable candidates for enteral feeding. In addition, no mechanical obstruction of the GI tract that cannot be bypassed with a feeding tube or GI hemorrhage should be present. With these exceptions, the provision of enteral feeding at home can be a viable option for meeting nutrient needs outside of the hospital.

Prior to initiating home enteral nutrition (HEN), the physician caring for the patient should discuss the benefits and obligations for the patient and/or care partner in managing HEN. Preparing the patient for discharge (Chapter 3) is important in assuring the success of the therapy at home. While HEN is less invasive than many other home infusion therapies, it does require an organized approach to daily care and management. For many pediatric patients, the parents or caregivers will provide all of the care while adults and older adolescents receiving HEN may provide their own care. Because the physician that places the enteral access may be different from the physician that manages the patient's enteral feeding on an ongoing basis, a thorough explanation of the therapy and its components may not be provided. A competent home care provider with the expertise of a skilled clinician in nutrition support is vital. Asking if a dietitian or nurse is a part of the home care team will help identify the best home care provider for a HEN patient.

ASSESSING NUTRIENT NEEDS

When it is determined that a patient will require home enteral nutrition, enteral access must be obtained. For many patients enteral access is placed in the hospital setting although enteral access may be placed in a clinic, or outpatient surgical center. Whether completed during hospitalization or in the home setting, the nutrition assessment will determine the patient's energy/calorie needs, enteral formula, goals of therapy and monitoring guidelines. Nutrition assessment is discussed in Chapter 3.

Energy and protein requirements are determined based on the patient's nutritional and medical status. When patients are in the hospital, their calorie needs are usually calculated by the dietitian or the nutrition support clinician based on the disease process, illness or injury status. Once the patient is at home, energy requirements may be different. An assessment of the activity level at home as well as needs for recovery is important to avoid over- as well as under-feeding. If weight gain or loss occurs, calories can be modified fairly easily if the patient and caregiver have a good understanding of the home enteral feeding regimen. Adequacy of wound healing and return or improvement in physical strength may be used as an indicator of protein status in the person receiving enteral nutrition in the home. Micronutrients, vitamins and minerals, are usually provided in adequate amounts through the enteral feeding formula as long as a minimum number of calories are provided. Patients requiring few calories or those who have increased vitamin or mineral needs may require supplementation to the enteral feeding.

ENTERAL ACCESS

Successful home enteral nutrition is often determined by the type and location of enteral access. A reliable, low-risk method of enteral access will obviate interruptions in therapy related to a displaced, occluded, broken, or painful enteral access device. Frequent or prolonged interruptions in therapy related to enteral access are frustrating for patients, caregivers, and clinicians and can be costly and negatively impact therapeutic goals. Well thought out decisions about the type and location of enteral access are necessary to minimize complications (see Chapter 7).

In determining the type of enteral access, the length of time the patient will receive the enteral feeding, that is, temporarily or permanently, as well as the type and viscosity of the feeding solution, volume of solution to be provided, the administration method and the risk of gastric or tube feeding aspiration must be considered. In general, enteral access is achieved via nasally placed tubes located in the stomach, duodenum, or jejunum or surgically or endoscopically placed tubes located in the stomach or jejunum.[5–7] Nasogastric or nasointestinal tubes are most suitable for short term therapy (<4 weeks). These tubes can be placed in an outpatient or home setting, however, their position should be confirmed radiologically after insertion to ensure proper placement.[8] Longer-term (>4 weeks) or lifetime enteral access is most often accomplished by percutaneous tube enterostomy placement of a feeding tube such as a percutaneous endoscopic gastrostomy (PEG) placed into the stomach and/or small bowel. The ability to place a tube using surgical techniques may be limited by scar tissue, intra-abdominal tumor, large abdominal wounds, stomas, or prior gastric resections and therefore a skilled physician with expertise in feeding tube placement is required.[8]

The risk of aspiration and the presence of potential or actual alterations in gastric function, such as gastroparesis or gastric ileus may necessitate post-pyloric placement of tubes.[8–9] Patients with gastroparesis from diabetes mellitus or neurological disorders and those with pancreatitis can often be fed via the intestine. Even patients with excessive vomiting, such as women with hyperemesis gravidarum, have been successfully fed via the intestine with nasointestinal tube placement.[10] In the home setting, enteral formula infused volumes can be gradually increased over time and decreased in frequency which will help avoid the risk of aspiration. When administering feedings at home, the patient should be sitting upright during the feeding and remain upright for 30 minutes after the feeding. If the patient is unable to sit up, then the head of the bed should be raised to 30 degrees and left there for 30 minutes after the feeding. It is further recommended that the head of the bed be placed on blocks to assure that the head remains raised as pillows can be unreliable as a means of head elevation and patients can inadvertently move over time.

ENTERAL DEVICE COMPLICATIONS

Mechanical complications of enteral access devices include displacement, occlusion, and breakage. Displacement is most often a problem for patients receiving a naso-enteric feeding which is why the use of these in the home is not optimal. It is important to recognize situations in which the tube is likely to become displaced, such as violent coughing, vomiting, and accidental tugging on the tube. Patients or caregivers should learn techniques to detect tube displacement, such as pH testing of secretions, monitoring tube centimeter markings, and checking the oropharynx for tube coiling, and perform these techniques prior to beginning formula administration.[11] In general, nasally placed tubes are not preferred for home enteral nutrition, but can be used with caution for patients who are meticulous in recognizing and reporting possible tube displacement. Tubes placed surgically, endoscopically, laporoscopically, and radiologically are less likely to become displaced than nasally placed tubes. Signs of displacement of percutaneously placed tubes include a change in the length of the external portion of the tube, difficulty in infusing or flushing, leakage of formula or flush solution from the exit site, and an immobile tube that is painful. When a long-term enteral feeding device is accidentally removed, it should be replaced as soon as possible as the tract in which the tube was placed can close quickly.[12] Patients and or caregivers should carefully document the type, brand, and size of their feeding tubes to give to their home care provider for replacement if needed. It is also helpful to develop a plan for replacement or repair of the tube should breakage occur. Most long term enteral access devices have replacement end adapters for leaks or breakage. Patients and or caregivers should contact their physician and/or the home care provider when there is a access device complication as soon as possible so that a solution can be devised. Home enteral nutrition patients or their caregivers can be taught to replace their enteral feeding device themselves. Alternatively, the home care clinician can re-insert the device or the patient may directed to the emergency room. Tube replacement should be done by the physician if the tube has been in place for less than 4 weeks or longer if the patient is malnourished or immunocompromised.[12]

TUBE MAINTENANCE

Prevention of feeding tube occlusion is key to tube maintenance. Factors contributing to occlusion include medication administration and inadequate flushing. Medications should be administered via another route or be provided in liquid form. Liquid medications should be evaluated for their potential osmolality as this will affect gastrointestinal tolerance of the medication and the feeding. Liquid oral medication in elixir form or containing sorbitol can cause diarrhea, bloating or cramping.[13] Some commonly used liguid medications with high osmolality (>300 mOsm/kg) include acetaminophen elixir (5400 mOsm/kg); cimetidine solution (5500 mOsm/kg), metaclopromide syrup (8350 mOsm/kg), theophylline elixir (6550 mOm/kg) and digoxin elixir (1350 mOsm/kg). Medications may be diluted to reduce osmolalty. The pharmacist can assist the patient or caregiver in evaluating the appropriate amount of water to utilize and the compatibility of the drug with dilution. Diluting medications with at least 30 ml of water is recommended although the patients fluid tolerance must be evaluated in light of water for flushing the tube, dilution of the medications and provision of free (non-tube feeding formula) water.[14] The pharmacist can also provide information on certain medications which should not be crushed, such as those for sustained release, and drug–nutrient interactions which may also occur.[13]

Water is the best flush solution. Many patients who receive home enteral nutrition do not receive adequate amounts of free (not in the tube feeding formula) water. Unless fluid is restricted, most patients should be advised to flush their tubes frequently with liberal amount of water (60 to 120 ml) and infuse additional free water. Fluid requirements may be calculated for adults as follows:[15]

Adults:

- 35 ml/kg body weight/day

Or

- 100 ml/kg/day for the first 10 kg body weight
- add 50 ml/kg/day for the second 10 kg of body weight
- For each additional kg of body weight add 20 ml/kg per day if ≤ to 500 years of age or 15 ml/kg if >50 years of age.

It is imperative to account for other losses from problems such as fever, diarrhea, and vomiting and to provide additional fluid replacement to meet these additional needs. Failure to account for fluid needs can lead to dehydration and rehospitalization. In addition, the enteral feeding will contain a percentage of free water from 84% in a 1.0 kcal/ml formula to 70% in a 2.0 kcal/ml formula.[16] This information is readily available from the enteral formula manufacturer on their website, informational materials and usually, on each individual can of formula.

CARE OF THE FEEDING SITE

Skin care around feeding ostomy site should be accomplished by cleaning with mild soap and water, rinsing and drying thoroughly. Mild soap and water can be used to cleanse around the tube exit site once it heals. Patients should be taught to clean carefully under external bolsters to remove debris and to check for excessive pressure. Routine use of antibiotic ointments is not advised, and dressings at the tube insertion site are not necessary unless there is drainage at the site.[17] The tube exit site and abdominal wound, if present, should be carefully assessed for edema, erythema, drainage, or necrotic material.[17, 18] This assessment becomes particularly important as hospital stays for insertion of enteral access have decreased and as outpatient enteral access placements are increasingly used. In most cases, it is better to avoid placing a dressing over the site once it has healed. Patients should learn to report any drainage, pain, bleeding, swelling, or irritation at the tube exit site.[19]

SELECTION OF ENTERAL FORMULAS

Considerations in the selection of enteral formulas include: digestive and absorptive capacity; nutritional status/medical therapy; renal function; fluid tolerance/electrolyte balance; route of delivery; and drug therapy. Standard enteral formulas are now available that can meet the needs of most patients. Formulas may also be calorically dense or disease specific. Most enteral formulas are lactose-free. Lactose, the primary sugar in milk, requires lactase an enzyme that breaks down lactose into glucose and galactose for absorption. Lactase deficiency is common in certain racial and ethnic groups and its frequency increases with age. To avoid lactose intolerance which is exhibited by gastrointestinal distress, such as pain, bloating and diarrhea, the majority of enteral supplements and tube feeding formulas are lactose-free or contain only a trace amount of lactose.

Functional status of the GI tract and absorptive capacity are the predominant factors in choosing an enteral formula. Because of this, enteral formulas are categorized according to their type and amount of protein

---

TABLE 6–1   Enteral Formula Categories

Standard Enteral Formulas
- 1.0–1.2 kcal/ml
- Whole/intact protein
- Fiber-containing

Concentrated Enteral Formulas
- 1.5–2.0 kcal/ml
- High protein—20–25% protein

Disease/Condition Specific
- Healing support
- Immune stimulating
- Glucose management
- Pulmonary disease
- Renal disease
- Hepatic disease

Modular enteral feeding components
- Protein
- Carbohydrate
- Fat

---

and calories as well as disease state or condition to make formula selection easier (Table 6–1).

ENTERAL FORMULAS

Standard whole protein or intact protein formulas contain a protein base (casein or whey protein) and provide 1.0 kcal per ml. Whole or intact protein formulas are usually administered to patients with a functioning gastrointestinal tract (ability to digest and absorb intact proteins) into the stomach or duodenum.

Standard whole protein formulas can be flavored or unflavored. Unflavored formulas are usually isotonic (concentration of all nutrients in the formula is the same as the concentration of the blood which is approximately 300 mOsm/kg water). Isotonic formulas (300 mOsm/kg) are well tolerated, but products with osmolalities greater that 300m/kg water may draw water into the GI tract causing diarrhea. The addition of sucrose to enteral formulas enhances the taste, but at the same time, increases the osmolality of the solution. Standard whole protein diets are useful in patients with functioning GI tracts who require oral supplements or tube feeding.

High calorie or calorically dense formulas also contain whole proteins but provide 1.5–2.0 kcal/ml. They are often used for patients with elevated calorie needs ranging from 25–35 kcal/kg, and/or require fluid restriction. Patients at home with cardiac or respiratory disease or those they have restricted fluid needs may benefit from the use of these products.

High protein formulas are designed for patients with increased protein requirements (1.5 to 2.5 gms/kg) and usually contain 20–25% of the calories from protein as compared to 14–16% of calories from protein in standard formulas. Patients with an increased need for protein are patients with wounds, decubitus ulcers, stress, and severe trauma.

Fiber containing formulas are useful in patients requiring bowel management. Fiber can be helpful in the management of diarrhea by absorbing excess water from the stool and in the management of constipation by providing bulk to the stool. Soy polysaccharide is the fiber used in the formulas and is provided in the range of 6–14 gms/1,000 kcals. It contains 95% insoluble and 5% soluble fiber. The use of soluble fiber in enteral formulas may provide benefits in blood glucose control, management of blood lipid levels, and the fermentation of short chain fatty acids (which may be trophic for colonocytes).

Elemental or hydrolyzed protein formulas are indicated for use in patients with a gastrointestinal dysfunction impairing their ability to digest and absorb nutrients. Elemental diets are composed of a protein source that contains a mixture of free amino acids and hydrolyzed protein in the form of small amino acid chains called peptides. The literature suggests that amino acids are absorbed more readily from a mixture of peptides and free amino acids than from free amino acids alone.[20] The carbohydrate source is usually a glucose chain in the form of glucose oligosaccharides or maltodextrin. Fat is provided from a blend of medium chain triglycerides (MCT) to enhance fat absorption and long chain triglycerides (LCT) to prevent essential fatty acid deficiency. There are elemental formulas available that are isotonic thus making them easier to tolerate and eliminate the need for dilution. Feedings can be initiated at full strength and infusion rates increased more quickly to reach optimal goal rates to meet nutrition requirements.

Enteral formulas have been developed for patients with specific disease conditions. These product formulations are based on current scientific evidence.

Enteral formulas are available that have been formulated to meet the needs of critically ill patients and for those with large open wounds or pressure ulcers. These formulas contain elevated protein and arginine for tissue synthesis. In addition, vitamin A, beta-carotene, vitamin C, and zinc have been added to promote collagen synthesis. Fish oil is added to several of these specialty formulas and is thought to enhance immune function. Glutamine is often added to enhance small bowel mucosal growth and maintenance.

Enteral formulas have been developed to provide nutrition support to patients who require glucose management. Ideally, the enteral formula should adhere to the American Diabetes recommendations which currently recommends that protein calories provide 10–20% of total calories; less than 10% of calories from saturated fats, no more than 10% of calories from polyunsaturated fats, and the remaining 60–70% of total calories to be distributed between monounsaturated fats and carbohydrates.[21, 22] In addition, soluble fiber may be included in the formulation to enhance blood glucose control. Often however, these patients can be successfully managed on a standard or fiber containing enteral formula with appropriate glucose monitoring to assure glucose control.

Enteral products are also available for patients with respiratory failure and chronic lung disease that are higher in fat and lower in carbohydrate.[23] This type of enteral formula is believed to help decrease the work load on the respiratory system by decreasing the amount of carbon dioxide produced. Pulmonary disease specific enteral formulas may contain as high as 55% of calories from fat and as low as 27% of calories from carbohydrate. To avoid fat intolerance, MCT can be used as a fat source as it may be better tolerated and result in less intolerance and diarrhea. Most pulmonary formulas are calorically dense (1.5 kcal/mL) as many of these patients have fluid restrictions.

Patients with acute or chronic renal disease may receive an enteral formula that are lower in protein content and that provides a high concentration of essential amino acids. It is believed that providing this high biological value protein in smaller quantities will help minimize the blood urea nitrogen (BUN). Modifications in the electrolyte profiles and elimination of fat soluble vitamins may be of benefit to patients with renal failure. Most of these formulas are calorically dense as patients with renal failure often require fluid restriction. In patients with renal failure receiving dialysis, it may be appropriate to utilize a standard protein formulation.

Patients with hepatic disease or hepatic failure who are suffering from encephalopathy (altered mental status) may benefit from a formula that contains a lower protein content and is derived from a source that is high in branched chain amino acids (BCAA).[24] It is believed that BCAA are taken up by the skeletal muscle and do not contribute to the production of false neurotransmitters causing encephalopathy. Hepatic formulas may provide up to 50% BCAA. In addition to lower protein levels, hepatic formulas also provide lower amounts of fat. MCT usually provide a major portion of the lipid content in the formulations as patients with liver disease may have bile insufficiency and fat malabsorption. Finally, these formulas are calorically dense providing greater than 1 kcal/mL to reduce the amount of fluid needed to meet nutritional requirements in patients with fluid restrictions.

Modular components of carbohydrate, fat, and protein are available in powder or liquid form for addition to enteral formulas or to enhance regular food. With the addition of a modular component to enteral formulas, it is essential to avoid contaminating the formula and to assure that a thorough mixing has occurred to prevent tube feeding occlusion.

Two other considerations in the selection of enteral formulas are the ease of use, and the cost of the formula. Because of the plethora of formulas available commercially, it should be relatively simple to find an easy to use formula. Products which have to be mixed with water or have modular components added often are the cause for mistakes and misuse. In addition, the cost as well as the reimbursement for the formula should be considered by the prescribing physician or consulting health care team. Enteral formulas are not always reimbursed and this varies by payor sources (insurance). Sometimes, the required enteral nutrition equipment is reimbursed while the feeding formula is not with the patient assuming the cost of the formula as he or she would have to assume the cost of normal daily eating. Fortunately, this is not always the case. For Medicare patients, documentation is required to initiate an enteral feeding including permanence and diagnosis and special documentation is required for specialized enteral feedings (see Chapter 16). It is important for the registered dietitian to be involved in the selection and substitution of products when necessary. Some home care providers and many hospitals have initiated preferred product enteral formulates to decrease cost, product variability and save storage space. These enteral formularies can be very successful when developed by a multi-disciplinary health care team.

TUBE FEEDING ADMINISTRATION

There are three ways to accomplish enteral feeding—through continuous drip or bolus feeding or with an enteral feeding pump. The continuous method of consists of enteral feeding that is administered via gravity or pump allowing the formula to "drip" in slowly over a long period of time such as over a 24-hour period. The use of a pump more accurately provides the feeding; however, the gravity drip method works very well. The gravity drip can be used with a larger amount of feeding but over a shorter period of time allowing some freedom from the feeding for the patients. The enteral formula is usually placed in an enteral feeding bag and allowed to drip in slowly using gravity. If a small amount is given, the gravity drip can be accomplished over a shorter period of time. Pump feedings can be convenient as well as many pumps are small and portable enough to comfortably fit in a backpack or even a fanny or waist pack. There are many types of enteral pumps including stationary pumps and portable pumps. Some are focused for pediatric patients and adults who are active while others may be more useful for the homebound patient. There are many pump manufacturers and suppliers. Accessing the world-wide web using a search engine to search "enteral feeding pumps" will provide information which can be used in evaluating enteral pumps including cost, size, portability and ease of use. The home care provider should also be able to suggest the appropriate enteral feeding pump to meet an individuals patient's needs.

Bolus feeding generally work better for those patients who would like some "time off" from the feeding during the day or night. Bolus feedings are as it sounds, a bolus or amount of tube feeding that is administered over a relatively short period of time. A syringe is usually used to administer the feeding so that it is received in a short amount of time. A large 60 ml syringe may be used and filled as many times as appropriate for the feeding time and amount. The bolus feeding method is done at specific intervals (like eating meals and snacks) and allows for freedom from the feeding administration since it is done a few times during the day over a short period of time (less than 30 minutes) allowing for work and activities. A combination of continuous drip (at night) and bolus feedings (during the day) can be used.

MONITORING

Follow up and monitoring at regular intervals provides assessment of adequacy of the nutrition regimen for the patient receiving home enteral nutrition. Home enteral patients are seen only occasionally by the primary physician or if a problem arises. Therefore, regular monitoring is not always accomplished if not done by the physician or the home care provider. Monitoring of home enteral patients; however, is essential to assure that therapeutic goals are met (Table 6–2). Some of the problems encountered in patients receiving home enteral nutrition include: poor understanding of the feeding regimen, inadequate administration of free water, too many or not enough enteral formula bag changes, significant but unrealized weight changes, exacerbated bed sores, and inadequate feeding regimens. These types of problems can only be uncovered if a qualified health care professional is monitoring the home enteral patient. Adequate monitoring is not achieved by inventory calls on a monthly basis for product need.[25]

In home care, enteral monitoring would ideally include a baseline chemistry profile for patients initiating therapy with correction of any abnormalities prior to or within a few days of therapy initiation. In patients receiving long term enteral therapy, follow up lab analyses may not be necessary other than those required to evaluate the underlying disease process. Body weight is useful to monitor nutritional status unless the patient is bed–bound and cannot be weighed. In these cases, a critical nutrition physical assessment is useful to identify signs of skin breakdown or deterioration. Some patients may require more intensive follow-up initially which can be accomplished telephonically and then monthly contact while a long term stable patient may require follow-up only once or twice per year.

The complications associated with enteral feeding fall into one of two categories for the most part: physiological or mechanical. Mechanical complications have been discussed previously as they are most associated with the enteral feeding apparatus-tube or equipment. Physiological

TABLE 6–2   Home Enteral Nutrition Monitoring

	Baseline	Daily	Weekly	Monthly
CLINICAL				
Intake/Output	X	X (progressing to)	X	
Temperature	X	X	X	
Weight	X	X	X	
Tube site care		X		
Urinary or Blood Glucose	X	(as needed)		
LABORATORY				
Electrolytes	X	(as needed)		
BUN/Cr	X	(as needed)		
Ca, PO4,Mg	X	(as needed)		
Albumin or Transferrin	X	(as needed)		
Liver Function Tests (bilirubin, alkaline phosphatase, aspartate aminotransferase, alanine aminotransferase)	X	(as needed)		
Complete Blood Count	X	(as needed)		
Prothrombin Time/INR	X	(as needed)		
Vitamin/Trace Mineral status	Evaluate and monitor as needed			

complications revolve around gastrointestinal (GI) intolerance manifested as nausea or vomiting, diarrhea, or constipation (Table 6–3). These GI symptoms may be caused by such things as inappropriate formula administration, lactose intolerance, or drug therapy.[26]

TABLE 6-3   Common Physiologic Complications of Enteral Nutrition Support

Complication	Possible Causes	Prevention/Therapy
Gastrointestinal —Diarrhea/cramping	Drug therapy including: antibiotic therapy or diarrhea-inducing medications	—Review medications with pharmacist and identify medications with causative agents (sorbitol-elixirs, magnesium, or laxatives).
	Fat malabsorption	—Repopulate normal gut flora with commercial lactobacillus granules. —Administer antidiarrheal medication as indicated. —Consider low fat or MCT containing formula.
	Formula administered too cold	—Administer at room temperature.
	Microbial contamination	—Assure that clean technique is used for preparation/administration. —Culture for C. difficile if on antibiotic therapy.
	Infusion rate too rapid	—Modify infusion rate to decrease.
	Hyperosmolar formula	—Dilute formula initially or decrease infusion rate. —Change to compatible formula with lower osmolality.
	Hypoalbuminemia	—Consider peptide containing formula until absorptive capacity of GI tract improved. —Initiate at low rate and increase gradually as tolerated.
—Constipation	Inadequate fluid intake/inactivity/medication	—Increase fluids or assure that adequate fluids are being infused. —Use fiber containing formula or add fiber to feeding. —Consider laxatives or stool softeners laxatives.

Complication	Possible Cause	Intervention
— Nausea, vomiting	Gastric retention Rapid infusion of formula or volume too large	— Consider small bowel feeding — Consider prokinetic agents — Small bowel feeding — Maintain HOB at least 30° — Modify rate of infusion (decrease or utilize low rate and gradually increase as tolerated).
— Abdominal distention, gas, bloating, cramping	— Rapid infusion of formula — Adjustment to feedings — Nutrient malabsorption	— Assure that air is removed from tubing before connecting set to tube and that tube is clamped when not in use. — Consider lower fat formula, formula composed of hydrolyzed nutrients.
— Dehydration	— Inadequate fluid intake — Increased losses due to fluid loss from diarrhea, vomiting, or gastric drainage	— Assess fluid status — Increase or supplement fluid intake as required. — Refer for treatment of GI condition.

Reprinted with modifications from Ireton-Jones C, Hennessy K, Orr M. Care of Patients Receiving Home Enteral Therapy. *Infusion.* 1996;2(6):30–43.

EDUCATING THE PATIENT AND FAMILY

When a patient is identified as a potential candidate for home enteral nutrition, education for the patient, family or caregiver should be initiated. Because of the decreased lengths of hospitalization, patient and family education may be initiated in the hospital and may be completed at home. The home enteral nutrition schedule may mimic that of a "normal" eating schedule, may be given in nocturnal cycles, or may be provided continuously, 24-hours per day. Training should be aimed at the permanent home feeding regimen. At the time of education it is important to be assured that the home care provider which will be providing the supplies and potentially nursing and nutrition services is well known to the patient and caregiver.[25] If the patient or family has been trained on enteral feeding techniques in the hospital, the home care provider may simply supply product and appliances (bags, tubing, pump).

The Oley Foundation is a patient support for long-term nutrition support patients (www.oley.org). In addition to support, the Oley Foundation has easy to read and understand charts on home enteral feeding complications and can provide patients with links to other patients receiving home enteral nutrition. This is important as well to the success of an home enteral nutrition patient's acceptance and compliance to the regimen in knowing they are not alone. Enteral nutrition therapy provided at home is an effective, relatively safe and common method of providing life sustaining nutrients to someone who cannot adequately consume nutrients orally. Although a less invasive type of nutrition support when compared to parenteral nutrition support, enteral nutrition support should be undertaken with the proper planning, patient education and monitoring to assure success.[26]

REFERENCES

1. Ireton-Jones CS, DeLegge MH, Epperson LA, et al. Management of the home parenteral nutrition patient. *Nutr Clin Pract.* 2003;18(4):310–317.
2. A.S.P.E.N. Board of Directors. Definition of terms used in A.S.P.E.N. guidelines and standards. *Nutr Clin Pract.* 1995;10(1):1–3.
3. Guidelines for the use of parenteral and enteral nutrition in adult and pediatric patients. American Society for Parenteral and Enteral Nutrition. *J Parenter Enteral Nutr.* 1993;17(suppl 4):1SA-52SA.
4. Cisler JJ, Buchman AL. Intestinal adaptation in short bowel syndrome. *J Investig Med.* 2005;53(8):402–413.

5. Minard G. Enteral access. *Nutr Clin Pract.* 1994;9(5):172–182.

6. Lazarus BA, Murphy JB, Culpepper L. Aspiration associated with long-term gastric versus jejunal feeding: a critical analysis of the literature. *Arch Phys Med Rehabil.* 1990;71(1):46–53.

7. Vanek VW. Ins and outs of enteral access: part 2—long term access—esophagostomy and gastrostomy. *Nutr Clin Prac.* 2003;18(1):50–74.

8. DeLegge MH. Enteral access in home care. *J Parenter and Enteral Nutr.* 2006;30(suppl 1):S13-S20.

9. Davis AE, Arrington K, Fields-Ryan S, et al. Preventing feeding-associated aspiration. *Medsurg Nurs.* 1995;4(2):111–119.

10. Boyce RA. Enteral nutrition in hyperemesis gravidarum: a new development. *J Am Diet Assoc.* 1992;92(6):733–736.

11. Baskin WN. Acute complications associated with bedside placement of feeding tubes. *Nutr Clin Pract.* 2006;21(1):40–55.

12. Guenter P. Nursing care of patients with enteral feeding devices. In: Guenter P and Silkrowski M, eds. *Tube Feeding. Practical Guidelines and Nursing Protocols.* Gaithersburg, Md: Aspen Publishers; 2001:69–80.

13. Magnuson BL, Clifford TM, Hoskins LA, et al. Enteral nutrition and drug administration, interactions, and complications. *Nutr Clin Pract.* 2005;20(6): 618–624.

14. Guenter P. Mediciation administration. In: Guenter P, Silkrowski M, eds. *Tube Feeding. Practical Guidelines and Nursing Protocols.* Gaithersburg, Md: Aspen Publishers; 2001:98–99.

15. Lysen LK. Calculation of daily water requirements. In: Lysen LK, ed. *Quick Reference to Clinical Dietetics.* Boston, Mass: Jones and Bartlett Publishers; 2006:297.

16. Lysen LK. Percent of free water in enteral formulas. In: Lysen LK, ed. *Quick Reference to Clinical Dietetics.* Boston, Mass: Jones and Bartlett Publishers; 2006:325.

17. McClave SA, Neff RL. Care and long-term maintenance of percutaneous endoscopic gastrostomy tubes. *J Parenter Enteral Nutr.* 2006;30(suppl 1):S27-S38.

18. Grant JP. Anatomy and physiology of the luminal gut: enteral access implications. *J Parenter Enteral Nutr.* 2006;30(suppl 1):S41-S46.

19. DeLegge MH. Consensus statements regarding optimal management of home enteral nutrition (HEN) access. *J Parenter Enteral Nutr.* 2006;30(suppl 1):S39-S40.

20. Heimburger DC, Geels VJ, Bilbrey J, et al. Effects of small-peptide and whole-protein enteral feedings on serum proteins and diarrhea in critically ill patients: a randomized trial. *J Parenter Enteral Nutr.* 1997;21(3):162–167.

21. Executive Committee of the American Diabetes Association. Nutrition recommendations and principles for people with diabetes mellitus. *J Am Diet Assoc.* 1994;94(5):504–506.

22. Tinker LF, Heins JM, Holler HJ. Commentary and translation: 1994 nutrition recommendations for diabetes. Diabetes Care and Education, a Practice Group of the American Dietetic Association. *J Am Diet Assoc.* 1994;94(5): 507–511.

23. al-Saddy NM, Blackmore CM, Bennett ED. High fat, low carbohydrate, enteral feeding lowers PaCO2 and reduces the period of ventilation in artificially ventilated patients. *Intensive Care Med.* 1989;15(5):290–295.

24. Marchesini G, Bianchi G, Rossi B, et al. Nutritional treatment with branched-chain amino acids in advanced liver cirrhosis. *J Gastroenterol.* 2000; 35(suppl 12):7–12.

25. Ireton-Jones CS. Home enteral nutrition from the provider's perspective. *J Parenter Enteral Nutr.* 2002;26(suppl 5):S8-S9.

26. McMahon MM, Hurley DL, Kamath PS, Mueller PS. Medical and ethical aspects of long-term enteral tube feeding. *Mayo Clin Proc.* 2005;80(11): 1461–1476.

Vascular Access in the Home Parenteral Nutrition Patient

Ikenna Okereke, MD, Ezra Steiger, MD, FACS, CNSP

INTRODUCTION

Home parenteral nutrition (HPN) is a valuable resource for the management of many gastrointestinal disorders that interfere with oral or enteral nutrition for prolonged periods of time (see Table 7–1). The safe use of parenteral nutrition (PN) support in the outpatient setting depends on obtaining and maintaining safe prolonged vascular access. Selection of vascular access catheter type, location of insertion, and method of placement are important considerations in selecting an appropriate access device for the HPN patient. The complications associated with obtaining and maintaining vascular access are the leading cause of rehospitalization in these patients and is associated with significant morbidity.[1,2] It is important to recognize the signs and symptoms of complications associated with the insertion and use of HPN vascular access devices in order to minimize the associated morbidity.

TABLE 7–1   Common Indications for Home Parenteral Nutrition in Adults

Chronic mesenteric ischemia
Crohn's disease
Dysmotility syndrome
Enterocutaneous fistula
Graft versus host disease
Hyperemesis gravidum
Malabsorption
Malignant bowel obstruction
Nonmalignant chronic bowel obstruction
Pancreatitis
Pseudo-obstruction
Radiation enteritis
Scleroderma
Short bowel syndrome

VASCULAR ACCESS DEVICES

Several types of vascular access devices may be used for delivery of parenteral nutrition solutions. Patient co-morbidities, body habitus, history of previous surgeries in the neck and chest, personal patient preferences, and need for multiple intravenous therapies are important determinants of the most suitable type of device. The initial access procedures for HPN patients involved the use of the external jugular vein[3] or the creation of an arterio-venous shunt.[4,5]

Development of bio-compatible silastic catheters and subcutaneous ports in the 1970's allowed for placement of the devices which could remain within the central veins for an extended periods of time.[3] Today, these indwelling venous catheters and ports are used routinely to provide venous access for patients on HPN. In retrospective studies, there were no significant differences between the use of tunneled cuffed catheters (Figure 7–1A) and subcutaneous ports (Figure 7–1B). The Dacron velour cuff on the external surface of the catheter in the subcutaneous tunnel anchors the catheter in place once scar tissue has grown into its interstices. In addition, the fibrous connective tissue around the cuff

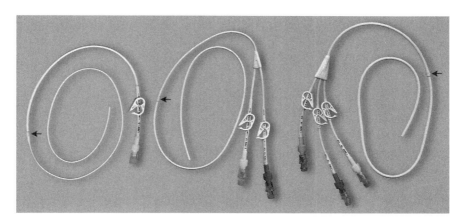

FIGURE 7–1A   Vascular Access Devices for Home Parenteral Nutrition; Shows a single, double, and triple lumen tunneled cuffed catheter used for long term central PN in the outpatient setting. The arrows note the location of the Dacron velour cuffs that are positioned in the tunnel near the exit site and serve to anchor the catheter in place and prevent tunnel infections.

theoretically prevented ascending infections of the catheter. An advantage of a port is that the device lies under the skin and when not cannulated no special care is needed. It does, however, require as much care as an external cuffed tunneled catheter when cannulated. Prior to placement the vascular access devices are shown to the patient and the risks and benefits of their placement and use are discussed. An exit or cannulation site convenient for the patient and or caregiver is chosen and marked to guide the interventional radiologist or surgeon in placing the port or catheter. Peripherally inserted central catheters (PICCs) (Figure 7–1C) are being used with increasing frequency to provide parenteral nutrition to patients in the hospital setting, but thus far have not been used routinely for long term HPN patients. Peripherally inserted central catheters were associated with an increased incidence of thrombosis and catheter dysfunction when used in the outpatient setting for various types of home intravenous therapies.[6]

OBTAINING ACCESS

Vascular access devices can be inserted either percutaneously by interventional radiology or surgically in the operating room. The percuta-

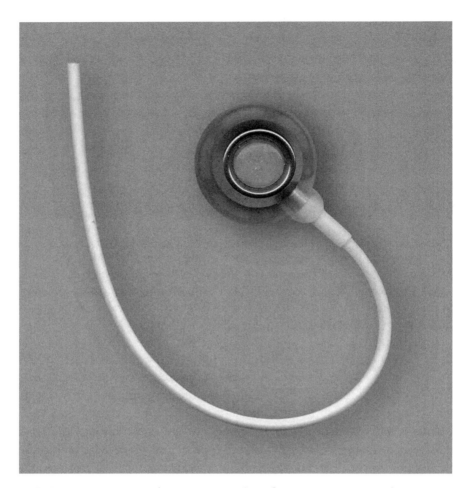

FIGURE 7–1B   Vascular Access Devices for Home Parenteral Nutrition; Shows a chest port.

neous approach, using ultrasound guidance in the radiology suite under sterile conditions, is safe, convenient and relatively inexpensive.[4] Placement in the operating room is mandatory when a venous cutdown is needed (i.e., cephalic or saphenous veins—see Figure 7–2) or when the patient requires a general anesthetic. The exit site is always tunneled away from the cut down or percutaneous site of venous entry to minimize risks of infection.

There are several different veins that can be used for introduction of the venous access device. The internal jugular vein approach is preferred by some because it has a lower incidence of pneumothorax[7] and many

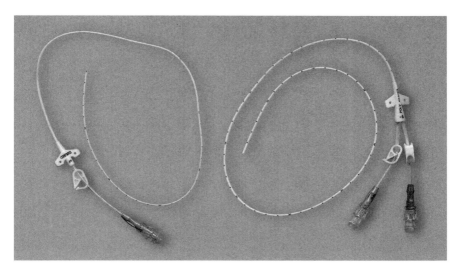

FIGURE 7–1C Vascular Access Devices for Home Parenteral Nutrition; Shows a single and double lumen PICC that can be used for central PN in the hospital or at home.

clinicians have an increased level of comfort in accessing this vein. Access to the internal jugular vein may be very difficult in obese patients or patients with short necks. Patients who have had carotid surgery or cervical lymph node dissections have scarring in this area and may have additional risk of injury to the carotid artery on attempted insertion of the catheter. Access to the internal jugular vein is also complicated in patients with tracheostomies or cervical esophagostomies. If the internal jugular vein is used, then the right side should be preferentially used, because the angle that the right internal jugular vein makes with the superior vena cava is nearly a straight line and therefore has a reduced chance of catheter malposition.

The subclavian vein approach has several advantages over other routes. Firstly, the distortion of landmarks is less marked in the subclavian vein area versus the internal jugular vein. Secondly, the incidence of catheter infection is lower with subclavian venous catheters than with internal jugular catheters in non-tunneled catheters,[8] probably due to the relative ease of maintaining sterile dressings over subclavian catheters. However, cannulating the subclavian vein is associated with an increased incidence of pneumothorax,[7] and, if bleeding ensues, it is difficult to control with direct pressure as opposed to the internal jugular vein. The tortuosity of the external jugular vein makes it difficult to pass catheters

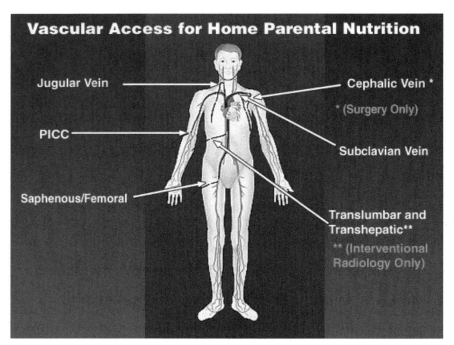

Reprinted from Sands MJ. Vascular access in the adult home infusion patient. JPEN, 2006;30(suppl 1):S58 with permission from the American Society for Parenteral and Enteral Nutrition (A.S.P.E.N.) A.S.P.E.N. does not endorse the use of this material in any form other than its entirety.

FIGURE 7–2   Vascular Access Sites for Home Parenteral Nutrition.

through but the use of this vein reduces the risk of pneumothorax compared to the subclavian vein or the internal jugular veins.

Occasionally, veins other than the subclavian and the internal jugular will be required especially when major venous thromboses have occurred. Though the risk of infection may be higher,[9] percutaneous access of the femoral vein or a saphenous vein cutdown is a good option for patients who have major upper torso venous thrombosis. The translumbar and transhepatic approaches should be considered as a last resort for venous access in the patient who has major upper torso venous thrombosis in whom a saphenous or femoral vein approach is not feasible.[10]

COMPLICATIONS OF VASCULAR ACCESS DEVICE INSERTION

Complications related to vascular access device insertion can be life threatening. Cardiac arrhythmia occurring during introduction of the catheter usually indicates that the catheter tip has been advanced into the right atrium or ventricle. Pulling the catheter back typically relieves the arrhythmia. Pneumothorax occurs approximately one percent of the time in most centers[11] and can either cause a shift of the mediastinum toward the injured lung or, in the case of tension pneumothorax, a shift the mediastinum away from the injured lung. In either circumstance, significant cardiovascular compromise can occur. Treatment with immediate tube thoracostomy is required to relieve the mediastinal shift and restore normal cardiovascular dynamics. A small pneumothorax, less than 15%, which is not associated with cardiovascular compromise or tension, can be followed without thoracostomy intervention. In this case, serial chest x-rays should be performed to ensure that the pneumothorax is not expanding.[11]

Vessel injury occurs rarely but can be associated with massive bleeding and the need for operative intervention. If an arterial injury is suspected and the catheter is in an aberrant position, a surgical consultation should be obtained prior to removing the catheter because catastrophic arterial bleeding can occur. Perforation of a central vein around the pericardial space may result in the pericardial tamponade. Signs and symptoms of cardiac tamponade include hypotension, diminished heart sounds, and sudden increase in jugular distension (Beck's triad). Diagnosis can be obtained with transthoracic echocardiogram, but if the patient is acutely decompensating, then immediate pericardiocentesis should be performed.

COMPLICATIONS OF PROLONGED VENOUS ACCESS

Infections

Long term complications include infection, thrombosis, and catheter occlusion. Catheter infections are either local or systemic. Local infections can be at the port or exit sight, subcutaneous tunnel, or at the venous entry sight. Symptoms of local infections are erythema, tenderness, and swelling. Purulent drainage may also be present. If the exit site alone is involved, then the patient can usually be managed with antibiotics and local wound care, without having to remove the catheter. If the port site or the subcutaneous tunnel and cuff is involved, then the device usually should be removed to prevent progression of infection. The combination of an antibiotic and device removal is usually necessary to allow for resolution of port pocket or subcutaneous tunnel and cuff infections. Temporary catheters, such as PICCs, should always be removed in the setting of local infection.

Catheter infections are probably produced by bacterium occupying the bio-film layer on the inner aspect of the catheter or its hub.[12] Patients classically develop fever, chills, nausea, and generalized malaise during PN infusion. Patients may also present with fever without an apparent source of infection. Patients at home with indwelling catheters who develop fever with no obvious source should be hospitalized. Their workup should consist of blood cultures drawn both peripherally and through the catheter. Quantitative culture differentials between blood drawn through the catheter versus peripheral blood or time to first growth help differentiate a primary catheter infection from other causes of sepsis.[13] The catheter should be used only for administration of antibiotics while other sources of sepsis are excluded. The most frequent responsible organism is *Staphylococcus epidermidis* and it can usually be treated with antibiotics without having to remove the catheter. Catheter infections caused by fungal species such as *Candida* usually require removal of the catheter. Septic shock, persistence of fever, or positive blood cultures despite intravenous antibiotics are indications for removal of the catheter as well. Endocarditis, osteomyelitis, and renal failure can also result from vascular access device catheter infections[14] and should be suspected in patients with recurrent or persistent catheter related infection. The catheter can be replaced after the patient no longer has a fever and blood cultures remain negative for at least 48 hours.

Measures taken to limit the incidence of catheter-related infections include using occlusive sterile dressing or plastic membranes over the catheter exit site, hand washing, avoiding touch contamination, and providing good patient training.[13] Multilumen catheters in the hospital setting are associated with an increased risk for infection and should be avoided in the home PN patient unless necessary for multiple intravenous therapies. The single lumen catheter should be ideally limited to use for PN only and not for blood draws. Other measures such as the use of prophylactic antibiotics and routine changing of catheters have not been shown to decrease infection rates.[15]

Thrombosis

Another frequent complication of vascular access devices is catheter occlusion. This is most commonly a result of an occluding thrombus within the catheter. When this occurs, the flow rate through the catheter steadily diminishes, and eventually fluid can not be infused and blood cannot be aspirated (withdrawal occlusion) from the catheter. Thrombotic occlusion affects up to 50 percent of indwelling catheters used for parenteral nutrition.[16] To treat catheter occlusion, the catheter should be flushed with saline or heparinized saline several times. If this does not restore patency then tissue plasminogen activator can be instilled and left to dwell in the catheter for 1–12 hours. If the catheter blockage is due to medication that had been infused through it, or precipitated mineral salts or lipid coagulum then sodium hydroxide, hydrochloric acid, or alcohol may be able to restore patency[17] (Table 7–2). Catheter associated venous thrombosis is more likely to occur when the catheter tip is malpositioned or in the upper part of superior vena cava.[18] Catheter-associated thrombosis can occur in the jugular and subclavian veins and in the superior vena cava. The patient may develop swelling and edema in the ipsilateral arm. Tenderness in the axilla over the axillary vein may be present and ipsilateral chest wall venous distention may be noted. Patients with jugular vein or superior vena cava thrombosis may be present with neck pain and swelling, headache, rhinorrhea, excessive tearing, and the appearance of collateral veins on the thorax. Once catheter associated thrombosis has been diagnosed, patients should be anticoagulated, unless a contraindication exists. Intravenous heparin should be initiated, followed by administration of oral warfarin to achieve an International Normalized Ratio (INR) between 2.0 and 3.0 for at least three months.[17] Thrombolysis may help to restore venous patency if instituted early in the clinical course. If septic thrombus is suspected, then thrombolytic agents should avoided.

TABLE 7–2   Algorithm for Treating Catheter Occlusions

Difficulty infusing solutions or withdrawing blood
↓
flush with saline or heparinized saline

patency restored—use device as before   persistent difficulty
↓   ↓
                                                    instill tissue plasminogen activiator
                                                    (tpa) for 2 hours
patency restored—use device as before   persistent difficulty
↓   ↓
                                                    check catheter position by
                                                    chest x-ray and/or dye injection
↓   ↓
catheter malpositioned?   Chest x-ray ok
                                            ↓   ↓
Change catheter   history of recent   history of recent
                                    medication infusion   lipid infusion
                                            ↓
                                    instill HCl or NaOH   instill EtOH
                                            ↓   ↓
                            patency   patency   persistent
                            restored   restored   difficulty
                                ↓   ↓   ↓
                            use device   use device   no history of
                            as before   as before   recent
                                                            medication or
                                                            lipid infusion
                                                                ↓
                                                            instill tpa and
                                                            leave in
                                                            overnight
                                                                ↓
                                                            persistent
                                                            difficulty
                                                                ↓
                                                            **Change
                                                            catheter**

CONCLUSION

Parenteral nutrition is an important supportive treatment for the management of patients with severe gastrointestinal disorders. An increasing number of patients are receiving PN at home and require appropriate safe prolonged vascular access. Selection of the most suitable venous access device will vary according to patient characteristics and needs. Short term complications are infrequent but can be life threatening. Long term complications occur more often and in the case of sepsis especially can also be life threatening. Adherence to recognized techniques of vascular access insertion and care can help reduce the incidence of these adverse events.

REFERENCES

1. Howard L, Hassan N. Home parenteral nutrition. 25 years later. *Gastroenterol Clin North Am.* 1998;27(2):481–512.
2. Steiger E. Home parenteral nutrition. Components, application, and complications. *Postgrad Med.* 1984;75(6):95–102.
3. Dudrick SJ. History of vascular access. *JPEN* 2006;30(suppl 1):S47–S56.
4. Sands MJ. Vascular access in the adult home infusion patient. *JPEN 2006;30(suppl 1):S57-S64.*
5. Tesio F, Panarello G, De Baz H, Canzi M, De Mattia T, Pasut R. Central vascular access: rational and results. *G Ital Nefr.* 2003;20(suppl 22):S30-S34.
6. Steiger E. Dysfunction and thrombotic complications of vascular access devices. *JPEN* 2006;30(suppl 1):S70-S72.
7. Plewa MC, Ledrick D, Sferra JJ. Delayed tension pneumothorax complicating central venous catheterization and positive pressure ventilation. *Am J Emerg Med.* 1995;13(5):532–535.
8. Williams DN, Rehm S, Tice AD, Bradley JS, Kind AC, Craig WA. Practice guidelines for community-based parenteral anti-infective therapy. *Clin Infect Dis.* 1997;25(4):787–801.
9. O'Grady NP, Dezfulian C. The femoral site as first choice for central venous access? Not so fast. *Crit Care Med.* 2005;33(1):234–235.
10. Rajan D, Croteau D, Sturza S, Harvill M, Mehall C. Translumbar placement of inferior vena caval catheters: a solution for challenging hemodialysis access. *Radiographics.* 1998;18(5):1155–1167.
11. Bowdle, T. Complications of invasive monitoring. *Anesthesiol Clin North America.* 2002;20(3):571–588.
12. de Jonge RC, Polderman KH, Gemke RJ. Central venous catheter use in the pediatric patient: mechanical and infectious complications. *Pediatr Crit Care Med.* 2005;6(3):329–339.
13. BCSH guidelines on the insertion and management of central venous lines. *Br J Haematol.* 1997;98(4):1041–1047.
14. Shah SS, Smith MJ, Zaoutis TE. Device-related infections in children. *Pediatr Clin North Am.* 2005;52(4):1189–1208.
15. Pearson ML. Guideline for prevention of intravascular device-related complications. Hospital Infection Control Practices Advisory Committee. *Infect Control Hosp Epidemiol.* 1996:17(7):438–473.

16. Dollery CM, Sullivan ID, Bauraind O, Bull C, Milla PJ. Thrombosis and embolism in long-term central venous access for parenteral nutrition. *Lancet.* 1994;344(8929):1043–1045.

17. Kerner JA Jr, Garcia-Careaga MG, Fisher AA, Poole RL. Treatment of catheter occlusion in pediatric patients. *JPEN* 2006;30(suppl 1):S73-S81.

18. Petersen J, Delaney J, Brakstad M, Rowbotham R, Bagley CM Jr. Silicone venous access devices positioned with their tips high in the superior vena cava are more likely to malfunction. *Am J Surgy.* 1999;178(1):38–41.

CHAPTER 8

Home Parenteral Nutrition in Adults

Cynthia Hamilton, MS, RD, LD, CNSD
Douglas L. Seidner, MD, FACG, CNSP

INTRODUCTION

The need for parenteral nutrition (PN) therapy in the home was recognized in the 1980s, after the establishment of safe and effective hospital PN practices. The growth and development of the homecare market is attributed to the availability of medical insurance reimbursement for a variety of home health services including home parenteral nutrition (HPN). Technological advances in equipment and formulas, the development of nutrition support as a specialty practice in the field of medicine, as well as the organization of national and international support societies, has made the use of HPN in the home a viable option for those with intestinal failure.

There is currently no established national registry in the United States that tracks patients on HPN. However, it was estimated in 1992 that 120 patients per million population, or 40,000 patients were receiving HPN based on Medicare data from the Health Care Finance Administration and Blue Cross/Blue Shield of South Carolina.[1]

Several important steps must be taken initially to establish a patient on HPN. Candidates should be identified by the etiology and expected duration of intestinal failure, and must be medically stable and able to care for themselves or have a willing, capable caregiver. Due to the complex nature of intestinal failure and the procedures used in providing

HPN therapy, a multidisciplinary team of nutrition support experts including a physician, dietitian, nurse, pharmacist, psychiatrist, social worker and discharge coordinator should be utilized to help establish this therapy.

INDICATIONS FOR HOME PARENTERAL NUTRITION

One of the most important features of establishing HPN is to identify the appropriate indication for this therapy. Inappropriate use of HPN can unnecessarily expose patients to the various risks associated with HPN and may result in a lack of reimbursement from insurance providers.

The most widely used guidelines that outline appropriate indications for HPN are published by the American Society for Parenteral and Enteral Nutrition (A.S.P.E.N.).[2] This organization is comprised of healthcare professionals representing the disciplines of medicine, nursing, pharmacy, dietetics, and nutrition science. These established guidelines, using an evidence-based approach, were designed for use by healthcare professionals who provide nutrition support services in the inpatient and outpatient settings.

According to the A.S.P.E.N. Guidelines,

- HPN is used when the gastrointestinal tract is not functional or cannot be accessed and in patients who cannot be adequately nourished by oral diets or enteral nutrition.
- HPN should be initiated in patients with inadequate oral intake for 7 to 14 days, or in those patients in whom inadequate oral intake is expected over a 7 to 14 day period.

The indications for HPN are the same as those for hospitalized patients requiring PN but whose intestinal failure continues when hospitalization is no longer required. Common diagnoses for which HPN is required include:[2]

- inflammatory bowel disease
- high output intestinal fistula
- nonterminal cancer
- pancreatic fistula

TABLE 8–1   Short-Term HPN Indications

Prolonged Post-Operative Ileus

Post-Operative Bowel Obstruction

Graft versus Host Disease

Enterocutaneous Fistula

Temporary Diverting Jejunostomy/Ileostomy

Chylothorax/Chylous Ascites

Hyperemesis Gravidarum

Malabsorptive Diarrhea with Enteral Feeding

TABLE 8–2   Long-Term HPN Indications

Crohn's Disease

Short Bowel Syndrome

Massive Bowel Resection Secondary to Mesenteric Infarction/Volvulus

Radiation Enteritis

Intestinal Pseudo-Obstruction

Adhesive Bowel Obstruction

- ischemic bowel
- small bowel volvulus
- radiation enteritis
- hyperemesis gravidarium
- motility disorders
- protein-losing enteropathy
- severe pancreatitis
- bowel obstruction

HPN may be provided as short-term or long-term treatment. Short-term HPN is frequently used for patients recovering from surgery, or for those who will require further surgery within a few months time and are then expected to resume oral nutrition with discontinuation of HPN.

Patients with chronic bowel diseases with malabsorption of enteral nutrients, patients with small bowel motility disorders, or patients who have suffered traumatic injury or surgical resection of the small bowel with inadequate bowel remaining for absorption are expected to require HPN long-term or even life-long.

In addition to guidelines provided by A.S.P.E.N., Medicare has established guidelines to identify appropriate HPN candidates.[3]   Medicare policies are administered by the Centers for Medicare and Medicaid Services within the US Department of Health and Human Services. Policies for HPN benefits fall under Part B of the Durable Medical Equipment Regional Carrier of Medicare services. Medicare guidelines may also be used by private medical insurance payors, whereas, individual state Medicaid agencies reimbursement policies will vary.[4] Medicare requires the establishment of permanent gastrointestinal (GI) failure, defined as therapy required for at least 90 days, and requires specific documentation of GI failure before approving the use and reimbursement of HPN.

Contraindications to HPN

HPN should not be given to patients who are imminently terminally ill, have major organ failure, are not clinically stable, or can tolerate and absorb enteral nutrients.[5] Patients who require long-term HPN but who cannot be safely discharged to home should be placed in a skilled nursing facility.

EVALUATING AND TRANSITIONING PATIENTS FROM HOSPITAL TO HOME

Once a patient's medical diagnosis or condition has appropriately identified the need for HPN, a thorough and complete evaluation process by a multidisciplinary team of nutrition support experts should ensue. The hospital discharge coordinator, physician, dietitian, nurse, pharmacist, social worker, and psychiatrist each make a significant contribution in the evaluation and transition process. The nutrition support team should establish a care plan prior to the patient's hospital discharge and make sure that the patient and caregiver understand all aspects of HPN therapy and accept the risks prior to implementation. Once the evaluation process is complete, all homecare needs have been identified with a homecare agency established, the patient has a stable HPN formula with a permanent venous access device in place, and the patient is well educated in their HPN therapy and venous access device (VAD) care, then the patient can safely be transitioned to home.

TABLE 8-3   Medicare Guidelines for Home Parenteral Nutrition

CRITERIA	DOCUMENTATION
Massive Small Bowel Resection	Operative Report
<5 ft of SB beyond ligament of Treitz	X-ray Report Physician letter documenting condition and need for PN
Short Bowel Syndrome —GI losses exceed oral intake by 50% —urine output <1 liter	same as above
Bowel Rest for 3 Months —symptomatic pancreatitis —regional enteritis exacerabation —proximal enterocutaneous fistula and cannot tube feed distal to the fistula	same as above
Mechanical Bowel Obstruction —inoperable	same as above
Severe Malnutrition with Weight Loss > 10% **Serum Albumin < 3.4 gm/dL** —severe fat malabsorption —motility disturbance unresponsive to prokinetics	Nutrition Assessment report by physician or RD Fecal Fat Test report Gastric empty study or barium x-ray report

Other
—unable to maintain weight and strength after:
  —diet modification
  —pharmacologic interventions
  —enteral feeding (failed)
	Nutrition Assessment report
	
	Results of tests/studies
	List of medications

Discharge Coordinator

The hospital discharge coordinator should be involved early in the patient's evaluation process. Verification of the patient's insurance benefits for HPN coverage are essential and may include restrictions as to the choice of providers including the physician and homecare agency. The hospital discharge coordinator usually makes the referral to homecare

---

New Home PN Patient

Preparing for Initial Discharge of Cleveland Clinic Foundation Patient

Staff Physician Approval
↓
Evaluations by:
Discharge Coordinator
Social Work
Psychiatry
Nutrition Support Vascular Access RN
Home TPN Clinician
↓
Arrange Permanent Venous Access Placement
↓
Order Trace Elements– "serum Chromium, Copper, Selenium, Zinc, whole blood Manganese "and "Phospholipid Fatty Acids"
↓
Stabilize Formula (electrolytes, blood glucose, fluid)
↓
Cycle Formula (goal 12 hours)
↓
Address Other Medical Issues (i.e., medications, pain control, anticoagulation)
↓
Discharge to Home

FIGURE 8–1   Home Parenteral Nutrition Algorithm

agencies, identifies all homecare needs, and coordinates all discharge aspects of HPN.

Dietitian

The home care dietitian performs a nutrition assessment, establishes calorie, protein, micronutrient, and fluid requirements, and a goal weight (see Chapter 4 for determining nutrient requirements). Some patients on HPN will still consume small amounts of liquids or solid foods, and any dietary restrictions should be discussed with the patient. Depending on professional licensure or clinical privileges of an institution the dietitian may be responsible for writing PN orders and adjusting electrolytes.[6]

Nurse

The nutrition support nurse is an expert in the selection and care of long-term central VADs and should work with each patient to identify the most suitable device considering the established care plan and patient preference. In addition, the nurse provides education and assesses the ability of the patient and caregiver(s) to learn and safely perform all procedures and tasks related to the HPN infusion.[7]

Pharmacist

The pharmacist provides expertise in compounding, storage, delivery route, and compatibility of HPN formulas. Medications to be added to the HPN should first be evaluated for stability and compatibility. Other medications taken by mouth or intravenously need to be evaluated for pharmacokinetic properties (absorption and metabolism) to avoid the risk of developing complications of drug interactions. Depending on institutional guidelines, the pharmacist may be involved in writing HPN orders and making electrolyte adjustments.[8]

Social Worker

The social worker can help identify those patients who may or may not be appropriate candidates for HPN based on psychosocial issues. An assessment includes information regarding the patient's personality, level of functioning, current stresses, and resources in his or her life situation.[9] The social worker may assess the home situation for general cleanliness and should ensure availability of electricity, refrigeration, telephone, and water. Alternatively, this may be done by the home care provider prior to initiating therapy. Patients with mental disorders, depression, and substance abuse may be poor or unsafe candidates for HPN and may require placement at an alternate site such as a skilled nursing facility. The social worker can provide information to patients and their families on support groups such as the Oley Foundation (800-776-Oley, www.oley.org) or the Crohn's and Colitis Foundation (800-932-2423, www.ccfa.org).

Psychiatrist

The psychiatrist may be consulted along with the social worker to help identify psychosocial issues related to a patient's ability to cope with HPN therapy.[10,11] The psychiatrist may administer the mini-mental state exam, a standardized test used to help assess cognitive skills, identify major mental, psychiatric, or depression disorders that require treatment, and assess for drug interactions, which can alter a patient's functional ability.[12]

Physician

The physician has the ultimate role of care coordinator by writing the orders under which the clinical teams function. Physicians may be well skilled in nutrition support and able to manage this therapy in the home or may need significant assistance from colleagues or the home infusion provider's clinical staff.

PATIENT EDUCATION

The education process begins in the hospital and continues in the patient's home.

Patient training should be performed by qualified staff who have specialized training and experience in the field of HPN.[13] The goals of educationare to provide the patient and caregiver with knowledge and skills to perform all HPN procedures. The training process can take several weeks before independence is established. Patients and caregivers must master new techniques and skills involving aseptic technique, pump operations, and manipulation of tubes, and they must understand their fluid and nutrient balance and be aware of emergency procedures.[14] Repeated demonstration is used during the training process to assure competence in techniques.

Training should be individualized according to the patient's and caregiver's needs and abilities. A number of educational aids or tools may be used during the training process including written materials with clear concise wording and graphics, mannequins or vests with vascular access devices, videos, and Web sites. A notebook or instruction manual should be provided to the patient and caregiver for reference to all procedures. Educational materials may have a positive impact on patient outcomes. In a randomized controlled trial, interactive and videotaped educational interventions have been shown to reduce catheter-related blood stream infections and reactive depression and to improve the ability of patients to problem solve with healthcare professionals.[15] Once the patient or caregiver has demonstrated competence in all areas of HPN care, homecare visits may be decreased or discontinued.

TABLE 8–4 Cleveland Clinic Foundation Home TPN Teaching Checklist

Patient's Name: _____

Instructor's Name/Pager Number: _____

	Discussed or RN Demonstrated	PT/Caregiver Returned Demonstration
1. Principles of Aseptic technique		
—Surface preparation		
—Hand washing		
2. Central venous catheter dressing change		
3. Central venous catheter cap change		
4. Central venous catheter flushing		
5. Central venous catheter guidelines		
(Do's and Don'ts)		
6. Complications of central venous catheters		
a. Infection: exit site & systemic		
b. Clotting/blockage of catheter		
c. Thrombus		
d. Catheter dislodgment		
e. Catheter breakage		
f. Blood back-up		
g. Emergency repair		
7. TPN Administration		
a. Infusion pump battery		
b. Infusion pump programming		
c. Infusion pump troubleshooting		
d. Infusion pump alarms		
e. TPN additives		
f. TPN set up		
g. TPN hook up		
h. TPN disconnect		
8. TPN Self-Monitoring		
a. Intake and Output Record Keeping		
b. Daily Weight		
c. Daily Temperature		
d. Urine glucose or Accuchecks		
e. TPN metabolic complications		
9. Home TPN phone numbers and resources		

VENOUS ACCESS DEVICES

Placement of a permanent VAD is essential prior to discharging a patient on HPN therapy. Patients should not be sent home with a temporary catheter for HPN use. Vascular access devices must be placed in the central vascular system in order to accommodate hyperosmolar HPN solutions. Factors to be considered when determining the type of permanent VAD include:[16,17]

- Length of Therapy
- Patient Preference
- Patient Available Venous Access
- Patient/Caregiver Ability to Care for Device
- Technical Skills of Practitioner Placing Device

There are three devices to select from, each with distinct advantages and disadvantages. (Table 8–5) The device selected should be placed by a skilled qualified surgeon, interventional radiologist, or, for peripherally inserted central catheters (PICC), a specially trained nurse. Guidelines have been developed by the Healthcare Infection Control Practices Advisory Committee of the Centers for Disease Control for practitioners who insert catheters and monitor for infectious complications in the hospital and home settings.[18] These guidelines are evidence-based and should be incorporated into the practices of healthcare professionals involved with providing HPN. (See Chapter 7 for more detailed information on VAD.)

TABLE 8–5 Venous Access Devices Used for HPN

TYPE	DESCRIPTION	ADVANTAGES	DISADVANTAGES	USE
Tunneled Central Venous Catheter (Hickman, Broviac, Groshong)	Placed under skin with external device on chest wall. Placed in surgical suite by skilled surgeon/ interventional radiologist. Indicated for daily IVF/PN.	Available with multi-lumens. Easy self-care. Decreased risk of dislodgement. Can repair external lumen in case of breakage. Removed in physician office.	Affects body image.	Long-term
Implanted Port	Silicone catheter with titanium disk placed under skin. Ideal for intermittent IV therapies. Placed in surgical suite by skilled surgeon/interventional radiologist.	Minimal body image alteration.	Requires frequent needle sticks. Requires removal to repair and treat infections. Removed in surgical suite.	Long-term
Peripherally Inserted Central Catheter (PICC)	Semi-permanent device placed in peripheral vein. Ideal for short-term IV therapies.	Placed by specially trained nurse at bedside or by a radiologist. Can be removed in home. Lower cost of placement. Less risk of insertion complications.	Higher incidence of catheter malfunction. Patient requires help for site dressing care. Affects body image.	Short-term (1–2 months)

TABLE 8–6   Macronutrient Stock Solutions for Parenteral Nutrition
Preparation

	Concentration	Grams/L	kcals/L
Dextrose	20%	200	680
	50%	500	1700
	70%	700	2380
Amino Acids	8.5%	85	340
	10%	100	400
	15%	150	600
	20%	200	800
Modified Amino Acids			
Renal Failure (Nephramine©)	5.4%	54	216
Hepatic Failure (Hepatamine©)	8.0%	80	320
Lipids	10%*	100	1100
	20%*	200	2000
	30%	300	3000

*may be administered intravenously as separate infusion

HOME PARENTERAL NUTRITION FORMULAS

HPN formulas are composed of dextrose, amino acids, lipids, vitamins, minerals, electrolytes, and sterile water to be infused via a permanent centrally placed VAD. The osmolarity of the solution will depend upon the concentration of the solution but usually is hypertonic with an osmolarity >900 mOsm/L.[19]

Dextrose

The major ingredient in HPN solutions, which usually provides the bulk of energy, is dextrose. Dextrose provides 3.4 kcals/g and is commercially available in multiple concentrations ranging from 3% to 70%. Higher concentrations of dextrose are generally used to compound HPN solutions.

Amino Acids

The protein source used to formulate PN solutions is crystalline amino acids, which yields 4 kcals/g and is available in a variety of concentrations. Most HPN formulas are made from concentrations ranging from 8.5% to 20%. Standard amino acid solutions contain a mixture of essential and nonessential amino acids. Modified amino acid solutions are available for certain disease states (i.e., renal and hepatic disease), although these are generally used in the critically ill patient and not in the HPN patient. There are some differences among the various amino acid solutions electrolytes and buffers that require consideration when adjusting formulas. The homecare pharmacist can provide information in this regard when preparing a HPN solution.

Lipids

Intravenous lipids are an oil-in-water isotonic emulsion product used in HPN formulas to provide energy (9 kcals/g) and a source of the essential fatty acids (EFA) linoleic and linolenic acid. The fat source is either soybean oil or a combination of safflower and soybean oil. In order to meet the requirement for EFAs, HPN should provide approximately 10% of the calories from intravenous fat.[20] This can be met by admixing lipids daily in the HPN solution or by infusing 500 mL of 20% fat emulsion once per week or in divided doses of 250 mL twice per week. Egg phospholipids are used as an emulsifier in lipids and therefore patients with egg allergies should not receive intravenous (IV) lipids. Cutaneously applied or orally ingested oils to prevent EFA deficiency may be necessary. Lipid emulsions are available as 10% (1.1 kcals/mL), 20% (2 kcals/mL) and 30% (3 kcals/mL) concentrations. Ten percent and 20% concentrations can be infused peripherally and centrally, whereas 30% concentrations are utilized only as a part of an overall HPN solution.

2-in-1 versus 3-in-1 Parenteral Nutrition Solutions

HPN is compounded as either 2-in-1 (dextrose + protein) or 3-in-1 (dextrose + protein + lipids) solutions. Dextrose-based solutions can be given to patients who can tolerate high carbohydrate concentrations with lipids admixed once or twice per week to meet EFA requirements. Daily 3-in-1 solutions may be given to any HPN patient and are especially useful for patients who have difficult blood glucose control. Typical 3-in-1 solutions will contain 30% to 60% of calories from lipids.

Concerns with 3-in-1 solutions include compatibility with other HPN nutrients, immunosuppression, and potential liver function abnormalities. Patients receiving >1 g/kg of lipid per day have been associated with a higher incidence of cholestatic liver disease.[21]

TABLE 8–7   Comparison of a 2-in-1 and 3-in-1 Parenteral Nutrition Solution for an Average Sized Adult*

		2-in-1	3-in-1
Distribution of Dextrose/Fat kcals		100%/0%	70%/30%
Amino Acids	gms	105	105
	kcals	420	420
Dextrose	gms	391	274
	kcals	1330	931
	Final concentration	20%	14%
Lipids	(20%)	1–2×/week	daily
	mL	250 2×/week	100/d
		or 500 1x/week	
	kcals	1000/wk	200/d
Total Volume mL		2000	2000
Total kcals		1750	1750

*70 kg patient, 1.5 gms pro/kg, 25 kcals/kg

The use of 3-in-1 solutions is common with home care companies and home infusion pharmacies because of the simplicity and convenience of the therapy for the patient.

Parenteral Nutrition Compatibility

HPN formulations are complex mixtures containing multiple components. Improper compounding can lead to unstable, incompatible mixtures, which can lead to serious harm or even death. Incompatible amounts of macro and micronutrients can cause *creaming* or *cracking* of 3-in-1 solutions. Excess amounts of cations, particularly divalent cations such as calcium and magnesium and the trivalent cation iron dextran, can result in destabilization of the emulsion. Precipitate formation can occur from excess amounts of calcium and phosphorus and from inappropriate amounts of macronutrients.[22] Table 8–8 provides figures used by our pharmacy for compatibility ranges of macro and micronutrient amounts. These have been tested and are safe for HPN compounding. Consult your pharmacist with questions and concerns regarding compatibility. In addition, A.S.P.E.N. has developed "Safe Practices for Parenteral Nutrition Formulations" which provides further guidelines.[23]

TABLE 8–8 Common Causes of Parenteral Nutrition Incompatibility

Problem	Description	Prevention
Intravenous Lipid Emulsion Disruption	Creaming/cracking Visible milk layer on surface or free oil droplets seen.	Limit nutrient ranges for 3-in-1 PN: amino acid 20–60 g/L dextrose 35–253 g/L lipids 13–67 g/L
Calcium/Phosphate Precipitation	Improper compounding or excess amounts of Ca and PO₄. May be visible as "white snow" precipitate in 2-in-1 PN. Not visible in 3-in-1 PN.	Maintain calcium/phosphate product below threshold: Ca mEq/L × PO₄ mEq/L = <200

TABLE 8–9 Steps to Determine Fluid Requirements in an Adult

1. Provide 1000 to 1500 mL fluid daily to support adequate urine output (in absence of renal failure).
2. Provide additional fluid to account for other fluid losses (ostomy, emesis, diarrhea, fistulas, wounds, drains).
3. Substract daily fluid intake other than PN.
4. Provide additional 500 to 1000 mL to account for insensible fluid losses.

Fluid

Normal fluid requirements for most adults is approximately 35 mL/kg.[24] Sterile water is added to HPN solutions to meet determined fluid needs and can provide full requirements if a patient does not absorb enteral fluid. One method used to determine fluid requirements in patients receiving HPN is described in Table 8–9.

Micronutrients-Vitamins, Minerals, Electrolytes, Trace Elements

Electrolytes, minerals, vitamins, and trace elements are essential for normal cellular function and are added to HPN daily. Requirements have been established for electrolytes and micronutrients, but it is important to assess the clinical and nutritional status of each patient and to alter these micronutrients as necessary.[25,26] Vitamin preparations are available as injectable multivitamins or as single entity products with the exception of biotin, pantothenic acid, riboflavin, vitamin A, and vitamin E. Trace element preparations are available in various combinations or as

TABLE 8–10   Average Daily Electrolyte Requirements During
Parenteral Nutrition*

Sodium 1–2 mEq/kg/day	
Potassium	1–2 mEq/kg/day
Chloride	As needed to maintain acid-base balance
Acetate	As needed to maintain acid-base balance
Calcium	10–15 mEq/day
Magnesium	8–20 mEq/day
Phosphorus	20–40 mmol/day

*A.S.P.E.N. Board of Directors. Guidelines for the use of parenteral and enteral nutrition in adult and pediatric patients. *JPEN*. 2002;26:22SA.

single-element products. Home parenteral nutrition patients should have trace element levels measured at the initiation of therapy and as needed while continuing HPN. We don't agree with saying "as needed" and recommend "at least every 6 months. "As needed" is not definitive enough for practitioners. Monitoring of HPN patient's trace element deficiencies or toxicities is usually based on a patient's clinical symptoms. (Clinical symptoms related to deficiencies or toxicities show up after tissue levels are affected. Therefore, it is important follow trace elements closely and make PN adjustments before clinical symptoms are apparent.)

Iron is not part of trace element preparations and must be added separately to HPN solutions. If iron deficiency anemia is diagnosed and the patient cannot tolerate or absorb oral iron preparations, then a test dose of IV iron dextran must first be administered to rule out anaphylactic reaction. Iron dextran is not compatible with 3-in-1 solutions and may only be added to 2-in-1 solutions.[20]

Additives

Some medications need to be added to the HPN formula by the patient or caregiver prior to each infusion because they are not stable in HPN solutions for extended periods of time.[20] Medications that may be routinely added to HPN include:

- heparin
- insulin
- histamine$_2$-receptor antagonists

TABLE 8–11   Parenteral Vitamin and Trace Element Requirements for Adults

Vitamins*	
A (mg)	1
D (mcg)	5
E (mg)	10
K (mcg)	150
Ascorbic Acid (mg)	200
Folic Acid (mcg)	600
Niacin (mg)	40
Riboflavin (mg)	3.6
Thiamin (mg)	6
B_6 (mg)	6
B_{12} (mcg)	5
Pantothenic acid (mg)	15
Biotin (mcg)	60
Trace elements**	
Chromium (mcg)	10–15
Copper (mg)	0.3–0.5
Manganese (mcg)	60–100
Zinc (mg)	2.5–5.0
Selenium (mcg)	20–60

* Food and Drug Administration. Parenteral Multivitamin Products; Drugs for Human Use; Drug Efficacy Study Implementation; Amendment: Federal Register. April 20, 2000. Vol 65 (77)21:21200–21201.
** A.S.P.E.N. Board of Directors. Guidelines for the use of parenteral and enteral nutrition in adult and pediatric patients. *JPEN*. 2002;26:23SA.

- octreotide
- corticosteroids
- metoclopramide

Heparin is added in a low dose to prevent catheter-related venous thrombosis. Its use is contraindicated in patients with heparin-induced thrombocytopenia. Regular insulin is effective in controlling blood glucose when added in appropriate amounts. Insulin may be used to keep blood glucose levels <150 mg/dL. Histamine 2-receptor antagonists such as famotidine, ranitidine, or cimetidine are used to decrease gastric acid secretions especially after extensive small bowel surgery or in patients with peptic ulcer disease and gastroesophageal reflux disease.

Octreotide can be helpful in controlling severe diarrhea or high output enterocutaneous fistulas.

Less common additives include corticosteroids for patients prescribed these agents who cannot take oral corticosteroids, and metoclopramide for patients with gastroparesis.

Some medicines can be co-infused with HPN and a pharmacist should be consulted prior to administration.

Cycling

Once a patient's HPN formula is stabilized as a 24-hour infusion, including fluid, electrolytes and macronutrients, then cycling of the formula should begin. Infusion of HPN for only part of the day provides both metabolic and psychological benefits. A "free" period off of PN infusion allows the liver to mobilize stored glycogen and may decrease the incidence of fatty liver and promote better nitrogen retention.[27] A period of time free from IV equipment allows a more normal lifestyle.

Cycling should be done in a stepwise fashion to allow adaptation to the dextrose load. Cycling can take several days until the desired infusion cycle is reached (usually 10 to 12 hours overnight). Blood glucose should be maintained below 150 mg/dL by adding insulin, by reducing the dextrose calories or by adjusting the taper schedule. Tapering is a technique in which the rate of delivery of the HPN solution is gradually increased or decreased at the beginning or end of the infusion period. Tapering up at the beginning of the infusion for 1 or 2 hours is done to avoid hyperglycemia that occurs in the first couple of hours of infusion and tapering down at the end of the infusion for 1 or 2 hours is done to avoid rebound hypoglycemia after the HPN has been stopped.[28]

Latex Allergy

Patients with a latex allergy require special precautions in the preparation and infusion of HPN. The homecare pharmacy should be notified of the patient's latex allergy and should compound the HPN formula in a latex-free environment. Home parenteral nutrition bags and tubing should be free of latex ports. Injectable medications, added daily to HPN by the patient, need to be provided in pre-filled latex-free syringes. Latex-free gloves should be used.

TABLE 8–12   Two Examples of Infusion Rates for Cycling a HPN Formula

1. Volume: 2400 mL, 12-hr cycle with 1 hr taper down
   Main rate = Total volume ÷ cycle hrs – ½ hr
       209 mL = 2400 mL ÷ 11 ½ hrs
   1 hr taper rate = Main rate ÷ 2
       104 mL = 209 mL ÷ 2 = 104 mL
   Infuse PN for 209 mL × 11 hrs, then 104 mL × 1 hr, then stop PN, flush catheter.

2. Volume: 2400 mL, 14-hr cycle with 1 hr taper up and 1 hr taper down
   Main rate = Total volume ÷ cycle hrs – 1 hr
       185 mL = 2400 mL ÷ 14 hrs – 1 hr
   Taper rates =Main rate ÷ 2
       92 mL = 185 ÷ 2
   Infuse PN for 92 mL × 1 hr, 185 mL × 12 hrs, 92 mL × 1 hr, then stop PN, flush catheter.

TABLE 8–13   Typical Supplies Required to Manage Parenteral Nutrition at Home

Refrigerator	Syringes
PN pump and tubing	Tape
Injectable additives (i.e., insulin, multi-vitamins)	Urine glucose strips
Catheter flushing supplies (heparin, saline)	Batteries
Catheter dressing change kit	IV pole
Gloves	Sharps container
Alcohol wipes	Hand/Nail scrub solution and brush

Delivery and Storage of Supplies

Patients on HPN must receive periodic shipments of all necessary supplies. The patient's home must be clean and must have electricity and a safe place to store all equipment away from children and pets. The patient should have designated refrigerator storage for HPN bags and injectable medications. The patient may have this separate refrigerator provided by the homecare pharmacy. Supplies for HPN can be quite extensive as shown in Table 8–13.

MONITORING OF HPN

Patients discharged on HPN require diligent follow-up to ensure a successful course of therapy and to minimize complications associated with HPN. Monitoring of HPN includes regular laboratory testing, assessment for development of long-term complications, assurance of compliance with infusion procedures and consistent follow-up with the HPN physician. Monitoring and management of HPN patients should be coordinated between the physician, nutrition support clinicians, and the homecare organization. Established protocols and procedures should be in place to appropriately care for HPN patients. A.S.P.E.N. has developed standards for home nutrition support and adults in long-term care facilities that can be used to establish all aspects of care for patients on PN outside of the hospital.[29,30]

Laboratory Testing

A regular schedule of laboratory testing needs to be established to determine tolerance and effectiveness of therapy and to ensure that nutritional goals are being met. The HPN formula should be stabilized for macronutrients, electrolytes, and the infusion cycle prior to hospital discharge. Patients should be stable enough at the time of discharge so they only require laboratory testing on a weekly basis. Once stable at home, patients may require laboratory testing less frequently. Table 8–14 provides a schedule of monitoring parameters for HPN patients. Clinical parameters include daily patient record keeping of intake and output, temperature, weight, and urinary or blood glucose. Daily monitoring of these parameters can lead to early recognition and treatment of problems related to hydration, infection and blood glucose control. See Table 8–15 for an example of a home patient monitoring form.

TABLE 8–14   Home Parenteral Nutrition Monitoring

	Daily	Weekly	Monthly	Other
CLINICAL				
Intake/Output	X			
Temperature	X			
Weight	X			
Urinary or Blood Glucose	X			
LABORATORY				
Electrolytes		X	X	
BUN/Cr		X	X	
Ca, PO$_4$, Mg		X	X	
Albumin or Transferrin			X	
Liver Function Tests (bilirubin, alkaline phosphatase, aspartate aminotransferase, alanine aminotransferase)			X	
Complete Blood Count			X	
Prothrombin Time/INR			X	
OTHER STUDIES				
DXA Scan				initially every 1–2 years
24-hour urine for Ca, Mg Trace Elements				every 6–12 months
Trace Elements				baseline then every 6–12 months
Essential Fatty Acids*				baseline then every 6–12 months
Iron studies (iron, ferritin)				every 3–6 months during repletion

*when fat emulsion only given 1–2 × per week

TABLE 8–15 The Cleveland Clinic Foundation Home Nutrition Support

Daily Intake/Output Record

Date									
Weight									
Goal Weight									
Temperature (F°)									
INTAKE (ml)									
Oral Fluid									
PN									
IV Fluid									
TOTAL INTAKE									
OUTPUT (ml)									
Urine									
Stoma									
OTHER OUTPUT (ml)(circle)									
GT JT PEG									
Drain Fistula									
Emesis Diarrhea									
TOTAL OUTPUT									
Urine glucose Accu-check (circle)									

Patient Name: _____   PN Physician: _____

Laboratory testing provides information on electrolyte, macro- and micronutrient tolerance of the HPN formula. Visceral proteins such as albumin and transferrin indicate adequacy of protein provided in the HPN formula. Twenty-four hour urine collections for calcium and magnesium are used to monitoring adequacy of these nutrients in the HPN formula, especially in patients at risk of developing metabolic bone disease. Other studies including dual-energy x-ray absorptiometry (DXA), trace elements and essential fatty acids are indicated as discussed later in the Chapter. Hepatic and renal complications are discussed in Chapter 12.

Home Visits

When a patient is first discharged to home, a home care nurse should be available beginning the first night to train the patient and/or caregiver in all HPN procedures. Visits should be scheduled around hook-up and disconnect times and should continue until training is complete and competence and independence is demonstrated for all procedures. Periodic visits by the homecare nurse are recommended to ensure compliance. Problems found in the home should be reported to the HPN physician. Patients should be given a 24-hour contact number of a homecare clinician involved in their care to address problems and emergencies.

Physician Follow-Up

A return visit to the HPN physician should be scheduled within several weeks of hospital discharge and then at established periodic intervals. Visits should include a review of the nutrition care plan, medical plan, physical exam, problems associated with the HPN infusion and the venous access device, development of long-term complications and psychosocial concerns.

RECOGNITION AND MANAGEMENT OF COMPLICATIONS

Complications associated with HPN can be divided into catheter and metabolic complications. Clinicians involved in the care of patients receiving HPN should be aware of these complications and the proper methods to address them. Some complications require immediate action.

TABLE 8–16   Patient Guide to Contact Home Parenteral Nutrition Clinician

PROBLEM	ACTION PATIENT SHOULD TAKE
Catheter breaks, cracks or leaks	Clamp catheter above problem area Call HPN clinician to arrange repair
Catheter has withdrawal/infusion occlusion	Call HPN clinician to arrange for catheter restoration
Fever, chills with PN infusion	Stop PN, immediately call HPN clinician or go to emergency room for hospital admission
Drainage, pus, tenderness, redness at catheter exit site or along catheter tract	Call HPN clinician for proper treatment
Chest pain, shortness of breath, loss of conciousness	Clamp catheter, call 911, lay on left side
Pump malfunction	Check electrical source, battery Call HPN clinician or homecare pump provider for repair/replacement
Elevated glucose in urine or blood	Call HPN clinician for adjustment of PN infusion rate or insulin
Low blood glucose with sweating, headache, shakiness, blurred vision	Drink juice, cola beverage or sugar water if permitted to take fluid. If oral fluid restricted take hard candy or glucose gel. Call HPN clinician for adjustment of PN infusion rate or insulin
Increased thirst, decreased urine output, Increased ostomy output, muscle cramps	Call HPN clinician with intake/output record and adjustment of PN fluid volume or additional IV hydration fluids
Rapid weight gain, swelling of hands, feet, ankles, short of breath	Call HPN clinician for adjustment of PN fluid volume

Patients should be made aware of HPN associated complications and provided with instructions on how to solve these problems.

Catheter Complications

Catheter complications include mechanical and infectious problems:[31]

Mechanical	Infectious
• catheter breakage	• catheter related blood stream infection (CRBSI)
• withdrawal/infusion occlusion	• tunnel infection
• air embolism	• exit site infection
• pump malfunction	• HPN solution/equipment contamination
• vein thrombosis	

Some catheter related problems are of a very serious nature that can be life threatening. Catheter-related sepsis was the cause of death in 20% of patients who died while on HPN at one large center.[32] Recognition of catheter-related problems and the need for appropriate treatment is imperative. For a complete discussion on catheter complications and management see Chapter 7.

Metabolic Complications

Several metabolic complications are associated with HPN. Laboratory data along with clinical data must be evaluated and appropriate changes must be made to the patient's HPN formula when metabolic complications occur. These complications may include:

- electrolyte abnormalities
- vitamin deficiencies and toxicities
- trace element deficiencies and toxicities
- EFA deficiency
- iron deficiency
- liver disease
- metabolic bone disease

Electrolyte Abnormalities

Electrolyte abnormalities are usually associated with a change in the patient's medical condition. Extra fluid losses from the gastrointestinal tract (ostomy, fistula, diarrhea, vomiting, drains), changes in renal and liver function, and changes in medications can lead to electrolyte abnormalities. Major changes in electrolytes may necessitate medical intervention and alteration of the HPN formula.[33] Managing some of the more common metabolic complications associated with HPN are presented in Table 8–17.

TABLE 8–17 Common Metabolic Complications in HPN Patients

Problem	Clinical Signs/Symptoms	Possible Etiology	Treatment
Hyperglycemia	BS >150 mg during PN infusion or positive urine glucose with first void after stopping PN Nausea, headache, polyuria	Excess dextrose kcals Overfeeding Inadequate insulin in PN Infection	Assess kcal needs Increase insulin in PN Change from 2–1 to 3–1 solution Lengthen infusion cycle or taper Assess for infection (i.e., catheter, wound, urinary)
Hypoglycemia	BS <60 mg during PN infusion Sweating, paleness, nausea, headache, shakiness, blurred vision	Excess insulin in PN Abrupt discontinuation of PN Rapid taper	Take sugar-rich food or instant glucose Decrease insulin in PN Increase taper from 1 to 2 hours at end of infusion
Hyperkalemia	Serum K+ above NL Listlessness, weakness, confusion, tingling	Excess amount of K+ in PN Change in renal function, meds Specimen hemolyzed	Reduce K+ in PN Assess renal function, review meds. Repeat serum K+
Hypokalemia	Serum K+ below NL Weakness, tingling, muscle spasms, vomiting	Inadequate amount of K+ in PN Extra GI/Urinary losses K+ wasting meds	Increase K+ in PN Review output losses Review meds Repeat serum K+
Dehydration	Elevated/abnl BUN/Cr, electrolytes Thirsty, weight loss, tired, weak, vomiting, decreased urine output	Inadequate PN fluid Excess GI losses Change in renal function Change in meds	Increase PN fluid and/or provide extra IVF Review changes in medical status Review meds
Overhydration	Abnormal electrolytes Rapid weight gain, edema,	Excess PN fluid Excess IVF/oral fluid	Decrease PN fluid Decrease sodium in PN

Problem	Clinical Signs/Symptoms	Possible Etiology	Treatment
	shortness of breath, increased urine output	Change in medical status	Consider diuretic
Hypomagnesemia	Serum Mg+ below NL Muscle cramps, twitching, confusion	Inadequate Mg+ in PN Excess GI, renal losses Change in meds	Increase Mg+ in PN Review output losses Review meds
Hypophosphatemia (Refeeding?)	Serum PO4 below NL. Muscle weakness, perioral, fingertip paresthesia	Inadequate PO4 in PN Excess GI, renal losses Changes in meds	Increase PO4 in PN Review output losses Review meds

Vitamin and Trace Element Deficiencies and Toxicities

Clinicians caring for patients on HPN should be aware of the signs and symptoms of vitamin and trace element deficiencies and toxicities. Vitamin deficiencies are generally not common as long as a multivitamin injection is added to the HPN daily. Specific vitamin requirements may be increased or decreased in a variety of conditions including stress, inflammation, disease process, or increased losses or retention. Assessing for vitamin deficiencies or toxicities serum levels may be helpful.[34] More detailed information on vitamin deficiencies is provided in Chapter 3.

Several case reports of trace element deficiencies and toxicities in patients receiving HPN have been reported in the literature. Manganese toxicity has also been reported in this patient population. Trace element recommendations for patients on HPN have been established for chromium, copper, manganese, selenium and zinc. Trace element levels should be checked at baseline then every 6 to 12 months when a maintenance dose is given and every 3 months during repletion if deemed clinically necessary.[35] See Chapter 3 for more information on trace elements.

Essential Fatty Acid Deficiency

Essential fatty acid deficiency can occur within days to weeks if an inadequate supply of EFA is not supplied. Essential fatty acids are necessary for platelet function, prostaglandin synthesis, wound healing, immunocompetence, and maintenance of skin, hair and nerve integrity. Jeppesen and associates [36] reported HPN patients not receiving IV lipids had significantly lower plasma levels of linoleic and linolenic acids compared to controls. When 500 mL of 20% IV lipid was given once per week plasma EFA levels returned to normal. Biochemical evidence of EFA deficiency can be determined by a triene:tetraene ratio of more than 0.2.[37] These levels can be drawn every 6 to 12 months to monitor for EFA deficiency if deemed clinically necessary.

Iron-Deficiency Anemia

Iron deficiency anemia has been reported to occur in 31% to 54% of adults on HPN who have inadequate enteral iron intake or absorption.[38,39] Patients with iron deficiency anemia may present with fatigue, dyspnea on exertion, tachycardia, headache, listlessness, paresthesia, altered attention span, pallor, inability to maintain body temperature, and pica. Anemia is recognized in the laboratory when a patient's hemoglobin or hematocrit falls below the normal range. Iron deficiency anemia is diagnosed by a low serum iron and ferritin. Other common causes of anemia in this patient population are recent blood loss and anemia of chronic disease. Anemia of chronic disease is diagnosed when there is a low serum iron with a normal ferritin. Less common causes include vitamin B_{12}, folate, and copper deficiencies. However, addition of daily multivitamins and trace elements make these latter causes of anemia less likely.

Iron deficiency anemia should be treated with iron replacement therapy. Patients who are able to absorb oral medications can be given iron supplements as a tablet or elixir. If patients cannot absorb oral medications, then they will require IV iron. The repletion dose for iron should be calculated when the IV route is used. The dose can be calculated using the following equation:[40]

$$\text{Replacement iron (mg)} = 0.3 \times \text{weight (pounds)}$$
$$\times (100 - [\text{Actual hemoglobin} \times 100 \div \text{desired hemoglobin}])$$

Iron dextran can be added to 2-in-1 HPN solutions *after* the patient has been given a test dose of iron dextran to rule out anaphylaxis.[40] A dose of 10 to 20 mg per day can be given or a total repletion dose may be given. Serum iron and ferritin levels should be monitored routinely every 3 to 6 months if a repletion dose is added to the HPN to document repletion of iron stores and to avoid hemosiderosis.

Liver Disease

Liver abnormalities in HPN patients can occur and ranges from mild fatty infiltration to life threatening cirrhosis and liver failure requiring liver transplantation. The most predominant HPN associated liver disease is steatosis and less frequently, cholestasis.[41] The prevalence of liver enzyme abnormalities has been reported to occur in 25% to 100% of patients on long-term HPN and the prevalence of end-stage liver disease in such patients is between 15% and 40%.[21,42,43] The exact etiology of liver abnormalities has not been identified although several causes have been proposed including:[41]

- hepatotoxins
- malnutrition (kwashiorkor)
- dextrose overfeeding
- choline deficiency

- lipid overfeeding
- bacterial overgrowth
- EFA deficiency

Patients with elevated liver enzymes should be evaluated to exclude secondary causes of this abnormality. A review of all medications is important including those added to HPN formulas. Histamine-2 receptor antagonists and octreotide can cause cholestasis and may be removed from the HPN solution with evidence of increasing liver abnormalities. Laboratory studies should be obtained to exclude viral hepatitis, autoimmune liver disease, and inherited forms of liver disease such as hemachromatosis, alpha 1-antitrypsin deficiency and Wilson's disease. An abdominal ultrasound or computed tomography should be done to exclude biliary tract disease. Hepatology consultation should be considered when enzyme elevation is increasing or present for over 6 months.

Preventative measures should be taken to minimize the incidence of HPN associated liver disease. Regular monitoring of liver function blood tests, and avoidance of known hepatoxins, overfeeding, and nutrient deficiencies are important. (See Chapter 12 for more details.)

Metabolic Bone Disease

Metabolic bone disease (MBD) is abnormal bone metabolism resulting in osteoporosis or osteomalacia. Bone pain, back pain, loss of height and atraumatic fractures are symptoms of patients with MBD, though patients may be asymptomatic. Metabolic bone disease associated with PN was first described in the 1980s in patients receiving HPN for 3 months or more.[44,45] The incidence of MBD in long-term HPN patients has been reported to range from 42% to 100%.[46,47] Though the exact cause of MBD in patients on long-term HPN is unknown, the origin is thought to be multifactorial including factors such as the underlying disease (Crohn's disease, ulcerative colitis), medications (glucocorticosteroids), and factors related to the HPN formula.[48] Adequate amounts of calcium, phosphorus, magnesium, and acetate for acid-base balance are important. Excess amounts of protein have been shown to contribute to hypercalcuria and should be avoided.[49]

Dual-energy x-ray absorptiometry (DXA) is a relatively inexpensive, noninvasive study that can accurately measure bone mineral density (BMD). It cannot differentiate osteoporosis from osteomalacia. Most patients with low BMD will have osteoporosis. The DXA study result is given as a T-score, which classifies the risk of bone fracture. Osteoporosis is defined as a T-score of −2.5 or below; osteopenia is a T-score of −2.5 to −1 and a T-score of −1 or above is normal.[50]

Patients with MBD should be referred to an endocrinologist for treatment, which may include supplementation of calcium, vitamin D, hormone replacement therapy, antiresorptive drugs such as bisphosphonates, or anabolic agents. Clinical trials of pharmacologic treatment in patients with MBD on HPN are limited to one trial, to date. A prospective, randomized, double-blinded, controlled trial comparing the effects of intravenous clodronate, a bisphosphonate, with placebo in patients receiving long-term HPN with MBD showed biochemical markers of bone resorption is correct, (reabsorption is not) were statistically lower in the bisphosphonate group with a significant increase in bone mineral density of the forearm. Bone mineral density of the spine and hip was increased, but not significantly.[51] Recent advances in drug treatment for osteoporosis include the use of parathyroid hormone analog which was shown to significantly increase BMD in post-menopausal women.[52] Its use in HPN patients has not yet been studied.

Clinicians caring for patients on long-term HPN should include monitoring for MBD as part of the routine care and clinical management of these patients. Table 8–18 provides guidelines for monitoring and managing HPN-associated MBD.

OUTCOMES

Technological advances have made the use of long-term HPN a life sustaining therapy for those with GI failure. However, HPN has a significant impact on the quality of life, and the mortality and morbidity of those undergoing this therapy.

Patients on HPN may experience reduced physical strength, sleep deprivation, depression, anger, anxiety, loss of identity, loss of employment, reduced social interactions, and loss of friends.[53,54] No specific tools used to assess quality of life in HPN patients have been developed, but two common tools used in patients with chronic disorders include the Short Form 36 (SF-36) and Euroquol index.[55] Repeat administration of the SF-36 to HPN patients has shown worsening quality of life scores associated with the deterioration of intestinal failure, increased number of infusions, need for a liquid diet, decreased body mass index, worsen-

TABLE 8–18   Suggested Guidelines for Monitoring and Managing PN-Associated MBD

1. All patients on long-term PN (>1 year) should be evaluated for MBD.
2. Monitor for physical signs of MBD such as loss of height and bone or back pain.
3. Provide adequate amounts of minerals in the PN solution necessary for bone remodeling including at least minimum requirements of calcium (~ 15 mEq) and phosphorus (~ 15 mmol) and magnesium (adjust amount per serum and urine levels).
4. Adjust higher protein doses to 1 gm/kg/day once nutritional status improved and proteins repleted.
5. Treat metabolic acidosis with adequate amounts of acetate in the PN solution to avoid calcium carbonate mobilization from bone to buffer excess acid.
6. Monitor blood studies (at least monthly) to include calcium, phosphorus, magnesium, and acetate. Maintain normal serum levels by adjusting amounts in the PN solution. Specific markers of bone metabolism may be of further diagnostic help.
7. Obtain 24-hour urine collection for calcium and magnesium every 6–12 months. Adjust PN to maintain positive balances.
8. Obtain DXA measurement and refer to endocrinologist for evaluation and pharmacologic treatment for low bone mineral density (T-score <–1). Initially repeat DXA every 1–2 years.
9. Minimize steroid use and all medications known to cause bone resorption.
10. Promote exercise or refer to physical therapist.
11. Encourage cessation of smoking.

ing HPN tolerance by presence of nocturia and a greater incidence of catheter complications with increased hospitalization.[56] Home parenteral nutrition patients affiliated with a national patient education and support group have shown higher quality of life scores, less incidence of depression and decreased incidence of catheter related blood stream infections compared to patients not involved with a support group.[57] Chapter 19 provides insight by HPEN patients/consumers and their caregivers.

The duration of therapy is influenced by the primary disease, length of bowel and age. Most patients require HPN for less than a year. The majority of cancer patients die at one year due to progression of their malignancy, whereas patients with Crohn's disease may return to full or partial oral nutrition within one to two years.[58] Patients with short bowel (<50–100 cm), end enterostomy, or bowel infarction have decreased survival rates. The presence of the terminal ileum and/or colon improves survival rates and increases the chances of weaning from HPN.[59,60] Younger patients have been shown to have better survival rates on HPN, a greater likelihood of resuming full oral nutrition and experience more complete rehabilitation than older patients.[1]

The rate of HPN related-deaths is generally low. One large center reported 9% of their patients died due to HPN complications in a 20-year period with catheter related sepsis and liver failure as the leading causes of death.[32]

THERAPEUTIC OPTIONS TO HOME PARENTERAL NUTRITION

Treatment for patients with short bowel syndrome (SBS) should include dietary modifications to help maximize absorption of fluid and nutrients and minimize fecal output.[61] Medications used to slow down intestinal transit time or increase absorption may also be prescribed. These include antidiarrheal medications, histamine 2-receptor antagonists, proton pump inhibitors, pancreatic enzymes, and oral antibiotics for bacterial overgrowth. Recently, growth hormone has been approved by the FDA as a treatment option in the management of SBS.[62]

Surgery should be considered in patients when a portion of the bowel is not in continuity with the fecal stream. This may decrease one's reliance on HPN. On the forefront of medical treatment of patients with GI failure is the development of intestinal transplantation. This surgical option is reserved for patients with life threatening complications of HPN therapy including repeated catheter sepsis, thrombosis of major venous access routes and liver failure.[63] Survival rates of this mode of therapy are improving but intestinal transplantation is not yet considered a replacement therapy for patients who are tolerating HPN.

CONCLUSIONS

HPN is a life-saving therapy for those with intestinal failure. Identification of appropriate candidates, patient education provided by a multidisciplinary team of nutrition support experts, and coordination of care with the homecare organization are essential steps that should be taken to provide treatment in a safe and effective manner. Complications can be either catheter and/or metabolic related and can be serious or life threatening. The establishment of routine monitoring protocols and procedures for treating complications is imperative so morbidity and mortality is kept to a minimum. Surgery should be considered for patients when a portion of the bowel is out of continuity with the digestive tract. In the near future, growth factors and intestinal transplantation may allow a significant number of patients who rely on HPN to decrease or discontinue HPN.

REFERENCES

1. Howard L, Ament M, Fleming CR, Shike M, Steiger E. Current use and clinical outcome of home parenteral and enteral nutrition therapies in the United States. *Gastroenterology*. 1995;109:355–365.
2. A.S.P.E.N. Board of Directors and the Clinical Guidelines Task Force. Guidelines for the use of parenteral and enteral nutrition in adult and pediatric patients. *JPEN*. 2002;26:1SA-138SA.
3. Palmetto Government Benefits Administrators, LLC. Parenteral Nutrition Therapy. In: ed. *Region C Durable Medical Equipment Regional Carrier Supplier Manual*. Autumn/1998.
4. Reddy P, Malone M. Cost and outcome analysis of home parenteral and enteral nutrition. *JPEN*. 1998;22(5):302–310.
5. Barrera R. Nutritional support in cancer patients. *JPEN*. 2002;26(5):S63-S71.
6. A.S.P.E.N. Board of Directors. Standards of practice for nutrition support dietitians. *Nutr Clin Prac*. 1990;5(2):74–78.
7. A.S.P.E.N. Board of Directors: Standards for nutrition support nurses. *Nutr Clin Pract*. 1996;11(3):127–134.
8. A.S.P.E.N. Board of Directors. Standards for nutrition support pharmacists. *Nutr Clin Pract*. 1999;8(3):124–127.
9. Roncagli T, Sharp J. Defining high psychosocial risk in home nutrition support. *Support Line*. 1994;6(5):10–12.
10. Gulledge A, Srp F, Sharp J, et al. Psychosocial issues of home parenteral and enteral nutrition. *Nutr Clin Prac*. 1987;2(5):183–194.
11. Engstrom I, Bjornestam B, Finkel Y. Psychological distress associated with home parenteral nutrition in Swedish children, adolescents, and their parents: preliminary results. *J Pediatr Gastroenterol Nutr*. 2003;37(3):246–250.
12. Folstein MF, Folstein SE, McHugh PR. "Mini-mental state". A practical method for grading the cognitive state of patients for the clinician. *J Psychiatr Res*. 1975;12(3):189–198.
13. Gorski L. Effective teaching of home IV therapy. *Home Healthc Nurse*. 2002;20(10):666–674.

14. Silver HJ, Wellman NS. Family caregiver training is needed to improve outcomes for older adults using home care technologies. *J Am Diet Assoc.* 2002;102(6):831–836.

15. Smith CE, Curtas S, Kleinbeck SV, et al. Clinical trial of interactive and videotaped educational interventions reduce infection, reactive depression, and rehospitalization for sepsis in patients on home parenteral nutrition. *J Parenter Enteral Nutr.* 2003;27(2):137–145.

16. Orr ME. Vascular access device selection for parenteral nutrition. *Nutr Clin Prac.* 1999;14(4):172–177.

17. Steiger E. Obtaining and maintaining vascular access in the home parenteral nutrition patient. *J Parenter Enteral Nutr.* 2002;26(suppl 5):S17-S20.

18. O'Grady NP, Alexander M, Dellinger EP, et al. Guidelines for the prevention of intravascular catheter-related infections. *Infect Control Hosp Epidemiol.* 2002;23(12):759–769.

19. Barber JR, Miller SJ, Sacks GS. Parenteral feeding formulations. In: Gottsclich MM, ed. *The Science and Practice of Nutrition Support, A Case-Based Core Curriculum.* Dubuque: Kendall/Hunt Publishing Company; 2001:251–268.

20. Mirtallo JM. Parenteral formulas. In: Rombeau JL, Rolandelli RH, eds. *Clinical Nutrition, Parenteral Nutrition,* 3rd ed. Philadelphia, Pa: W.B. Saunders Co; 2001:118–139.

21. Cavicchi M, Crenn P, Beau P, et al. Prevalence of liver disease and contributing factors in patients receiving home parenteral nutrition for permanent intestinal failure. *Ann Intern Med.* 2000;132:525–532.

22. Lennon E, Speerhas R. Parenteral nutrition. In: Parekh, N and DeChicco RL, eds. *Nutrition Support Handbook.* Cleveland, Ohio: The Cleveland Clinic Foundation; 2004:78–92.

23. Safe practices for parenteral nutrition formulations. National Advisory Group on Standards and Practice Guidelines for Parenteral Nutrition. *JPEN* 1998;22(2):39–66.

24. Whitmire SJ. Fluid and electrolytes. In: Gottsclich MM, ed. *The Science and Practice of Nutrition Support, A Case-Based Core Curriculum.* Dubuque, Iowa: Kendall/Hunt Publishing Co; 2001:53–83.

25. Food and Drug Administration. Parenteral Multivitamin Products; Drugs for Human Use; Drug Efficacy Study Implementation; Amendment: Federal Register, April 20, 1965(77), 21200, 2000.

26. A.S.P.E.N. Board of Directors and the Clinical Guidelines Taskforce. Guidelines for the use of parenteral and enteral nutrition in adult and pediatric patients. *JPEN* 2002;26(suppl 1):1SA-138SA.

27. Maini B, Blackburn G, Bistrian BR. Cyclic hyperalimentation: an optimal technique for preservation of visceral protein. *J Surg Res.* 1976;20;515–525.

28. Hamilton C, Lennon E, Saylor K, et al. Home nutrition support. In: Parekh N and DeChicco RL, eds. *Nutrition Support Handbook.* Cleveland, Ohio: The Cleveland Clinic Foundation; 2004:162–178.

29. A.S.P.E.N. Board of Directors. Standards for specialized nutrition support: home care patients. *Nutr Clin Prac.* 2005:20:579–589

30. A.S.P.E.N. Board of Directors. Standards for nutrition support for adult residents of long-term care facilities. *Nutr Clin Prac.* 1997;12:284–293.

31. Grant J. Recognition, prevention, and treatment of home total parenteral nutrition central venous access complications. *JPEN* 2002;26(5):S21-S28.

32. Scolapio JS, Fleming R, Kelly DG, et al. Survival of home parenteral nutrition-treated patients: 20 years of experience at the Mayo Clinic. *Mayo Clin Proc.* 1999;74:217–222.

33. Howard L, Ashley C. Management of complications in patients receiving home parenteral nutrition. *Gastroenterology.* 2003;124:1651–1661.

34. Fuhrman MP, Parker M. Micronutrient assessment. Support Line. 2004; 26(1):17–24.

35. Kelly D. Guidelines and available products for parenteral vitamins and trace elements. *J Parenter Enteral Nutr.* 2002;26(suppl 5):S34-S36.

36. Jeppesen PB, Hoy C, Mortensen PB. Essential fatty acid deficiency in patients receiving home parenteral nutrition. *Am J Clin Nutr.* 1998;68:126–133.

37. Holman RT, Smythe L, Johnson S. Effect of sex and age on fatty acid composition of human serum lipids. *Am J Clin Nutr.* 1979;32:2390–2399.

38. Forbes GM, Forbes A. Micronutrient status in patients receiving home parenteral nutrition. *Nutrition.* 1997;13:941–944.

39. Khaodhiar L, Keane-Ellison M, Tawa NE, et al. Iron deficiency anemia in patients receiving home total parenteral nutrition. *JPEN* 2002;26:114–119.

40. Kumpf VJ. Update on parenteral iron therapy. *Nutr Clin Pract.* 2003;8(4):318–326.

41. Buchman A. Total parenteral nutrition-associated liver disease. *JPEN* 2002;26(suppl 5):S43-S48.

42. Fulford A, Scolapio JS, Aranda-Michel, J. Parenteral nutrition-associated hepatotoxicity. *Nutr Clin Pract.* 2004;19(3):274–283.

43. Chan S, McCowan KC, Bistrian BR, et al. Incidence, prognosis, and etiology of end-stage liver disease in patients receiving home parenteral nutrition. *Surgery.* 1999;126:28–34.

44. Klein GL, Targoff CM, Ament ME, et al. Bone disease associated with total parenteral nutrition. *Lancet.* 1980;2(8203):1041–1044.

45. Shike M, Harrison JE, Sturtridge WC, et al. Metabolic bone disease in patients receiving long-term total parenteral nutrition. *Ann Intern Med.* 1980;92:343–350.

46. Hurley DL, McMahon MM. Long-term parenteral nutrition and metabolic bone disease. *Endocrinol Metab Clin North Am.* 1990;19(1)113–131.

47. Pironi L, Labate AM, Pertkiewicz M, et al. Prevalence of bone disease in patients on home parenteral nutrition. *Clin Nutr.* 2002;21:289–295.

48. Haderslev KV, Tjellesen L, Haderslev PH, et al. Assessment of the longitudinal changes in bone mineral density in patients receiving home parenteral nutrition. *JPEN* 2004;28(5):289–294.

49. Hamilton C. Parenteral nutrition-associated metabolic bone disease. *Support Line*. 2003;25(5):7–13.

50. Assessment of fracture risk and its application to screening for postmenopausal studies. World Health Organization Technical Report Series 843. Geneva, Switzerland: World Health Organization; 1994.

51. Haderslev KV, Tjellesen L, Sorensen HA, et al. Effect of cyclical intravenous clodronate therapy on bone mineral density and markers of bone turnover in patients receiving home parenteral nutrition *Am J Clin Nutr.* 2002;76:482–488.

52. Neer RM, Arnaud CD, Zanchetta JR, et al. Effect of parathyroid hormone (1–34) on fractures and bone mineral density in postmenopausal women with osteoporosis. *N Engl J Med.* 2001;344:1434–1441.

53. Jeppeson PB, Landholz E, Mortensen PB. Quality of life in patients receiving home parenteral nutrition. *Gut.* 1999;44:844–852.

54. Malone M. Longitudinal assessment of outcome, health status, and changes in lifestyle associated with long-term home parenteral and enteral nutrition. *JPEN* 2002;26(3):164–168.

55. Howard LJ. Length of life and quality of life on home parenteral nutrition. *J Parenter Enteral Nutr.* 2002;26(suppl 5):S55-S59.

56. Pironi L, Paganelli F, Mosconi AM, et al. The SF-36 instrument for the follow-up of health-related quality-of-life assessment of patients undergoing home parenteral nutrition for benign disease. *Transplant Proc.* 2004;36:255–258.

57. Smith C, Curtas S, Werkowitch M, et al. Home parenteral nutrition: does affiliation with a national support and educational organization improve patient outcomes? *J Parenter Enteral Nutr.* 2002;26(3):159–163.

58. North American Home Parenteral and Enteral Nutrition Patient Registry: Annual report with outcome profiles 1985–1992. The Oley Foundation, Albany, NY, 1994.

59. Carbonnel F, Cosnes J, Chevret S, et al. The role of anatomic factors in nutritional autonomy after extensive small bowel resection. *JPEN* 1996;20:275–280.

60. Messing B, Crenn P, Beau P, et al. Long-term survival and parenteral nutrition dependence in adult patients with the short bowel syndrome. *Gastroenterology.* 1999;117:1043–1050.

61. Byrne T, Veglia L, Camelio M, et al. Beyond the prescription: optimizing the diet of patients with short bowel syndrome. *Nutr Clin Prac.* 2000;15(6):306–311.

62. Byrne TA, Lautz DB, Iyer KR, et al. Recombinant human growth hormone (rhGH) reduces parenteral nutrition (PN) in patients with short bowel sy-

drome: a prospective, randomized, double-blind, placebo-controlled study. *JPEN* 2003;27(1)A034:S17.

63. Iyer KR. Organ transplantation for intestinal failure. *JPEN* 2002;26(suppl 5):S49–S54.

CHAPTER 9

Home Enteral Nutrition in the Pediatric Patient

Connie Anastasio, MSc RD, CNSD
Robin Nagel, RD, CNSD

INTRODUCTION

Utilization of home enteral nutrition (HEN) has grown dramatically in the last few decades. Continuous advancements in practice and technology have made HEN easier and safer to administer outside the hospital environment helping make lengthy hospital stays for the sole purpose of administering nutrition support a thing of the past.[1] Data from the North American Home Parenteral and Enteral Nutrition Registry indicated that pediatric patients (0 to 18 years) had the highest survival rate and rehabilitation of all nutrition support patients.[2] Medically stable pediatric patients are, therefore, good candidates for HEN because they can be expected to have good outcomes and may require nutrition support for extended periods of time and during critical periods of growth.

Nutrition support in the pediatric patient is a complex therapy that requires diligence and attention to detail in order that these patients may receive optimal benefit. Pediatric patients are more susceptible to the adverse effects associated with starvation than their adult counterparts by virtue of their smaller nutrient reserves.[3] In stark contrast to the well-nourished adult with, theoretically, enough stored energy to sustain life for almost a year under conditions of semi-starvation, a premature infant will exhaust all energy reserves of glycogen, fat, and protein within about 2 to 10 days.[4] Similarly, the young pediatric patient is more susceptible to dehydration due to their large body surface area, high percentage of total body water and its rapid turnover, limited capacity for handling renal solute load, and inability to express thirst.[5]

Infants and children are metabolically more fragile than adults. Premature and full term infants are at increased risk for both hypoglycemia and hyperglycemia. In term infants, for example, approximately 60% of resting energy metabolism can be attributed to brain metabolism in comparison to about 25% for a normal adult. Because the primary energy source for the brain is glucose, infants are more susceptible to hypoglycemia and require more immediate intervention with carbohydrate.[6]

It is not uncommon for children to be receiving multiple nutrition support therapies simultaneously. Therefore, the issue of overfeeding or underfeeding is very important. Particular attention should be focused on any contribution made by absorbed oral nutrients or parenteral nutrition (PN) to ensure nutrient and fluid adequacy and prevent redundant or excessive delivery of specific nutrients.[7] Careful patient/caregiver selection and a multidisciplinary team to guide and monitor therapy are required for home nutritional therapy to succeed.[1] During the course of treatment at home assistance and emotional support may be required while problems are resolved and caregivers become comfortable with their routine.

GOALS OF HOME ENTERAL NUTRITION

All clinicians working with the pediatric patient at home must establish appropriate nutrition support goals and schedule regular monitoring to ensure that goals are being met. The main goals of HEN for pediatric patients are outlined in Table 9–1.[8]

Establishing realistic goals in the pediatric patient requires good clinical judgment and knowledge of the patient's disease state. Goals for growth may need to be modified as the specific disease state makes attainment of optimal weight and height for age unlikely. Furthermore, the home environment and caregiver status need to be assessed in order to develop realistic and achievable goals.

TABLE 9–1   Goals of Pediatric Home Enteral Nutrition Support

- Provide adequate nutrition for normal growth and development
- Preserve existing tissue stores
- Provide catch-up growth in malnourished patients
- Preserve age-appropriate oral motor skills
- Resolution of disease progression, wound healing, and rehabilitation of depleted patients
- Optimal gastrointestinal, metabolic, and mechanical tolerance to nutrition support
- Optimal psychosocial adaptation to home and school
- Weaning to an age-appropriate diet as medically feasible
- Strength, independence

INDICATIONS

Enteral nutrition (EN) is indicated in the pediatric patient with a functional gastrointestinal tract who is unwilling or unable to ingest or absorb sufficient nutrients and is likely to become malnourished.[9] Pediatric patients may require EN if they experience acute weight loss (wasting) or chronic growth retardation (stunting) due to neurological disorders, congenital anomalies, mechanical injuries that impair ingestion or propulsion of food, increased metabolic stress with anorexia, anorexia due to consequences of disease or treatment, altered absorption or metabolism of nutrients, or psychosocial disorders.[9] Table 9–2[5,10] lists commonly encountered conditions in which EN should be considered. The enteral route is contraindicated only when there exists an inability to digest, absorb, or propulse nutrients through the digestive tract.[11]

Early EN has been shown to promote intestinal adaptation and growth.[12] Trophic feedings, the provision of some nutrients into the gastrointestinal tract for the purpose of gastrointestinal priming are associated with enhanced gut motility and better mineral retention in comparison with enteral starvation after preterm birth. Gastrointestinal priming in preterm neonates has not been found to increase necrotizing enterocolitis (NEC) rates.[13]

Infants and children with bowel resections may exhibit malabsorption and the metabolic complications associated with short bowel syndrome (SBS). This may occur with even minimal or modest resections of the small bowel. Remaining intestinal length and functional differences between the proximal and distal small intestine have a major impact on a patient's overall clinical course, their nutritional management, and ultimate ability to adapt to enteral nutrition.[12]

TABLE 9–2   Conditions Under Which Enteral Nutrition Should be Considered

Inability to suck, swallow, or breathe due to injury or illness	
Prematurity (<34 weeks)	Cystic fibrosis
Orofacial malformations	Congenital heart disease
Anorexia or chronic disease	Chronic lung disease
Gastrointestinal tract disease or dysfunction	Renal disease
Hypermetabolic states	Trauma or burns
Aquired immunodeficiency syndrome	Neurological disorders
Failure to thrive—organic and nonorganic	Congenital metabolic abnormalities
Cancer treatment and bone marrow transplant	

Compared with the parenteral route, feeding by the enteral route is more compatible with normal physiology and consequently has fewer short-term and long-term complications. However, when the GI tract is non-functional due to illness or injury, the parenteral route is very appropriate to provide nutrient needs. Enteral more so than parenteral nutrition is associated with better preservation and restoration of the gastrointestinal mucosa by exposure to the trophic effect of nutrients, stimulation of the activity of non-luminal neuronal and hormonal factors, which stimulate bowel growth, and enhanced immunity through stimulation of liver production of secretory IgA and stimulation.[1,2,3,14,15]

NUTRITION ASSESSMENT CONSIDERATIONS

Failure to Thrive

In the pediatric patient failure to thrive (FTT) is used to describe instances of growth failure based primarily on attained weight or rate of weight gain in an infant or child. Table 9–3 provides guidelines to help the clinician and caregiver screen for FTT.

In chronic and severe cases of FTT growth stunting can occur in which head circumference, length, and developmental skills may also be affected. Failure to thrive is generally diagnosed as due to organic or nonorganic causes, but most often it is a complex interaction among medical, psychosocial, environmental, nutritional, neurologic, and anatomic factors.[16] There are three distinct criteria (Table 9–4), that utilize

TABLE 9–3   Screening Mechanism for Slow Weight Gain vs FTT

Characteristic	Slow Weight Gain	Failure to Thrive
Weight Gain	Consistent	No gain or loss
Urine	Pale dilute, at least 6–8 wet diapers daily	Strong dark, fewer than 6 wet diapers daily
Feedings	At least 8 daily	Less than 8 daily
Muscle tone	Good	Poor
Skin turgor	Good	Poor
Stools	At least 4 daily, seedy	Infrequent, scant

Adapted from: Lessen R. Failure to Thrive in the Breast-fed Infant: A Case Study. *Building Block for Life.* Spring 2001; 24(3):1–10.

TABLE 9–4   Identification of Failure to Thrive[16]

Criteria:	Exceptions:
1.) A child younger than 2 years of age whose weight is below the 3rd or 5th percentile for age on more than one occasion	1.) Children of genetically short stature
	2.) Small-for-gestational age infants
2.) A child younger than 2 years of age whose weight is less than 80% of the ideal weight for age	3.) Preterm infants rate of weight gain decreases
	4.) "Overweight" infants whose rate of height gain increases while the rate of weight gain decreases
3.) A child younger than 2 years of age whose weight crosses two major percentiles downward on a standardized growth grid, using the 90th, 50th, 25th, 10th, and 5th percentiles as the major percentiles	5.) Infants who are normally lean

the 2000 standard growth charts of the Centers for Disease Control to describe the child with FTT.

Children who have either type of FTT, organic or nonorganic, are undernourished. Both groups respond equally well when the malnutrition is treated.[17] An infant who exhibits weight loss or poor weight gain should be fed aggressively to prevent irreversible cognitive deficits while the clinician is searching for the underlying etiology.[18]

DEVELOPING THE NUTRITION SUPPORT PLAN

A number of factors must be considered in developing a safe, adequate, and appropriate nutrition support plan in the pediatric patient. Macronutrient needs must be identified and the nutrient distribution monitored to maintain the formula within optimal ranges for carbohydrate (35–65%), protein (7–18%), and fat (30–55%).[19] Vitamin, mineral, and electrolyte provisions should be evaluated with respect to disease-specific risk factors. Fluid requirements, osmolality, and renal solute load in HEN should be monitored along with hydration status. Dietary fiber can be added to long-term enteral feedings as is deemed appropriate to the age and gastrointestinal function of the child. Growth and nutrient intake must be monitored regularly to prevent nutrient needs from exceeding intake as the child grows.[20]

ENERGY AND PROTEIN REQUIREMENTS

The Recommended Dietary Allowances (RDA), Table 9–5, are the most frequently used tools to estimate daily energy and protein needs for healthy infants and children. Adjustments in the estimates of daily intake are necessary when the patient is under/overnourished, has increased or decreased metabolic requirements due to injury or illness, or there is markedly increased or decreased physical activity.

In 2002 the Food and Nutrition Board of the National Institute of Medicine published dietary reference intakes for macronutrients. Table 9–6 provides the equations used to derive energy needs for the general pediatric population in the United States.[21] The equations are based on gender, age, height, weight, and physical activity (PA).

Children with developmental disabilities have unique nutritional requirements related specifically to their disease state. Genetic and neurological disorders may affect growth patterns and alter the metabolism of some nutrients. Standard growth charts may be used to plot serial measurements except when disease-specific growth charts are available (see Chapter 4).[22] Table 9–7 provides guidelines for calculating caloric requirements in some of the most commonly encountered developmental disabilities.

TABLE 9–5   Recommended Energy and Protein Intake for Age in Healthy Children

	Age (yr)	Average Energy Needs (kcal/kg/day)	Average Energy Needs (kcal/day)	Protein (g/kg/day)
Infants	0.0–0.5	108	650	2.2
	0.5–1.0	98	850	1.6
Children	1–3	102	1300	1.3
	4–6	90	1800	1.2
	7–10	70	2000	1.0
Males	11–14	55	2500	1.0
	15–18	45	3000	0.9
Females	11–14	47	2200	1.0
	15–18	40	2200	0.8

National Research Council: Recommended Dietary Allowances, 10th Ed. National Academies Press, Washington, DC, 1989.

CATCH-UP GROWTH

When the patient has wasting of tissue stores or stunting of growth, catch-up requirements are required and can be calculated using the following method.

$$\text{kcal/kg/day} = \frac{\text{RDA (kcal) for Weight Age} \times \text{Ideal Body Wt (IBW) for Age*}}{\text{Actual Weight}}$$

*where:

IBW for age: 50th percentile of weight-for-age (corrected age in prematurity) from growth chart.

RDA (kcal) for *weight age*: Find the age at which the child's actual weight would be at the 50th percentile then use the RDA kcal for this age (see Table 9–5).

Protein "catch-up" (g protein/kg/day) is calculated with the same equation.[23]

$$\text{Protein (g)/kg/day} = \frac{\text{RDA (g protein) for Weight Age} \times \text{IBW for Age}}{\text{Actual Weight}}$$

FLUID AND ELECTROLYTE REQUIREMENTS

Ensuring that the pediatric patient on HEN receives adequate hydration and electrolytes is one of the greatest challenges of home care nutrition

TABLE 9-6   Estimating Energy Requirements (EER) in Healthy Children

EER = TEE (Total Energy Expenditure)* + ED (Energy Deposition)
0–3 months: (89 × weight [kg] – 100) + 175 (kcal for ED)** 4–6 months: (89 × weight [kg] – 100) + 56 (kcal for ED)** 7–12 months: (89 × weight [kg] – 100) + 22 (kcal for ED)** 13–36 months: (89 × weight [kg] – 100 + 20 (kcal for ED)**
Males, 3–8 years: 88.5 – 61.9 × age [years] + PA × (26.7 × weight [kg] + 903 × height [m]) + 20 (kcal for ED) Males, 9–18 years: 88.5 – 61.9 × age [years] + PA × (26.7 × weight [kg] + 903 × height [m]) + 25 (kcal for ED) where PA is the Physical Activity Quotient: PA = 1.00 if PAL is estimated to be ≥ 1.0 and <1.4 (sedentary) PA = 1.13 if PAL is estimated to be ≥ 1.4 and <1.6 (low active) PA = 1.26 if PAL is estimated to be ≥ 1.6 and <1.9 (active) PA = 1.42 if PAL is estimated to be ≥ 1.9 and <2.5 (very active)
Females, 3–8 years: 135.3 – 30.8 × age [years] + PA (10.0 × weight [kg] + 934 × height [m]) + 20 (kcal for ED) Females, 9–18 years: 135.3 – 30.8 × age [years] + PA (10.0 × weight [kg] + 934 × height [m]) + 25 (kcal for ED) where PA is the Physical Activity Quotient: PA = 1.00 if PAL is estimated to be ≥ 1.0 and <1.4 (sedentary, bed rest) PA = 1.16 if PAL is estimated to be ≥ 1.4 and <1.6 (low active) PA = 1.31 if PAL is estimated to be ≥ 1.6 and <1.9 (active) PA = 1.56 if PAL is estimated to be ≥ 1.9 and <2.5 (very active)

*TEE is approximately 80% of the 1985 FAO/WHO/UNU recommendations for energy intake of infants and toddlers.
**No gender difference at these ages.

support. Pediatric patients are often at high risk of dehydration due to numerous factors which may increase their fluid requirements including fever, diarrhea, vomiting, chronic respiratory distress (such as is seen in cystic fibrosis), hypermetabolism, renal tubule defects, diuretic therapy, fistula and stoma output, and increased fiber intake.[20] The leading cause of readmission to the hospital in pediatric HEN patients is dehydration. When the micronutrient content of the formula is being concentrated to encourage growth, it is imperative to evaluate whether the child is receiv-

TABLE 9-7 Calorie Requirements in Children with Developmental Disabilities

Clinical Condition	Calorie Recommendations
Down's syndrome (boys 5-12 yr)	16.1 kcal/cm height (40.9 kcal/in)
Down's syndrome (girls 5-12 yr)	14.3 kcal/cm height (36.3 kcal/in)
Prader-Willi syndrome	Maintenance: 10-11 kcal/cm height for (26.7 kcal /in) Weight loss: 8.5 kcal/cm height (21.6 kcal/in)
Myelomeningocele (spina bifida)	Maintenance: 9-11 kcal/cm height (25.0 kcal/in) Weight loss: 7 kcal/cm height (17.78 kcal/in)
Cerebral palsy (age 5-11 yr)	Mild-Moderate activity: 13.9 kcal/cm height (35.3 kcal/in) Severe physical restrictions: 11.1 kcal/cm height (28.2 kcal/in)

Adapted from Ekvall SW, Bandini L, Ekvall V: Obesity. In: Evall SW ed.: Pediatric Nutrition in Chronic Diseases and Developmental Disorders. New York. Oxford University Press. 1993. p 168. In: Davis, AM. "Pediatrics" In: Matarese LE, Gottsclich MM (eds), WB Saunders, Contemporary Nutrition Support Practice, Philadelphia, Pa. 1998

ing their daily hydration needs and that all water and electrolytes losses are replaced daily. The patient may require parenteral fluid and electrolyte supplementation at home until their daily fluid requirement is tolerated enterally.

Table 9-8 provides methods of calculating fluid and electrolyte requirements in pediatric patients. The basic assumption underlying the Holliday-Segar Method is that for each 100 calories metabolized, 100 mL of water will be required. This formula was developed to address parenteral fluid needs in children. It can be useful in clinical practice when patients are on combination feedings of parenteral and enteral nutrition to ensure that fluid needs are met and when enteral feedings are concentrated.

Parents or caregivers should be trained to recognize the signs and symptoms of dehydration, such as decreased skin turgor, dry or cracked lips, reduced or absent tears, increased and weak pulse rate, and decreased urine output (<6 wet diapers/day). Oral rehydration solutions (ORS) can be used in place of, or in addition to HEN, in those infants and children with mild to moderate dehydration from diarrheal losses

TABLE 9–8   Daily Fluid and Electrolyte Requirements in Infants and Children

Preterm Infants (post-discharge–1 year):
120–160 mL/kg water[24]   2–3 mEq/kg/day of Na+, K+, Cl-[25]

0–6 months:
RDA: Water: 1.5 mL/kcal[26]
Est. Safe and Adequate Intake: Na+: 120 mg/day K+: 500mg/day

| Holliday-Seger Method:*[28] | | Electrolytes[27] |
Body weight	Water	mEq/100mL H_2O
1–10 kg	100 mL/kg	Na+ 3
11–20 kg	1000 mL + 50mL/kg for each kg >10	Cl- 2
> 20 kg	1500 mL + 20mL/kg for each kg >20	K+ 2

* Used when parenteral fluids are required.
Not suitable for use in neonates <14 days old because it overestimates their fluid needs.

Enterally feedings only: Child's Weight*	Total Fluid Needs in 24 hours
7 lbs.	2 cups (16 fluid ounces)
12 lbs.	3 ½ cups (28 fluid ounces)
21 lbs.	5 cups (40 fluid ounces)
26 lbs.	6 cups (48 fluid ounces)
36 lbs.	7 cups (56 fluid ounces)
44 lbs.	8 cups (64 fluid ounces)
63 lbs.	9 ½ cups (76 fluid ounces)
99 lbs.	10 ½ cups (84 fluid ounces)
119 lbs.	10 ½ cups (84 fluid ounces)

*Adapted from Lucas B ed. Children with Special Health Care Needs — Nutrition Care Handbook. American Dietetic Association, Chicago, Ill. 2004: p 106.

(<10 mL/kg/hr stool losses). We should provide approximately 10 mL/kg (or about 120 mL in older children) of rehydration for each diarrheal stool. As a general rule, pharmacologic agents should not be used in acute diarrheal illnesses. This decision is at the discretion of the treating physician. Probiotic agents are undergoing studies in children and may shorten the course of acute diarrheal illnesses.[27] Table 9–9 provides information on commercially available rehydration solutions that can be given orally or through an enteral feeding tube, either mixed with the feeding or given between feedings. Generally it is not recommended that HEN be stopped during episodes of acute diarrheal illnesses. Patients usually tolerate decreased feedings with ORS added to replace fluids and

TABLE 9–9 Oral Rehydration Solutions

Solution (Manufacturer) Osmolality (mOsm/kg H₂0)	Kcal/mL (kcal/oz)	Carbohydrate (g/L)	Sodium (mEq/L)	Potassium (mEq/L)
Ceralyte-70 (Cera)* 232	0.16 (4.9)	Rice digest 40	70	20
Ceralyte-50 (Cera) 200	0.16 (4.9)	Rice digest, gluc 40	50	20
Ceralyte-90 (Cera) 264	0.16 (4.9)	Rice digest, gluc, 40	90	20
Enfalyte (Mead Johnson)** 200	0.12 (3.7)	Rice syrup solids 30	50	25
Oral Rehydration Solution 330	0.06 (2)	Dextrose 20	90	20
(WHO) (Jaianas) † Pedialyte Unflavored 250	0.1 (3)	Dextrose 25	45	20
(Ross)†† Rehydralyte 305	0.1 (3)	Dextrose 25	75	20
(Ross)				

* Cera Products, Inc. Columbia, MD 21045, (12/3/04). 1–888-Ceralyte.

http://www.ceraproductsinc.com/productline/ceralyte.cfm.

** Pediatric Products Handbook (2004), Mead Johnson & Company, Evansville, Ind., 47721.

† Jaianas Bros. Packaging Co., 2533 SW Boulevard, Kansas City, Mo. 64108.

†† Pediatric Nutritionals Product Guide (2004) Ross Products Division Abbot Laboratories Inc., Columbus, Ohio, 43215.

electrolytes with gradual resumption of regular feeding schedule over the next 24–48 hours.

The benefits of ORS include better absorption of fluid than plain water, replenishment of electrolyte losses, and an additional source of carbohydrate calories (see Table 9–9).[29]

FORMULA SELECTION

Human Milk

Human milk is the "gold standard" of infant feeding and is always the preferred food for neonates and infants.[30] Ideally, term and some preterm infants should be able to nurse and establish lactation before discharge from the hospital. However expressed human milk can also be fed to the baby by tube and is often well tolerated. Protocols exist for collecting, storing, and feeding pumped human milk.[31] Advantages for the use of human milk include:

- Whey predominant protein (more digestible than casein)
- Improved digestion and absorption of fat, zinc, and iron
- Low renal solute load
- Presence of anti-infective factors
- Promotion of maternal–infant attachment
- Possible protection against necrotizing enterocolitis (NEC) and late-onset sepsis
- Neurodevelopmental advantages including advanced cognitive abilities.

Human Milk Fortifier

Preterm infants may often be discharged from the hospital at weights less than 2000 grams. Breastfed preterm infants weighing more than 1500 grams at birth who continue to have suboptimal growth may benefit from fortification of their breast milk. Commercial fortifiers include Ross Similac Human Milk Fortifier by Ross Labs™ and Mead Johnson™ Enfamil Human Milk. They may not be readily available for retail purchase. Both contain 3.5 kcal/pkt, added whey protein, and calcium phosphate. One packet mixed in 25 mL of breast milk brings the nutrient density to 24 kcals/oz. When fortifiers are used after discharge, intake should be monitored to avoid excessive consumption of nutrients as volumes increase beyond 360–400 mL/day.[32,25] Contraindications for the use of human milk include:[25]

- When the mother has an infectious disease, such as HIV or tuberculosis, which can potentially be transmitted to the child via the mother's breast milk,
- When the mother is on a drug or therapy that can be transferred into her breast milk supply, and
- When the infant has a medical contraindication which precludes the use of human breast milk such as galactosemia or inborn errors of metabolism.

Infant Formulas

If human milk is not available or indicated, then iron-fortified infant formula is recommended for the first year of life.[33] Standards for nutrient content of infant formulas have been established by the American Academy of Pediatrics (AAP) and the Infant Formula Act. The AAP recommends that all formulas fed to infants be fortified with iron at 10 to 12 mg/L (>6.7 mg/100kcal) as infant stores of iron become depleted within 4–6 months of birth.[33] Iron deficiency in infants must be avoided. Even when treated, iron deficiency in children is associated with continued developmental and learning disabilities at age ten.[34] In studies comparing iron fortified formulas to low iron formulas, no differences are seen in gastrointestinal tolerance or in behavioral abnormalities.[35] Relative to total calories, pediatric enteral formulas generally have less protein and more calcium, phosphorus, and vitamin D than those made for adults. Additionally, disease states which are more common in the pediatric population, such as inborn errors of metabolism and cystic fibrosis, all have unique nutritional issues which must be considered when designing the nutrition support regimen.[36]

Most commercial formulas contain adequate vitamin and mineral content to maintain long-term plasma and serum vitamin status for normal children.[37] However, because pediatric patients may have specific nutrient losses, due to their disease state and functional gut adaptation, the home care clinician should be familiar with signs and symptoms of micronutrient deficiencies and assess the patient periodically. Serum micronutrient levels should be assessed when deficiencies are suspected. The fluid restricted patient with modular energy components added to their formula to increase calories and protein should be assessed for micronutrient intake and multivitamin and mineral supplementation added as needed. For those patients receiving multimodality nutritional support (PN, EN, oral) special attention should be focused on the contribution of parenteral nutrition and absorbed oral intake, if any, to the nutrition support regimen to ensure adequacy of EN and to prevent excessive or redundant delivery of specific nutrients.[38]

Selection Criteria for Home Enteral Nutrition Pediatric Formula:[12,38,39]

- patient's age:
  - preterm infant formulas (<37 weeks gestational age*)

- ○ infant formulas (0 to 12 months)
- ○ child formulas (1 to 10 years)
- ○ older children (>10 years) adult formulas are used
- medical condition:
  - ○ lactase deficiency/intolerance
  - ○ severe fat malabsorption
  - ○ chylothorax
  - ○ IgE-mediated allergy to cow's milk formula
  - ○ diarrhea
  - ○ preterm/low birth weight (LBW) infants (see Table 9–11)
  - ○ former preterm/LBW infants (see Table 9–11)
  - ○ Inborn errors of metabolism
- organ function:
  - ○ malabsorption due to gastrointestinal disease
  - ○ malabsorption due to hepatobiliary disease
  - ○ renal disease
- gastrointestinal length and function:
  - ○ presence of the ileocecal valve (ICV)
  - ○ presence or length of remaining colon
  - ○ presence or length of remaining small bowel
  - ○ physiologic status of the remaining bowel
- access route and type:
  - ○ diameter of gastrostomy or jejunostomy feeding tube and formula viscosity
- nutrient needs:
  - ○ standard vs nutrient-dense
  - ○ fluid allowance

Standard Formulas

Commercial cow's milk-based formulas meet the nutrient needs of infants when used as the sole source of nutrition for the first six months of life and as the primary source during the second six months of life. When cow's milk formula is not tolerated, soy formulas promote growth and bone mineralization in a manner similar to breast milk and cow's milk formula.[13] In most children older than 12 months who will rely on HEN as their sole or predominant source of nutrition when discharged home, commercial formulas are available that can provide 100% of the RDA for all essential nutrients in an appropriate volume. Children older than ten years can generally tolerate adult enteral products. Children younger than ten years should not receive adult enteral formulas because their excessive amounts of protein and electrolytes and insufficient iron, vitamin D, calcium, zinc, and phosphorus.

Table 9–10 provides guidelines for choosing pediatric formulas, including age ranges and formula characteristics, and examples of commercially available formula options for each category. Docosahexanoic Acid (DHA), an omega-3 fatty acid, and Arachidonic Acid (ARA), an omega-6 fatty acid, are found in human breast milk and were approved by the US Food and Drug Administration in 2001 for addition to infant formulas.[40–43] The amount of DHA and ARA added to formulas are similar to those contained in breast milk. These formulas are designed for infants who are solely formula fed.

DHA and ARA have many key functions in infants including the support of retinal and brain development.[40–43] DHA is a prominent component of the phospholipids in the gray matter of the cortex and brainstem. DHA represents an even higher concentration of the fatty acids comprising the retina of the eye. DHA and ARA are identified as components of the formula ingredients *Crypthecodinium cohnii oil* and *Mortierella alpina oil*, respectively. Conventional formulas without DHA and ARA contain the essential fatty acids linolenic and linoleic acid, precursors to DHA and ARA. Studies are equivocal, however, whether DHA and ARA are superior to adding the essential fatty acids for supporting retinal and brain development. In light of the increased expense of formulas supplemented with DHA and ARA, it is argued that mothers should not be forced to purchase these formulas until their superiority is proven conclusively. DHA and ARA may enhance weight gain in premature formula-fed infants.

Nutrient-dense and Specialized Formulas

Infants and children with conditions that preclude the use of standard pediatric formulas must meet their nutritional needs through other means. Finding the correct formula that will allow full or partial use of the gastrointestinal tract can be a great challenge for the clinician working with these patients. It is not uncommon for many children with gastrointestinal disease to require extended periods of parenteral nutrition. Much trial and error may be necessary until the gastrointestinal tract adapts to enteral feeds and the correct formula is found. This process can

TABLE 9-10   Standard Infant and Child Formulas Suitable for EN

0-12 months	Infant Standard (20 cal/oz)	Tolerates milk based formula May be low iron or iron fortified May contain DHA and ARA Available in Lactose Free Form	Ross Similac Advance (1) Ross Similac Lactose Free Advance Nestle Good Start Essentials (2) Mead Johnson Enfamil Lipil Low Iron (3)
	Infant Soy Protein-Based (20 cal/oz)	When lactose-free formula is needed May be low iron or iron fortified May contain DHA an ARA Used in Galactosemia, IgE mediated cow's milk allergy, vegetarians. Contraindicated when birth weight >1800 g	Ross Similac Isomil Advance Mead Johnson Prosobee Lipil
9-24 months	Toddler Standard (20 cal/oz)	Iron fortified DHA and ARA Contains higher amounts of calcium and phosphate for older babies Available in milk and soy based	Ross Similac Advance Mead Johnson Enfamil Next Step Prosobee Lipil
1-10 years	Child Standard (30 cal/oz)	Tolerates milk-based formula Complete or supplemental With or without fiber May contain whey-protein for ease in gastric emptying	Ross Pediasure (4) Ross Pediasure with Fiber Nestle Nutren Junior (5)
	Blenderized (30 cal/oz)	Tolerates traditional foods including meat, fruit, and vegetables Contains fiber Designed for chronic long-term tube feeders	Novartis Compleat Pediatric (6)

(1) *Pediatric Nutritionals Product Guide* (2004) Ross Products Division Abbot Laboratories Inc., Columbus, Ohio. 43215.

(2) *The Baylor Pediatric Nutrition Handbook for Residents* (2003), Nestle Nutrition Institute.

(3) *Pediatric Products Handbook* (2004), Mead Johnson & Company, Evansville, Ind. 47721.

(4) *Medical Nutritional Products* (2004), Ross Products Division Abbot Laboratories Inc., Columbus, Ohio. 43215.

(5) *2004 Product Guide* (2004), Nestle Nutrition, Glendale, Calif. 91203

(6) *Novartis Nutrition Product Guide* (2004), Novartis Medical Nutrition, Minneapolis, Minn. 55440.

be quite lengthy and the clinician must decide whether the patient is sufficiently stable to be discharged home during this transition.

Table 9–11 describes nutrient-dense and special formulas that have been developed to meet the needs of infants and children who will not tolerate standard formulas.

Breast milk of mothers who deliver preterm is higher in protein and electrolytes and is more suited to the preterm infant's needs than term infants' mother's breast milk. Formulas for premature infants are specially made to simulate preterm human milk. Preterm formulas promote growth and bone mineralization at an intrauterine rate.[33] After hospital discharge, continued use of preterm formulas up to the age of 9 months is recommended by the AAP for preterm infants due to studies which show that their extended use results in greater growth and bone mineralization[13] and improved developmental outcomes up to the age of eight years.[44,45] In small preterm infants, preterm human milk will not be adequate to provide sufficient nutrition and commercial human milk fortifiers must be used (see Table 9–14). Studies show that multinutrient fortification of preterm human milk improves growth in preterm infants.[13] Infants with intact protein allergy can usually tolerate casein hydrolysate formulas.[46] Infants who are highly allergic to intact protein or even protein hydrolysates show symptom resolution and normal growth on amino acid elemental formulas.[47] Tube fed infants who are fluid sensitive may be fed with concentrated feedings. Commercial feedings for premature infants are available in 22 and 24 kcal per fluid ounce. Concentrated fluid formulas and powders are available so that formulas can be concentrated to between 24 and 30 cal/fluid oz. The ability of the infant to tolerate increased renal solute load and osmolality must be taken into consideration. Some infants may require calorie supplements added to their formula, rather than concentration of the formula, to avoid overfeeding of protein and electrolytes.[13]

TABLE 9–11   Nutrient-Dense and Specialized Formulas

Age	Type	Indication	Formula
<37 weeks gestation until specified weight	Premature 20 or 24 cal/oz	Rapidly growing premature infants Available in 20 and 24 cal/oz caloric densities Contain DHA and ARA Available in low iron or iron fortified Protein source whey-predominate Higher percentage protein, calcium, electrolytes, phosphorous, magnesium, and vitamin D than term or transition formulas	Mead Johnson Enfamil Premature with Iron (For use in infants up to 5.5 pounds) Ross Similac Special Care Advance with Iron (For use in infants up to 8 pounds)
>5.5 lbs up to 9 months	Nutrient Dense 22 cal/oz	Transition formula from premature to term-infant formula Contains lower levels of protein, minerals, and vitamins than premature formulas and higher level than term formula Contains DHA, ARA and iron	Ross Similac Neosure Advance Mead Johnson Enfamil Enfacare Lipil
0–12 months	Protein Hydrolysate	Milk-protein allergy Gastrointestinal disturbances May contain MCT oil, DHA, and ARA	Ross Similac Alimentum Advance Mead Johnson Enfamil Nutramigen Lipil Mead Johnson Enfamil Pregestimil
	Amino-Acid Based	Milk-protein allergy Gastrointestinal disturbances Sucrose, Lactose, and Galactose free	SHS Neocate

Age	Type	Indication	Formula
	Renal	Renal dysfunction Hypocalcemia 2nd hyperphosphatemia Low iron	Ross Similac PM 60/40
	Antidiarrheal	Short-term feeding for nutritional management of diarrhea in infants >6 months Contains soy fiber Lactose free Dual carbohydrate absorption	Ross Similac Isomil DF
	Carbohydrate Intolerance	Need for limitation in amount or type of carbohydrates (i.e., disaccharidase deficiency, or impaired glucose transport) May be indicated in treatment of diarrhea Not nutritionally complete: requires addition of carbohydrate in type and tolerated amount.	Ross Carbohydrate Free (RCF)
1–10 years	Malabsorptive Disorders/High MCT	Defects in intraluminal hydrolysis of fat, mucosal fat absorption, and lymphatic transport of fat.	Mead Johnson Portagen*

Age	Type	Indication	Formula
	Malabsorptive Disorders/ Peptide based	Impaired GI function Early enteral feeding transition from TPN Lactose and gluten free Low residue May contain fiber May contain partially hydrolyzed whey	Novartis Pediatric Peptinex DT Nestle Peptamen Junior
	Malabsorptive Disorders/ Amino-Acid Based	Milk-protein allergy Gastrointestinal disturbances Fructose, galactose, and gluten free	Ross Elecare Novartis Vivonex Pediatric

Pediatric Nutritionals Product Guide (2004), Ross Products Division, Abbot Laboratories Inc., Columbus, Ohio. 43215.
Pediatric Products Handbook (2004), Mead Johnson & Company, Evansville, Ind. 47721.
Neocate, SHS North America, Gaithersburg, Md. 20884.
Novartis Nutrition Product Guide (2004), Novartis Medical Nutrition, Minneapolis, Minn. 55440.
2004 Product Guide (2004), Nestle Nutrition, Glendale, Calif. 91203.

Concentrating Infant and Enteral Formulas

Many infants and children who receive HEN cannot meet their needs for growth and development with standard formulas and may benefit from concentrating the nutrient density of their feedings. The necessity for increased calories is the most common reason for concentrating a formula. It is important, however, to maintain an optimal range of macronutrient distribution to avoid deficiencies. It is, therefore, preferable to add less water to a commercially-prepared concentrated (40 kcal/ounce) or powdered formula than it is to add modular components. Concentration can be achieved this way up to caloric densities of 24 calories per ounce. When concentration rises above this amount modular fat and carbohydrate modules should be used to avoid excessive protein which is the major contributor of excess renal solute load. Once caloric density has reached 30 calories per ounce, however, the amount of calories provided as protein can drop to as little as 7% and adequacy will then need to be reassessed.[53] Formulas made for adults should never be used in infants and young children.

Commonly encountered reasons for using concentrated formulas in HEN patients include:

- Maintenance of a fluid restriction with or without increased energy needs
- Inability to tolerate sufficient volume of tube feeding formula with or without increased energy needs
- Increased energy expenditure
- Malabsorption of carbohydrate or fat
- Earlier transition from gavage feedings to nipple feedings.[25]

Modular components are not nutritionally complete and should only be added when additional calories or protein are needed but other nutrient requirements are met.[25] Caloric density should be advanced by 2–4 calories per ounce every 12–24 hours. The rates of infusion and concentration should not be advanced simultaneously.[48] Intolerance to an increase in concentration requires a return to the previously tolerated concentration. The final concentration of protein, fat, and carbohydrate should remain within recommended ranges. When the patient has progressed to enteral and oral intake alone, micronutrient intake should be assessed when modular components are added to increase caloric density in order to ensure that extra supplementation is not needed. Calculating micronutrient intake from both enteral and oral nutrition and comparing it to the Recommended Dietary Allowances will assist the clinician in deciding whether or not micronutrient supplements are indicated. Oral micronutrient supplements can be used in either liquid or chewable form. Liquid forms of micronutrients are preferable when they must be flushed through a feeding tube in order to avoid both mechanical destruction and tube clogs.

If a child presents with preexisting malnutrition, then refeeding syndrome can occur, which is described as a constellation of fluid and electrolyte disturbances, especially hypophosphatemia that occur as a result of reinstitution of nutrition to patients who are starved or severely malnourished[49] at a rate that exceeds the patients ability to metabolize the nutrients provided. When weight loss exceeds 20% of usual weight the risk of refeeding syndrome is elevated and initiating and advancing the feeding in the hospital may be the most prudent course. The feeding must be advanced more slowly than otherwise would be attempted. Monitor electrolytes, weight, and fluid status closely so that serious and life-threatening electrolyte and fluid imbalances can be avoided.

Children receiving feedings supplemented with high amounts of protein and inadequate fluid intake may develop "tube feeding syndrome" which is characterized by dehydration, azotemia, and hypernatremia. Decreasing the protein content and increasing the fluid is the required intervention.[50]

Whenever a formula is concentrated or a supplement is added the formula osmolarity is increased. The patient receives less volume of water per calorie of EN delivered. Caution should be used to avoid metabolic and gastrointestinal complications.

OSMOLARITY

Osmolarity is affected most by the carbohydrate and mineral content of the formula. Upper limits of 277 mOsm/L and 30–35 mOsm/100 kcal have been proposed for infant formulas.[51] Some infants and children may have difficulty tolerating hyperosmolar feedings. Generally, the osmolarity of a formula will increase by approximately the same percentage as the caloric increase.[52] Despite increasing osmolarity per volume of EN delivered to the child with an increase in caloric density, most infants will tolerate gradual changes.

It is essential to ensure that the caregiver has a thorough understanding of formula mixing and preparation and that the appropriate measuring devices are in the home. Use of commercially concentrated formulas in recipes takes precedence over powdered formulas when possible because they are easier to mix and are less prone to measurement errors.

POTENTIAL RENAL SOLUTE LOAD

Potential renal solute load (PRSL) refers to the solutes that must be excreted in the urine if not used for synthesis, storage, or lost through other nonrenal routes.[51] One of the major components of PRSL is protein. If children are allowed too little fluid and significant amounts of extra protein, then more water may be excreted with the protein than they can afford to lose.[53] The PRSL is expressed as mOsm/L or mOsm/100 kcal. Due to the difference in protein content between human milk (10g/L) and cow's milk (32.9g/L), the PRSL of human milk is 36 mOsm/L (13 mOsm/100 kcal) whereas cow's milk contains 120 mOsm/L (46 mOsm/100 kcal). Infant formulas contain approximately 48–67 mOsm/L (18–25 mOsm/100 kcal).[48]

Knowledge of PRSL is important when:

- Fluid intake is low or losses are high.
- Growth is suboptimal.
- Highly concentrated formulas are ingested.
- Renal concentrating ability is limited.

The PRSL can be calculated by use of the following formula:

PRSL (mOsm/L) = [Protein(g/L) ÷ 0.175] + [Na(mEq/L) + K(mEq/L) + Cl(mEq/L)] + [Pa*(mg/L ÷ 31]

Pa = Available phosphorus; that is, the total phosphorus of human milk and milk-based formulas, and two-thirds phosphorus of soy-based formulas.[51]

Premature infants appear to be able to concentrate urine up to 700 mOsm/L and full-term infants older than 2 months of age have a concentrating ability of up to 1200 mOsm/liter.[54] Concentrated infant formula preparation guidelines are provided in Table 9–12.

TABLE 9–12   Preparation of Infant Formulas for Standard and Soy Formulas*

Formula Type	Caloric Concentration (kcal/oz)	Amount of Formula	Water (oz)	Final Volume
Liquid concentrate	10 (0.34 kcal/mL)	13 oz	39	52 oz
	15 (0.50 kcal/mL)	13 oz	22	35 oz
	20 (0.67 kcal/mL)	13 oz	13	26 oz
(40 kcal/oz)	24 (0.80 kcal/mL)	13 oz	8.5	21.5 oz
	26 (0.87 kcal/mL)	13 oz	7	21 oz
	27 (0.90 kcal/mL)	13 oz	6	19 oz
	28 (0.93 kcal/mL)	13 oz	5.5	18.5 oz
	30 (1.00 kcal/mL)	13 oz	4	17 oz
Small volume preparation	10	1 scoop**	4	4.5 oz
of powder	15	2 scoop	5.5	6.0 oz
(44 kcal/scoop)	20	4 scoop	8	9.0 oz
	24	3 scoops	4.5	5.5 oz
	27	5 scoops	7	8.0 oz
	28	7 scoops	10	11.5 oz
	30	6 scoops	7.5	9.0 oz

*Does not apply to Enfacare, Neocate, Neosure, Elecare. Enfamil AR should not be concentrated greater than 24 kcal/oz. Use a packed measure for Similac PM 60/40, Lactofree, Similac Lactose Free, Portagen, Nutramigen, and Pregestimil.

**Check the can to determine the number of grams in each scoop and the number of scoops per can. This will indicate the patient "usage" or the number of cans that will be needed in any given time period. It is best to send a small amount (a week's worth perhaps) when a new formula is being tried so that excess formula is not wasted in case it must be changed. Once formula is shipped it cannot, by law, be returned to the provider. As soon as tolerance is established larger amounts can be sent that will last a longer time.

Adapted from Cox J, Chaffin-Jordan L. "Nutrition and Growth" In: The Harriet Lane Handbook 16th ed, Nutritional Care for High-Risk Newborns. Gunn VL, Nechyba C. (eds). Mosby, Philadelphia, 2002:p.466. and Kuzma-O'Reilly B. "Preparing Formulas with Various Caloric Densities". In: Groh-Wargo S, Thompson M, Cox J, eds. 2000. Precept Press, Inc., Chicago, Ill. p. 652

MODULAR COMPONENTS

The infant or child's clinical condition will determine which modular component is added. Table 9–13 provides guidelines for the use of energy-increasing modular components in particular situations.

Concentration of a base infant formula, by adding less water or more concentrate, is generally recommended up to 24 to 26 calories per ounce. Higher caloric densities require consideration of modular component addition, including formula concentrations of 1 cal/mL (30 calories per ounce) that do not have ready-to-feed formula equivalents or require nutrient additions that can not be met by any ready-to-feed product. Ta-

TABLE 9–13   Indications for Calorie Enhancement by Commonly Used Modulars

Carbohydrate	Long Chain Fats	Medium Chain Triglycerides
Congenital heart disease	Carbohydrate malabsorption	Chylothorax
Delayed gastric emptying	Diarrhea	Fat malabsorption
Failure to Thrive	Hypermetabolic states	Prematurity
Gastroesophageal reflux		Thoracic Duct Trauma
Hypermetabolic states		

Adapted and reproduced with permission from Davis A, Baker S. The use of modular nutrients in pediatrics. *JPEN* 1996;20:228–236.

ble 9–14 provides product information on the most commonly used modular components.

MICRONUTRIENTS

Adding carbohydrate or fat products to a pediatric formula will dilute the ratio of vitamins and minerals per calorie when the formula is concentrated above 24 kcal/oz.[53] Restricted volume itself may result in inadequate vitamin and mineral nutrition. An infant at 6 months of age with a fluid restriction of only 15 ounces of formula per day because of congenital heart disease will receive only about half the volume required to provide the RDA for vitamins and minerals. Concentrating the formula may increase this to 70% but still does not reach 100% of the RDA.[53] In addition, the infant with special health care needs may require selected micronutrients exceeding the RDA hence, supplemental vitamins and minerals may be indicated. Because liquid children's multivitamins do not contain minerals and folic acid it may be preferable to crush a pediatric chewable "complete" vitamin/mineral supplement. One to one-half tablet can be used, as indicated by the amounts provided in the infant's formula. Clinicians should check the content of the multivitamins for calcium, phosphorus, potassium, and magnesium and should provide added supplementation when needed by using liquid or chewable forms.[53]

Adding modular components to infant formulas to increase nutrient density above 26 calories per ounce avoids changing the total amount of daily fluid provided and is a common practice. However, this may compromise the nutrient integrity of the formula by increasing its osmolality and diluting the mineral and micronutrient content. These infants may benefit from use of a 30 kcal/oz ready-to-feed pediatric formula. Puangco[55] showed that fluid-restricted premature infants, at approximately 2–6 months of age, tolerated a 1 cal/mL (30 calories per ounce) of standard ready-to-feed pediatric formula well and grew better than infants fed an equal amount of calories from infant formula fortified with modular components. This option would also benefit caregivers at home in terms of cost, hygiene, and convenience. Of course, when choosing this option, consideration must be given to the total amount of protein and micronutrients provided in relation to the infant's medical condition so that safe limits are not exceeded.

TABLE 9–14 Common Modular Components

Type	Indication	Formula/Nutrient Content Dose	Na mg/Tbs	K mg/Tbs	Cl mg/Tbs	P mg/Tbs
Protein	Increased protein needs	Ross Promod ® 17 kcal/Tbs., 3g protein/Tbs.	15	27	13	21
	Inadequate protein intake	Mead Johnson Casec® 17 kcal/Tbs., 4g protein/Tbs.	<5	<2		35
Carbohydrate (CHO)	Supplemental calories Rapidly absorbed	Ross Polycose® 23 kcal/Tbs.	7	0.6	13	0.7
	Longer glucose polymers to minimize potential for osmotic diarrhea	Mead Johnson Moducal® 30 kcal/Tbs.				
Polyunsaturated Fat	Increased caloric requirements	Mead Johnson Microlipid® 4.5 kcal/mL, 68 kcal/Tbs.				
	Decreased carbohydrate tolerance	Vegetable oil[55] 8.3 kcal/mL, 120 kcal/Tbs.				
	Volume restriction					
CHO/Fat	Cornstarch, corn and coconut oil, MCT	SHS Duocal® 42 kcal/Tbs.	<20	<5	<20	<5
	Completely soluble in water					
	For use in protein and electrolyte restrictions					
	Does not alter taste					

Type	Indication	Formula/Nutrient Content Dose	Na mg/Tbs	K mg/Tbs	Cl mg/Tbs	P mg/Tbs
Medium Chain Triglyceride	Defect in intraluminal hydrolysis, mucosal absorption, or lymphatic transport of fat. Does not contain essential fatty acids Absorbed via the portal system Affects osmolarity	Mead Johnson MCT Oil® 115 kcal/Tbs.; 14 g fat/Tbs. 7.7 kcal/mL				
Human Milk Fortifier	Premature, low birth weight infants Milk-based powder used to increase protein, energy, calcium, phosphorus, and other nutrients in human milk (25)	Mead Johnson: Enfamil Human Milk Fortifier® to increase formula by 2 calories/oz: Add 1 packet to each 50mLs Formula to increase formula by 4 calories/oz: Add 1 packet to each 25mLs formula.				

Type	Indication	Formula/Nutrient Content Dose	Na mg/ Tbs	K mg/ Tbs	Cl mg/ Tbs	P mg/ Tbs
Fiber	Constipation, irritable bowel, short bowel syndrome (trophic effect) Requires adequate hydration	Novartis Resource Benefiber® 3 g soluble fiber/ Tbs. Pediatric dose by weight: 0.66 to 1.0 g/kg, up to 45 g/day[20] Pediatric dose by age and sex:[56] 1–3 yrs: 19 g/day 4–8 yrs: 25 g/day girls, 9–13 yrs: 26 g/day boys, 9–13 yrs: 31 g/day girls, 14–18 yrs: 36 g/day boys, 14–19 yrs: 38 g/day.	15	15		
Glutamine	Preferred fuel source for rapidly dividing enterocytes Improves nitrogen balance, reduces gut atrophy, and promotes healing. Contraindicated in liver disease and head injury; caution in CRF. Available in packets containing probiotics.[54]	Corpak GlutaPak-10® 40 kcal/pkt 10 g glu/pkt Corpak Glutapak R® (Lactobacillus Reuteri) 40 kcal/pkt 10 g glu/pkt Dose by weight: 0.285–0.57 g/kg/d (divided into 3 even doses) Standard pediatric dose: 15g per day or 5g TID[54]				

Type	Indication	Formula/Nutrient Content Dose	Na mg/Tbs	K mg/Tbs	Cl mg/Tbs	P mg/Tbs
Probiotics	Probiotic agent: Lactobacillus GG Maintains healthy intestinal flora Helps support natural resistance to infection	Con Agra Culturelle® Adolescent Dose: While on antibiotics + 7 days: 2 capsules BID Maintenance: 1 capsule/day Infants and Children: ½–1 capsule/day (open capsule and mix into water or formula)				

Medical Nutritional/Products (2004), Ross Products Division Abbot Laboratories Inc., Columbus, Ohio, 43215.

Medical Nutritionals Pocket Guide (2003), Mead Johnson & Company, Evansville, Ind., 47721.

Novartis Nutrition Product Guide (2004), Novartis Medical Nutrition, Minneapolis, Minn., 55440.

Pediatric Products Handbook (2004), Mead Johnson & Company, Evansville, Ind., 47721.

SHS Product Guide, P.O. Box 117, Gaithersburg, Md., 1-800-636-2283 (for recipes and information)

GlutaPak 10, Corpak Medsystems, Wheeling, Ill., 60090.

Culturelle Product Information, Dec 2004, Con Agra Functional Foods, Inc., Omaha, Nebr., 1-888-828-4242.

ROUTE AND METHOD OF ADMINISTRATION

Patients receive HEN through a tube or a stoma that delivers nutrients distal to the oral cavity.[56] The method of feeding chosen (see Table 9–15) must take into account the patient's gastrointestinal tolerance to the selected method, whether the patient is ambulatory or nonambulatory, convenience for the caregiver, and ease of mobility and travel. The least possible intrusion into the normal home life of the patient and caregivers should be chosen. Continuous feedings may be best tolerated at first, especially when the infant or child is weaning from parenteral nutrition, but progression to bolus feedings, combination feedings, and weaning to oral feedings, whenever possible, should be the ultimate goal. Every effort should be made to accommodate the emotional and practical needs of the family while still providing adequate nutrition support for normal growth and development. Regular sleep patterns, eating patterns, and daily routines, such as school and after-school activities, should be interrupted to the least extent possible. The home care team can often provide resources and suggestions that will make transition to home as accommodating to the family's needs as possible. Table 9–15 reviews methods of feeding pediatric patients by enteral tube.

Studies in preterm infants have shown that both continuous and bolus feeding methods result in similar outcomes of growth, micronutrient retention, length of hospitalization, and days to reach full feedings. In practice, however, continuous feedings may be better tolerated in infants with malabsorption.[13]

ADVANCING THE FEEDING

Enteral feedings must be introduced gradually. Infants and children who have not been fed in more than 24 hours, or with evidence of gastroesophageal reflux and malabsorption, may experience intolerance when feedings are advanced rapidly. Generally, it is advised that premature and full term infants and children with these conditions receive continuous feedings at a slow rate gradually working toward bolus intermittent, or oral feedings as tolerance allows.[8,11] Clinical judgment must be used during the transition process taking into account the age of the patient and condition and length of the small bowel. Generally, the feeding can be decreased from 24 hours per day by 2 hours each day as tolerance al-

TABLE 9–15   Methods of feeding pediatric patients by tube[56]

Method:	Characteristics:	Technique:
Bolus	An intermittent-type feed Most physiologic Most practical for HEN No need for feeding pump	Confirm tube placement in stomach Syringe or gravity drip administration over 15–20 minutes with syringe; up to 1 hr. with gravity-drip feeding bag on IV Pole
Intermittent	Feeding pump assisted Useful when slower infusion is desirable for reflux, decreased gastric motility	Administered over 2–4 hours into the stomach divided by periods of rest
Continuous	Small intestinal feedings Pump required Desirable for delayed gastric emptying decreased absorption, brittle diabetes, poor digestion, volume sensitivity	Slower infusion and longer time
Cyclic	Useful for nocturnal, continuous feedings pump May supplement daytime bolus or oral feedings.	Compression of formula into discreet time intervals.
Combination	May ensure optimal nutrition, Optimal advancement of feedings during pump bowel adaptation, and attention to lifestyle needs.	

lows. The rate is then increased for the remaining hours such that the total volume remains constant. Once nocturnal feedings are achieved, the number of hours can be gradually decreased and the remaining formula provided as a bolus, intermittent, or oral feedings spaced evenly during the day.

Standard preterm and infant formulas are isotonic and usually need not be diluted when initiating feeds.[57] Infants and children starting on tube feedings may be started at full strength formula given at low volumes. Children should be fed with head elevated 30–45 degrees during feeding and for 1 hour after to limit risk of aspiration.[58] The feeding rate may be advanced as suggested in Table 9–16 until the nutrition goal is met. Volume may be increased every 4–12 hours if the previous rate is well tolerated as defined by the absence of diarrhea, abdominal distention, vomiting, or gagging. If intolerance occurs, then return to the previously tolerated rate and allow more time for the child to adjust.[58]

When a hypertonic formula must be used, it should be initiated at one-half or one-fourth of the final concentration.[11] The concentration can be advanced thereafter, as tolerance allows, by one-half or one-fourth strength every 8–24 hours.[57] For patients not on parenteral nutrition or IV fluids, advance volume then increase concentration. Advancing both volume and concentration on the same day may provoke abdominal pain and diarrhea.[11]

Instructions on safe methods of HEN administration must be provided to the caregiver prior to initiation of feedings. Table 9–17 provides manufacturer guidelines for maximum tube feeding hang times. The hang time tells the caregiver the length of time the formula remains safe from bacterial contamination which can cause diarrhea and dehydration from enteric infection. In 2002 the Food and Drug Administration issued statements, based on findings of the Centers for Disease Control, pointing out the risk of bacterial contamination inherent in nonsterile powdered formulas. Later that year the FDA stated that the use of boiling water to reconstitute these formulas could destroy certain nutrients, could change the physical characteristics of the formula, might not kill the bacteria, and could result in injury during preparation.[59] Clinicians should ensure that caregivers are thoroughly familiar with the procedures which will maintain the safety of non-sterile, powdered formulas.

TRANSITIONAL FEEDINGS

The process of transitioning the pediatric patient can vary widely depending on the age and medical condition of the patient and the initial indications for enteral feedings.[11]

Often times the pediatric patient is discharged on home parenteral nutrition (HPN). During the subsequent weeks or months the infant or child can successfully make the transition from HPN to HEN once gut function improves and enteral access is in place. Recommendations for transitioning from HPN to HEN are listed in Table 9–18.

Once continuous feedings are well tolerated at the final goal rate, consideration can be given to changing the feeding schedule to best suit the

TABLE 9-16   General Guidelines for Advancement of Pediatric Enteral Feedings

Age	Initial Infusion	Advances	Goal
Continuous Feedings			
Preterm*	1-2 mL/kg/hr	10-20 mL/kg/d	120-175mL/kg/d
0-12 months	1-2 mL/kg/hr	1-2 mL/kg q 2-8 hr	6 mL/kg/hr
1-5 yr	1 mL/kg/hr	1 mL/kg q 2-8 hr	4-5 mL/kg/hr
>6yr	25 mL/hr	25 mL/hr q 2-8 hr	100-150 mL/hr
Bolus/Intermittent Feedings			
Preterm (>1200 g)	2-4 mL/kg/feed	2-4 mL/feed	120-175 mL/kg/d
0-12 months	10-60 mL/2-3 hr	10-60 mL/feed	90-180 mL/4-5 hr
1-6 yr	30-90 mL/2-3 hr	30-90 mL/feed	150-300 mL/4-5 hr
>6 yr	60-120 mL/2-3 hr	60-90 mL/feed	240-480 mL/4-5 hr
Cyclic Feedings			
0-12 months	1-2 mL/kg/hr	1-2 mL/kg/2 hr	60-90 mL/hr 12-18 hr/d
1-6 yr	1 mL/kg/hr	1 mL/kg/hr/2 hr	75-125 mL/hr 8-16 hr/d
>6 yr	25 mL/hr	25 mL/hr/2 hr	100-175 mL/hr 8-16 hr/d

Product information suggests that premature infant formula be diluted at first and increased gradually over 3-8 days. Hypertonic feedings should not be given to premature infants.[60]

Adapted from Davis A. "Pediatrics". In: Contemporary Nutrition Support Practice: A Clinical Guide. Gottsclich, M M., Matarese, L E., eds. W.B. Saunders Company, Philadelphia, Pa. 1998: 347-364.

Corrales KM, Bechard LJ, Kane KA, Kelleher DK. "Enteral Nutrition." In: Manual of Pediatric Nutrition, 3rd Edition. Hendrick KM, Duggan C, Walker WA, eds. Hamilton, Ontario, 2000:186-241.

TABLE 9–17 Tube Feeding Hang Time Recommendations for Infants Maximum Hang Time (HT) at Room Temperature (hours)

Feeding Type	Infants who are not immunocompromised	Immunocompromised infants
Feedings prepared from powder	4	Powdered formulas are not recommended due to their compromised sterility once opened. Cannot be reconstituted with boiling water due to adverse effects on nutrients.* If no other alternative, HT should **not** exceed 2 hours.
Feedings prepared from liquid concentrates.	4	4
Feedings of Ready-to-Use liquid formulas	8	4
Feedings prepared from Concentrated Liquid or Ready-to-Use Liquid with Powder added.	4	2
Expressed Breast Milk with Enfamil Human Milk Fortifier© powder added.	4	4

needs of the child and the family environment. General guidelines for transitioning to bolus feedings include:[61]

- Patients may be gradually transitioned to nocturnal continuous feedings over 8 to 10 hours by decreasing the feeding time 2–4 hours each day with the remaining amount of feeding given as a combination of oral and/or bolus feedings during normal daytime eating times.
- Bolus feedings can be started at 1–2 times the hourly rate and gradually increased to the age-appropriate goal (see Table 9–16).
- Stop nocturnal feedings 2–3 hours before a bolus feeding to promote appetite.
- If tolerance to bolus feeds continues to improve they can gradually be increased while nocturnal feeds are decreased until no longer

TABLE 9–18   Recommendations for Transition from Parenteral to Enteral Nutrition

- Match PN caloric density with HEN caloric density when feasible so that fluid needs are met, and not exceeded, during the transition.
- When the initial HEN rate is tolerated, the PN rate can be decreased by approximately the same amount. Incremental increases in HEN rate should be accompanied by the same, or similar, decrease in PN rate. Changes in rate can be made on a daily basis as tolerance allows until the EN goal is reached and PN is discontinued. (see Table 9-16: Advancing Enteral Feedings in the Pediatric Patient)
- Once PN is discontinued the caloric density of the HEN formula can be increased as needed so that fluid allowance is not exceeded. Calorie requirements of enterally fed patients are generally >10% higher than parenterally fed patients and should therefore be adjusted to meet the RDA.
- In infants who do not tolerate the concentration or rate of HEN sufficiently to meet their caloric needs, parenteral lipids may be continued until the goal for HEN is met.
- Patients with chronic gastrointestinal disease may require slower transitions, special enteral formulas, and closer monitoring to ensure that fluid and nutrient intake remains adequate.

Adapted from Corrales KM, Bechard LJ, Kane KA, Kelleher DK. Enteral Nutrition. In: Hendrick KM, Duggan C, Walker WA, eds. Manual of Pediatric Nutrition, 3rd Edition. Hamilton,Ontario, 2000:186–241.

necessary. The goal is to mimic the eating of 3 meals and 2–3 snacks during the day as bolus feedings, or a combination of oral and bolus feedings. (Be patient. This process may take months.)

- Bolus feedings may need to be administered by gravity drip or by pump over ½–1 hour in those children with delayed gastric emptying.
- The total volume of feedings over 24 hours should be constant to meet calorie needs. Whatever volume is not consumed or infused during the day should be given during the night as a nocturnal infusion.

Until the child is stabilized on the final tube feeding regimen, frequent clinical assessments are necessary to ensure that both the child and family are adjusted to the feeding regimen. Once the formula is tolerated, there are no complications, and growth is appropriate, children will need regular, but less frequent, monitoring of tolerance and weight checks.

Growth monitoring can be checked as follows:[50]

- Infants need weight/growth checks and monitoring every 2–4 weeks.
- Toddlers, when stable, may have weight checks every 1–2 months.
- Older children can be evaluated every 3–4 months.

More frequent monitoring will be necessary if the child is, or becomes, unstable due to the disease process or an acute illness. It is wise for the home care clinician to maintain monthly contact with the family to ensure that all is going well.

Transitioning from tube feeding to oral eating is not a single event but a process that may take weeks, months, or years and is one that must be tailored to the individual child.[61] Psychomotor development may be impaired in children who have been maintained on tube feedings or PN for long periods.[62] When oral feedings are not possible at any point during the first year of life, the infant should have continuous oral stimulation, such as non-nutritive sucking (sucking on a nonfeeding nipple or finger), to prevent food aversions and developmental delay in feeding skills. In older children, periods of fasting may be necessary to elicit hunger as the amount of oral feedings is increased. Home enteral nutrition feedings following any oral intake or nighttime HEN supplementation may aid in the weaning process.[11] Oral meals and snacks can be offered before or during bolus feedings to facilitate the perception of eating by mouth and the alleviation of hunger. Bolus feedings must be scheduled at regular family meal times and the child should be with the family.[61]

During the transition to oral feedings a reduction in total calories by 25% is often needed to stimulate hunger. It is important for the child to be well nourished and be able to withstand a period of slow or no weight gain and possibly some weight loss. As oral intake increases, calories provided by tube feeding are incrementally reduced. When oral intake reaches 75% of daily needs for a sustained period of time such as one week, tube feedings can be withheld. It is recommended that the gastrostomy tube remain in place for a minimum of 3 months of non-use or through at least one acute illness before removal. The tube may also be kept in place for gastric decompression or for the administration of unpleasant medications or hydration.[61]

Some families eventually transition their child to homemade blended foods (HBF), or a mixture of commercial formula and HBF. Home blended foods may allow greater dietary diversity and increased fiber depending on the recipe used. With HBF, families report improved bowel function. Children are more willing to try a food by mouth that they have been given through the tube first. Tube sizes 14 French or greater seem to support the HBF best. It is easiest to start with jarred baby vegetables, fruits, or juice. Begin with a tablespoon of a single baby food mixed with the commercial formula. Adding an ounce of pureed foods to the bolus will not increase the volume but will increase the thickness. Add one new food at a time every 4–7 days. When individual foods are clearly tolerated they can be combined. When HBF is prepared in large batches, it is best to freeze each food separately. If there is a family history of food allergies, it is best to wait until after age 3 to introduce fish, shellfish, and peanuts. Honey should be avoided in all children younger than one year of age due to the risk of infant botulism. Introduce only 1–2 new foods per week to avoid GI upset. Gradually move toward the typical foods used by the family ensuring adequate nutrients and fluids are provided. Include food from all food groups to provide balanced nutrition.[63] For recipes and great suggestions read E. Duperret and associates' "Homemade Blenderized Tube Feedings."[63]

FEEDING DEVICES FOR USE IN THE HOME

The clinician transitioning the patient home should review the details of the enteral access device ordered as well as ensure the patient receives the appropriate supplies. The caregiver must understand the proper operation, care, and maintenance of the device. The choice of access device depends upon the estimated length of therapy, diagnosis, function of the gastrointestinal tract, risk of aspiration, need for abdominal surgery, pertinent social and family dynamics, and potential complications.[8] The experienced clinician must use clinical judgment in selecting the most appropriate route of administration of the feeding as guidelines can sometimes be conflicting. There are studies that suggest that the risk of aspiration may actually be increased with jejunal feedings because of increased gastric secretions. Some authors suggest that a fundoplication to prevent reflux and aspiration is more appropriate than jejunal feeds for individuals at high risk for aspiration.[64] This remains an area of discussion and controversy. Table 9–19 reviews guidelines for the selection of enteral access devices for use in pediatric patients.

TABLE 9–19 Pediatric Enteral Access Devices

Route:	Indications:	Advantages:	Disadvantages:
Orogastric	Used mostly in preemies (obligatory nose-breathers) Short-term use	Easily inserted Easy for residual checks.	Malposition Aspiration Discomfort
Nasogastric	Short-term (4–6 wks) or intermittent (nocturnal) use. Indicated only for children at low risk of aspiration.	Easily inserted Pt/family can insert Avoids surgery or endoscopy	Potential aspiration Nasal necrosis, sinusitus Otitis media, Esophagitis over long time with large-bore tubes
Nasoduodenal/ Nasojejunal/ Transgastrojejunal (TGJ)	For children at high risk of aspiration Best used for: gastroparesis, delayed gastric emptying, severe reflux. TGJ can be left in for long periods.	Decrease aspiration risk Surgery or endoscopy not required for ND, NJ, or GT conversion to a TGJ Can initiate early post-op feeds.	Placement may be difficult No bolus feeding. Potential for intestinal perforation Dumping syndrome or diarrhea possible Cosmetic issues

Route:	Indications:	Advantages:	Disadvantages:
Gastrostomy	Long-term GT-surgical PEG-endoscopic PEG - radiologic Low-profile GT ("button") inserted after GT site is fully healed. Sizes: 12–18 Fr.	Less likely to clog than JT due to larger diameter. Easy access to gut. Can check residuals. Can decompress stomach. Can bolus feed. Care partner can learn to replace tube. No interference with respiratory tract. Improved cosmetic issues	GT requires surgery, endoscopy or interventional radiology. Stoma care required. May have infection, peri-tubular leakage, skin breakdown, tube migration, tissue granulation.
Jejunostomy	Long-term patients with gastroparesis, gastric aspiration or gastric outlet obstruction. JT: Surgical. PEJ: endoscopic.	Can be placed at time of surgery or endoscopy and TF started soon after surgery or endoscopy	Clogs easily due to small bore tube.
Oral feedings	Children who are able and willing to swallow	Preserves motor skills and suck and swallow ability. Most physiologic.	Contraindicated for high aspiration risk.

Adapted from Klotz KA, Wessel JJ, Hennies GA. "Goals of Pediatric Nutrition Support and Nutrition Assessment". In: Merritt RJ, ed., The ASPEN Nutrition Support Practice Manual. The American Society for Parenteral and Enteral Nutrition, Silver Spring, Md, 1998: p23–1–14.

TUBE SELECTION

When planning for HEN, it is important to consider which method of administration will best suit the patient's medical condition, anatomy, and preference. Once the method of feeding is selected, proper tubes and feeding sets must be ordered that are compatible with the method.

The following includes characteristics and considerations for commonly used enteral access devices in the pediatric HEN patient.

NASOGASTRIC TUBES

Often in clinical practice, the pediatric patient will utilize nightly insertion of a nasogastric tube (NGT) for administering the daily feeding regimen. There are several clinical scenarios where feeding by NGT may be preferable to placement of a semi-permanent feeding tube (e.g., PEG). Children with temporary need for food supplementation of their diet are one group that may benefit from intermittent use of a NGT such as in patients with cystic fibrosis, exacerbation of Crohn's disease, and those who are undergoing cancer treatment. They may not be able to consume adequate quantities of food by mouth to maintain normal growth for finite periods of time and may prefer insertion of the NGT tube at night to semi-permanent feeding tube placement.

Another group that may utilize NGT at home are those patients on TPN and trophic feedings who are being evaluated to see whether TF will be tolerated before a GT or PEG is placed.

Nasogastric tubes come in a variety of types and sizes.[65] Materials commonly used include:

- polyvinylchloride (PVC)—Less flexible, potential for GI irritation, stiff for ease in insertion, exposure to gastric acid causes tube to become brittle, for short-term use of less than 3 days
- Polyurethane (PU)—More flexible, less potential for GI irritation, may require a stylet for ease in insertion, usually replaced once a month and as needed

French (Fr) size refers to the outer diameter (OD) of the tube. Inner diameter (ID) is determined by tube material—PVC has a larger ID than does PU. Pediatric NG tubes are generally No. 10 Fr or smaller. This measurement is the OD of the feeding tube. The actual ID of the

TABLE 9-20   Important Selection Characteristics of Nasoenteric
Feeding Tubes

Formula Category	Feeding Tube French Size	
	Gravity	Pump
Infant Formula	5-8	5-6
Blenderized	12-18	8-10
Milk-based	8-10	6-8
Lactose-Free	8	6-8
Fiber-enriched	10	6-8
Elemental	6	6
High Density	8-10	6-10

Common Feeding Tube Lengths:

Age (years)	Tube Length (inches)	
	Nasogastric	Transpyloric
<1	22	22-36
1-18	36	36-43

Adapted from Del Rio D, Williams K, Esvelt B: *Handbook of Enteral Nutrition: A Practical Guide to Tube Feeding.* Medical Specifics Publishing. ©1982, p.71.

tube is smaller. Various formula categories require a minimum Fr size for proper flow during administration (see Table 9–20).[65]

Nasogastric tubes are available in various lengths (see Table 9–20). The length of the tube required to reach the stomach can be estimated by measuring the distance from the tip of the nose to the ear lobe and then adding it to the distance from the ear lobe to the xyphoid process. This measurement tool is known as the NEX method.

Weighted and non-weighted NGTs are available. Weights are at the distal end of the tube. Typically weights are made of tungsten in 3, 5, or 7 g amounts. Controversy exists regarding the usefulness of weighted tubes in facilitating transpyloric placement (for nasojejunal tubes (NJT) and for maintaining the tube in proper position in the GI tract.

Nasogastric tubes are manufactured with and without wire stylets. Stylets are designed to ease placement of soft, flexible feeding tubes. Most stylets come preinserted in NG tubes and should not be re-inserted once removed after tube placement. This is to avoid the stylet from inadvertently leaving the tube on reinsertion and increasing the risk of puncture of the lungs or another organ. Stylet design should include *flow-through* which allows for attachment of a syringe at the proximal end of the stylet to allow withdrawing of stomach content, or for injecting air for auscultation to confirm proper NGT placement.

Other pediatric NG tube design considerations include:[65]

- Tip—location/number of eyelets (openings)
- Ports—compatibility with syringes and feeding sets
- Cm markings—for measuring depth of tube insertion
- Radiopaque—for placement verification on radiographs
- Lubrication—external/internal for ease in insertion and stylet removal, some tubes have lubrication that is water activated to reduce friction with placement
- Cost

GASTROSTOMY FEEDING TUBES

The gastrostomy feeding tube (GT) is the most frequently used access device in HEN. A GT can be placed at the time of surgery or in anticipation of treatment-related decreased nutrient intake. Gastrostomy feeding tubes are manufactured in silicone and polyurethane (which have a larger internal lumen). They may have a solid, flexible internal bumper or an inflatable balloon to maintain internal placement and an external retention bolster to prevent tube migration.[66] A GT with a jejunal extension can be used for transpyloric, small bowel feeding and the gastric portion of this tube may be used for simultaneous decompression ("venting") of the stomach.

Once inserted, GTs extend six inches or longer from the abdominal wall, for connection of a feeding set, or access via syringe. Generally, two to three ports extend from the proximal end of the tube, one port for feeding, one port for medication administration and one port for balloon inflation (if indicated). Catheter tip syringes, which have larger internal diameters for easy flow, are typically used for formula feeding, whereas Luer-Lok syringes are used for medications and balloon inflation.

Port configuration may be different in gastro-jejunal tubes in that there may not be a dedicated medication port, due to the need for dual access to the stomach and small intestine. Two ports are usually present, one for accessing the stomach and one for accessing the small intestine. Each port has a cover for closure when not in use.

Once the stoma (opening created between the gastric wall and the abdominal wall via surgical or endoscopic placement of the tube) has matured, the original GT may be replaced by a replacement GT or a

"Low Profile Feeding Device" also known as a "button." Low profile feeding devices, because of their flush position to the abdominal wall, provide a more aesthetic access in the pediatric population and may also prevent unintentional removal of the GT by the child. Low profile feeding device design eliminates the need for an external retention bolster to prevent tube migration. The majority of buttons are secured with an inflatable balloon internal bumper. However, nonballoon devices are also available.[66]

Replacement GTs come in a variety of French sizes ranging from 12–24 Fr, with the most commonly used sizes being 12, 14, 16, and 18 Fr in pediatrics. Graduated port adapters with covers are available to ensure appropriate connection to the feeding set or syringe and may aid in prolonging the life of ports that become worn from use.

Use of a button requires determination of the "shaft" size in centimeters. Shaft size is influenced by the thickness of the abdominal wall. This measurement will change as the child responds to nutritional intervention. Shaft size should be measured periodically by a trained professional to assure proper fit of the button. A "Stoma Measuring Device" is used by the clinician to take this measurement. The measurement obtained assists the practitioner in ordering the appropriate shaft size for the button. Shaft sizes may range from 0.8 cm to 5.4 cm. Low profile devices require extension sets (tubing) to work in conjunction with the button. Extension sets come in two types: "Straight" extension sets are used for bolus feeding, and "right angle" extension sets are used for continuous feeding. Both types of extension sets are available in 12-inch and 24-inch lengths.[66] Replacement low profile feeding devices extension sets may be purchased from the low profile feeding device manufacturer.

Extension sets may be specific with regard to Fr size, or they may be used in a wide variety of tube sizes depending on the manufacturer.

JEJUNOSTOMY TUBE

Jejunostomy tubes (J-tubes) are less commonly used than GT in the pediatric population. They are manufactured in silicone and PU. J-tubes are surgically or endoscopically placed and secured in place via suture wings, T-fasteners, or an external and internal bumper. The internal bumper is often an inflatable balloon. Like GT buttons, jejunostomy low profile buttons are also available and require similar extension sets as gastrostomy buttons. Determination of shaft size is also necessary. Sizes of J-tubes vary from 5 to 8 Fr for needle catheter jejunostomies[67] and from 12–24 Fr for other standard J-tubes.[68]

Di(2-ethylhexyl)phthalate (DEHP) is one of a family of chemicals that are used as softeners for polyvinylchloride (PVC). Nasogastric tubes and enteral nutrition feeding bags are devices which may include DEHP.[69] However, DEHP can leach from PVC medical devices. Leaching of DEHP can cause damage to the liver, kidneys, lungs and reproductive system, particularly the developing testes, according to animal studies. The amount of DEHP that will leach out depends on the temperature, the lipid content of the liquid, and the duration of exposure to the plastic.[70] The Food and Drug Administration (FDA) issued an FDA Safety Assessment and a Public Health Notification urging health care providers to use alternatives to DEHP-containing devices for more vulnerable patients, such as pediatrics. PVC-free and DEHP-free alternatives are available for almost every use of PVC in the health care setting. Alternatives to PVC and DEPH-containing enteral feeding sets and enteral feeding nasogastric tubes are listed in Table 9–21. The manufacturer of the medical device may also be contacted.

A specialized gastric tube for use in neonates, pediatrics, and adults with conditions such as delayed gastric emptying, abdominal distension/discomfort or gastro-esophageal reflux is available. The specialized tube works simultaneously with enteral administration equipment (syringe, gravity, or pump fed) to prevent interruption in the feeding schedule and works to continuously decompress the stomach[40] ("FARRELL Valve," CORPAK MedSystems, www.corpakmedsystems.com/products/enteral/farrell.htm).

PEDIATRIC ENTERAL FEEDING PUMPS

Bolus feeding with a syringe is always the optimal goal for the older pediatric patient because of its simplicity and ease of use, convenience, lower cost, and ability to provide more physiologic feedings. However, infants and children with severe gastrointestinal or neurologic disease are frequently not able to tolerate bolus gastric feedings and must utilize an enteral feeding pump in order for HEN to succeed. Pediatric patients have special needs that must be addressed when selecting an enteral feeding pump. Children with high risk of aspiration, low gastric capacity,

TABLE 9–21 DEHP-Free Enteral Feeding Products

Products	Manufacturer	Material	Comments	Telephone	Web Page
Enteral Feeding Sets	Children's Medical Ventures	Non-DEHP PVC	Enteral feeding bag and tubing	800-377-3449	www.childmed.com[1]
	CORPAK MedSystems	Nylon, Ethylene vinyl acetate, Polypropylene	Enteral feeding bag and tubing	800-323-6305	www.corpakmedsystems.com
	CORPAK MedSystems	Nylon, Ethylene vinyl acetate, Polypropylene	Farrell valve for enteral gastric pressure relief: PVC-free bag with tubing made from PVC with DEHP	800-323-6305	www.corpakmedsystems.com
	CORPAK MedSystems	Silicone	Cubby button gastrostomy device (CorFlo)	800-323-6305	www.corpakmedsystems.com
	Zevex International, Inc.	Non-DEHP PVC	Enteral feeding bag	800-970-2337	www.zevex.com[2]
	Kendall Healthcare (Tyco)	Non-DEHP PVC	Non-DEHP bag and tube	800-962-9888	www.kendallhq.com
Enteral Feeding-Nasogastric (NG) Tubes	CORPAK MedSystems	Silicone	Gastrostomy tube-neonates and adults	800-323-6305	www.corpakmedsystems.com
	CORPAK MedSystems	Polyurethane	PEG tube, Nasoenteric feeding tube, Jejunal tube-neonates and adult	800-323-6305	www.corpakmedsystems.com

Products	Manufacturer	Material	Comments	Telephone	Web Page
	C.R. Bard, Inc.	Polyurethane	Pediatric clear straight catheter	800-545-0890	www.bardmedical.com
	Kendall Healthcare (Tyco)	Polyurethane	Nasogastric tube, PEG tube, Nasojejunal	800-962-9888	www.kendallhq.com
	Kendall Healthcare (Tyco)	Silicone	Replacement skin level g-tube	800-962-9888	www.kendallhq.com
	Kendall Healthcare (Tyco)	Silicone	Gastrostomy tube	800-962-9888	www.kendal.hq.com
	Kimberly-Clark (Ballard Medical Devices)	Silicone	PEG feeding tube, Gastrostomy feeding tube, Jejunal feeding tube	800-524-3557	www.kchealthcare.com
	Klein-Baker Medical	Silicone	Feeding tube for neonates.	210-696-4061	www.neocare.com
	Ross (Abbott Laboratories)	Polyurethane	Gastrostomy tube, Nasoenteric feeding tube, Nasojejunal feeding tube	800-231-3330	www.ross.com

(1) "Alternatives to Polyvinyl Chloride (PVC) and Di (2-Ethylhexyl) Phthalate (DEHP) Medical Devices (Part 2 of 7)". *Healthcare Without Harm.* Dec 10 2004 http://www.noharm.org/detals.cfm?type=cocument/d=591.

(2) "Enteral Delivery Sets by ZEVEX Therapeutics. Dec 14 2004 http://www.zevex.com/therapeutics/delivery/

TABLE 9–22   Product Support

Manufacturer	Phone Number	Web Site
ROSS Products	800-323-6305	www.ross.com
Corpak Medsystems	800-551-5838	www.corpakmedsystems.com
Ballard Medical Products	800-528-5591	www.kchealthcare.com
Applied Medical Technology	800-869-7382	www.appliedmedical.net
Kendall	800-962-9888	www.kendallhq.com
C. R. Bard, Inc.	800-826-2273	www.bardendoscopy.com

gastrointestinal dysmotility, or feeding into the jejunum are good candidates for use of a pump. Enteral feeding pumps can deliver a continuous flow and a large volume of formula at a constant rate with less risk of accidental bolus feeding than with gravity drips. In patients who must receive hypertonic formulas, such as with completely elemental feedings, enteral feeding pumps have been shown to reduce the occurrence of osmotic diarrhea and help patients reach their nutritional goals faster.[71]

Pumps are made for either ambulatory or nonambulatory patients and operate by either a rotary peristaltic mechanism or a volumetric cassette. Advantages of cassette pumps over rotary pumps may include a decreased risk of free formula flow, less risk of improper setup, automatic priming, and a reduced number of false occlusion alarms.[71] However, when powdered formulas must pass through cassettes or bellows they may cause clogs and frequent alarming of the pump due to formula occlusions. If blending the powder does not resolve this problem, then the pump may need to be changed to one that does not utilize a cassette or bellows in the feeding mechanism.

Pediatric patients often live an active lifestyle and benefit from the lighter portable pumps which come with a variety of features that are ideal for children who are mobile. These pumps come with a carrying case that can be worn as a backpack, over the shoulder or wheelchair, or around the waist. Their batteries have a long life and can be recharged.[71] Table 9–23 compares the features of several commercially available ambulatory enteral feeding pumps that are suitable for use in the pediatric population.

There are many advocacy organizations for children that may be able to assist those in need for advice on supplies and services required by HEN patients, such as The Oley Foundation and The Cystic Fibrosis Foundation (see the resource list at the end of chapter).

TABLE 9–23 Comparison of Commonly Used Ambulatory Enteral Feeding Pump Comparison in Pediatrics

	Ross Embrace	Ross Flexiflo-Companion	Kendall PET	Zevex EnteraLite
Pump type	Volumetric cassette	Volumetric cassette	Rotary peristaltic	Rotary peristaltic
Battery type	NiMh	Sealed lead acid	NiCd	NiMh
OP time, hrs*	18 hrs at 125 ml/hr	8 hrs at 150 ml/hr	14 hrs	24 hrs at 125 ml/hr.
Recharge time	6 hrs	1½ hr per hr of use	8 hrs	5 hrs
Sight Chamber	Optional	Yes	Yes	No
Memory retention	24 hrs	Yes, unlimited	14 hrs	Yes, unlimited
Weight (lbs)	1.5 lbs (pump)	1.5 lbs (pump) 2.5 lbs (charger)	1.4 lbs (pump)	1.3 lbs (pump)
Generic sets available	No	No	No	Not recommended
Accuracy	+/– 5%	+/– 10%	+/– 10%	+/– 5%
Priming	Automatic or Manual	Manual	Manual	Manual
Age <1 year	Yes	No (>12 months) (rate: >25ml/hr)	Yes	Yes
One-hand set loading	Yes	Yes	Yes	Yes
Dose setting	Yes: 1–9,999ml	Yes: 1–9,999ml	Yes: 1–2000ml	Max 3000ml, 10ml increments
Flow rate	1ml increments from 1–500 ml/hr	5 ml increments from 1–300 ml/hr	1 ml increments from 1–75 ml/hr 5 ml increments from 76–400 ml/hr	1 ml increments from 1–600 ml/hr
Special features	Battery indicator Free flow protection clamp	Automatic clog clearing at rates of 30 ml/hr and above. Free-flow protection.		Free flow protection Runs when turned in any position.

*Pump run times are dependent on many variables including the rate and viscosity of the solution.

Adapted from: Minard G, Lysen LK. "Enteral Access Devises". In: Gottsclich MM, ed. The Science and Practice of Nutrition Support. The American Society for Parenteral and Enteral Nutrition. Kendal/Hunt, Iowa: 2001. p.181.

SUPPLIES

Some feeding tubes, especially jejunal tubes and low profile gastrostomy tubes require brand-specific adapters and extension sets to allow patients to use them. This allows the tube to be connected to a syringe or feeding bag and pump.[1] Some tubes are interchangeable with adapters from other tube brands and others can use "universal adapters." When a tube or button is changed to a new or better brand that cannot use parts from a model other than itself, the corresponding parts should be ordered and delivered to the patient before the new tube or button is placed so that feeding is not delayed. Part numbers and ordering information can be obtained from the manufacturer. It is important that insurance verification be made before a new device is ordered. Insurance companies will also pay periodically for associated supplies. They may require prior authorization if the limit is exceeded.

Extension tubes that are provided with a low profile gastrostomy device should always be rinsed immediately after use with cold water and then followed by hot, soapy water. A tablespoon of vinegar or a couple of drops of chlorine bleach can be added to help maintain a newer looking appearance. Thorough rinsing is required to remove all formula residue. The extension tubing should be replaced whenever it looks cloudy or unclean. Good care will help avoid more frequent replacements than are allowed by the insurance company. Usually, one extension tube per week is adequate depending on the medication being administered and the type of formula.[50]

Daily change of the feeding bag is standard care to avoid bacterial growth. Occasionally, reimbursement issues make it necessary to reuse the feeding bag for 2–3 days and the parent must be instructed to thoroughly clean the bag and tubing and to store them in the refrigerator between feedings.[50]

TRANSITIONING THE PATIENT TO HOME

Pediatric nutrition support patients should be considered for home nutrition support early in their hospital course, and provisions should be made in advance for their home care so that discharge is not delayed. Home tube feeding should be arranged:[48]

- Once the child is medically stable for discharge

- When the child tolerates the tube feeding
- When the child is expected to require tube feeding for longer than one week.

Caregivers will require familiarity with the nutrition support regimen and systems well before the patient is discharged. Reinforcement of teaching efforts should be provided by the home care team once the patient is home. The team should be capable of providing clinical assessment and intervention when needed and of supporting the caregivers regarding questions and concerns that arise during the course of home care.

Table 9–24 provides guidelines for the home care provider to ensure that all necessary information is obtained before discharge from the hospital so that transition to home is as trouble-free as possible. Referral sources working with the home care team will also benefit from knowing in advance that their assistance will be required in providing some of this information before the patient's discharge.

MONITORING

Monitoring of the long-term HEN patient is required to prevent unnecessary setbacks in the provision of care and to ensure optimal growth and nutrition outcomes. Table 9–25 provides suggestions for frequency of monitoring gastrointestinal, metabolic, anthropometric, and mechanical tolerance to HEN in infants and children.[38] The clinician must determine when and how the monitoring schedule should be implemented, taking into account the patient's medical condition, nutrition goals, and past history of deficiencies and intolerance. Monitoring may need to be more frequent when the child's medical condition or tolerance to the tube feeding changes, growth is not optimal, the infant or adolescent is in a period of rapid growth, or an acute illness occurs. Conversely, monitoring schedules may be decreased during long periods of stability in patients whose condition and feeding regimen are not expected to change.

TOLERANCE AND COMPLICATIONS

Tolerance to enteral feedings is determined by gastrointestinal, mechanical, and metabolic factors. Routine monitoring of these factors is vital to minimize complications that can delay attainment of feeding goals and

---

TABLE 9–24   Pediatric Home Enteral Nutrition Order Essentials

- Patient's Name
- Date of Birth
- Date of Order/Start of Care Date
- Medicare/Insurance Identification Number and/or Medicaid Authorization Number (as applicable)
- Insurance approval
- Physician: name, address, phone, fax numbers, e-mail address
- Diagnoses: include those with relevance to the need for tube feeding, nutritional implications and supporting ICD9 codes
- Formula: name, usage (total volume per day), strength, daily calories provided
- Method of Administration: Pump—specify: ambulatory vs. stationary, name/manufacturer gravity, syringe/bolus, oral
- Administration Specifications:

    Continuous: pump rate: ml/hr, number of hours per day, specify intermittent or continuous and hang times or schedule of feedings (Parents often appreciate being given a timetable of feedings)

    Gravity: volume per feed; number of feedings per day, infusion time, schedule

    Syringe/Bolus: volume per feed; number of feedings per day, schedule

    Oral: volume per feed; number of feedings per day, schedule

- Free water: mls/flush, number of flushes per day, timing (before, after, between feedings and following medication instillation
- Identify additional products/usage/method of administration for modular components, oral rehydration solutions, etc.
- Feeding tube: type, French size, length
- Pump/Gravity/Syringe/Bolus Supplies: carrying case, IV pole, feeding bags (Feeding bags are manufactured to match the feeding pump used and may not be interchangeable with other feeding bags). Provide 1 feeding bag per day, syringes, tube adaptors*
- Supplies: tape, gauze, instructional support materials, etc.*
- Nursing education/Registered Dietitian home consultation (Obtain MD order)
- Duration of EN therapy
- Home care clinician's signature (date/time)—the clinician's signature indicates that the above order has been reviewed with the physician or her agent and is safe, accurate, and appropriate for the patient.
- Physician's signature (date/time)—The physician's signature indicates that the above order is safe, accurate, and appropriate for the patient's care. It is required for legal and insurance purposes in order that the patient can receive services from the home care company.

---

*The Homecare Company may have pre-established supply templates specific for the method of administration of the feeding that may be used in filling the order.

impact the child's growth. It begins when the nutritional assessment has been completed, enteral access is established, and the feeding is initiated.

The most frequently reported complications of enteral feedings are:[72]

TABLE 9–25   Pediatric Monitoring Parameters for HEN

Parameter	Long-term Frequency
Gastrointestinal	
Gastric residuals	When indicated: Prior to each bolus feeding; Every 2–4 hours
Abdominal distention	When indicated
Stool output	When indicated
Metabolic	
Glucose	Every 1 to 3 months
Electrolytes	Every 1 to 3 months
BUN, creatinine	Every 1 to 3 months
Calcium, phosphorus	Every 1 to 3 months
Magnesium	Every 1 to 3 months
Transaminases, bilirubin	Yearly
Hemoglobin, hematocrit	Yearly
Iron, TIBC, ferritin	Yearly
Folate, vitamin B_{12}	Yearly
Trace elements	Yearly
Anthropometric	
Weight	Weekly for infants Monthly for children
Length/Height	Monthly for infants Bi-annually for children
Mechanical	
Tube position	Daily
Tube site	Daily
Formula preparation technique	When indicated
Equipment use	Every 1–3 months

Adapted from Weckwirth, JA. Monitoring Enteral Nutrition Support Tolerance in Infants and Children. *Nutr Clinic Prac.* October 2004;19:496–503.

- diarrhea,
- vomiting,
- occlusion of the feeding tube

DIARRHEA

Horn and Chaboyer define diarrhea in children as the passage of 3 or more loose or liquid stools in a 24-hour period.[73] The causes of diarrhea are mutifactorial and constitute one of the most immediate and obvious signs of enteral feeding intolerance. In pediatric patients diarrhea is most often related to the underlying disease state, altered GI anatomy, immaturity of the GI tract, or substrate allergy or intolerance and is patient specific.[74] Unrecognized disorders of the small bowel, liver, or pancreas may result in carbohydrate or fat malabsorption. Once identified, continuous rather than intermittent infusion of the formula may be helpful, or a change in formula, appropriate to the specific malabsorptive disorder, may be required.[72] Most pediatric practitioners test for carbohydrate malabsorption by checking the stool for reducing substances and pH. It is perhaps most accurate to check these parameters at predefined intervals during the day rather than at random. Carbohydrate malabsorption is characterized by a low (acidic) pH and positive stool-reducing substances (>0.25% to 0.5%).[38]

Long-chain fat can be malabsorped in children with biliary, pancreatic, or intestinal diseases and may be detectable through a Sudan III stain for fecal fat. Medium-chain triglyceride oil can be useful in providing calorie supplementation while avoiding the need for pancreatic lipase or bile salts for absorption.[38] The clinician should keep in mind that any type of fat added to the formula as a modular component has a tendency to separate and may be, unintentionally, administered as a bolus. A large bolus of lipid may overwhelm the absorptive capacity of a child's intestine, resulting in diarrhea in much the same fashion as a dose of mineral oil.

Strategies to prevent diarrhea due to unintentional infusion of a large fat bolus include:

- Making up and utilizing only small volumes at a time of the formula-lipid mixture during continuous feedings,
- Decreasing the concentration of lipid, and
- Adding an emulsifier to continuous feedings (such as Tween)[75] (Tween 80, UniQema, Inc. 800–424–2024).[72]

Although the incidence of *Clostridium Difficile (C.Difficile)* colitis is far less prevalent in pediatric patients than adult patients,[76] diarrheal stool should be examined for evidence of *C.Difficile* and other enteric pathogens when antibiotic medications are being administered and no other cause is apparent.[72] The clinician may need to work through an outpatient lab when stool examinations and cultures for home HEN patients are required.

Another cause of gastrointestinal infection that can cause diarrhea is bacterial contamination during feeding.[50] The tops of formula cans should be cleaned before opening.

- All open cans of formula must be kept refrigerated and discarded according to the manufacturer's instructions—usually 24 hours.
- Cold formula should be warmed to room temperature before administering to prevent cramping.

When a hyperosmolar formula enters the duodenum the child may experience a "dumping" type of diarrhea caused by a rapid shift of fluid into the bowel lumen—usually within 30 minutes of the feeding.[38] Dumping can also be experienced when a rapid rate of administration exceeds the ability of the intestine to absorb the volume infused.

Intervention for complications caused by hyperosmolar feedings or a rapid infusion rate may include:[50]

- Switch to an isotonic formula.
- Dilute the current formula to isotonic strength and then gradually increase to goal.
- Check to ensure that the formula is properly mixed.
- Avoid adding other foods to the formula (baby food, powdered milk, flavorings).
- Avoid adding medications to the formula; give medications between feedings with water or juice. Medications that may cause diarrhea include antibiotics, GI or neurologic stimulants, beta blockers, stool softeners, and liquid medications with sorbitol. Medications should be reviewed and changed if possible.
- For continuous feedings, return infusion rate to previously tolerated rate, then gradually increase more slowly or over longer time.
- For bolus feedings, increase length of time for feedings. Allow short break during feedings. Offer smaller, more frequent feedings.

When the infant or child has rapid GI transit time, or when diarrhea is not caused by any of the factors mentioned previously, adding fiber to the formula or selecting a fiber-enriched formula can be useful.[50,72]

VOMITING

Aspiration of regurgitated gastric contents is a potentially life-threatening complication and all measures to avoid it in HEN pediatric patients must be taken.

Vomiting may also be due to:[72]

- Mechanical obstruction of the gastric outlet due to forward migration of the internal bumper of the G-tube through the pylorus or edema and spasm of the pylorus due to a stress-related peptic ulcer or gastritis. Radiographic or endoscopic evaluation and medical treatment is necessary if suspected and confirmed.
- Intraabdominal adhesions should be considered in those patients with previous abdominal surgery.
- Functionally delayed gastric emptying may respond to continuous feedings rather than bolus feedings. Reduction of nutrients that delay gastric emptying, such as hypercaloric, hyperosmolar, or high-fat formulas can be useful. In the absence of mechanical obstruction, a prokinetic agent such as metoclopramide to enhance gastric emptying should be administered, or transpyloric, continuous feedings initiated.

GASTRIC RESIDUAL VOLUME

For most HEN patients with gastrostomy tubes, there is no need to check gastric residual volumes once they have been stable for at least 48 hours—no more so than if they were on oral feedings.[74] When enteral feedings are being started in the home, however, patients may need to be monitored for gastric residuals, especially in those patients who are at risk for aspiration.

Clinical factors associated with increased aspiration risk include:[38]

- Decreased level of consciousness
- Vomiting/regurgitation
- Neuromuscular disease
- Previous aspiration
- Delayed gastric emptying

The following is a sample of guidelines that have been proposed for monitoring of gastric residual volume in infants and children in the hospital that may be applicable in the home if necessary:[38]

For continuous gastric feedings:

- Check residuals every 4 hours.
- Hold feedings if the residual is greater than or equal to the hourly rate, or greater than twice the hourly rate.

For intermittent feedings:

- Check residuals before each feeding.
- Hold the feeding if the residual is greater than half of the prior feeding volume.

MECHANICAL COMPLICATIONS

Inquiry of family members administering HEN should be made periodically to ensure proper use and handling of pumps and response to alarms. Proper use of feeding bags, tubing, and syringes should be reinforced. When gastrointestinal intolerance develops in the absence of obvious cause, formula mixing and administration techniques should be reviewed and observed as necessary.[38] Common technical complications of enteral feedings are reviewed in Table 9–26 with suggestions for intervention.

Excess granulation tissue at the site of a PEG of J-tube is a complication of HEN which can cause significant pain and bleeding at the site.[77] Silver nitrate, colloidal silver, and antibiotic ointment are the usual treatments, but they can be accompanied by extended periods of healing. Corticosteroid cream has been reported to decrease the time required for healing of the granulation tissue and can help to abate pain.[78]

FEEDING TUBE OBSTRUCTIONS

Occlusion of feeding tubes occurs in 6–10% of patients. Tubes smaller than 8–10 French obstruct more easily. Declogging methods can be time consuming, can delay the feeding, and may not result in clearing the occlusion. Prevention is, therefore, the best line of defense.[79] Prompt attention to a feeding tube occlusion will provide the best chance of unclogging the tube. Understanding the most common causes of enteral tube

TABLE 9-26 Common Mechanical Complications of Tube Feeding

Complication	Possible Tube Cause	Intervention
Leakage of gastric contents	Improper positioning Tube migration Breakdown of stoma	Place child upright for feeding Ensure GT is firmly in place Stabilize tube with gauze, adjust crosspiece Remeasure stoma, insert new tube as needed Keep skin around stoma clean and dry, use protective ointment and gauze Refer to physician
Bleeding around stoma	Excessive movement or pressure on tubing	A small amount of bleeding is normal Tape tube securely in place to avoid irritation from movment Secure tube under child's clothing Refer to physician
Infection of stoma	Gastric leakage around tube Stoma site not clean Allergic reaction to soap	Correct cause of leakage Carefully cleanse and protect stoma Use plain water, change soap used Refer to physician for culture and medication
Granulation tissue	Body rejecting foreign body Poorly fitting tube causing friction Use of antiseizure meds	Keep area clean and dry Adjust snugness of PEG tube with friction crosspiece Stabilize tube using tape, bandnet, ace bandage, tube top blouse Prevent child from pulling on tube Apply silver nitrate as directed by physician

Adapted from Appendix N – Technical Aspects of Enteral Feeding (Tube Feeding). In: Nutrition Interventions for Children with Special Health Care Needs, Washington State Department of Health, 2nd ed. May 2002: 319–321. and Frederick A. Practical Tips for Tube Feeding. *Nutrition Focus*, January/February 2003;18(1):1–8.

occlusions will help to avoid clogs and to effectively resolve them when they occur without resorting to the need for changing the tube. Caregivers should be well-trained upon discharge to care for the enteral feeding tube and to take appropriate action when occlusions do occur. Routine flushing with warm water is the single most effective way to avoid occlusions and maintain patency.[1] The following are remedies for enteral feeding tube clogs:

1. Manufacturers of enteral feeding tubes recommend warm water to unclog feeding tubes. A 60 cc syringe filled with lukewarm water can gently be inserted into the feeding tube and the water released as close to the site of the clog as possible. Clamp the tube for several minutes to allow the clog to soak up the water. A gentle and firm push and pull on the syringe plunger may dislodge the clog. The procedure may need repeating a few times. This should resolve the majority of clogs.
2. Manufacturers do *not* recommend flushing or removing clogs with the use of carbonated beverages and similar fluids because they can accelerate degradation of the feeding tube material with more frequent changing of the tube.
3. When feeding tubes clog repeatedly, cannot be unclogged, or are hard to replace, consider having a commercially made tube declogger in the home, or readily available, through the home care company. This will prove especially useful when conventional techniques have failed to unclog the tube and could save the patient a trip to the emergency room or doctor's office to unclog or replace the tube. Cleaning devises are also available.

WORKING WITH THE HOME CARE TEAM

The home care company providing HEN supplies and services to pediatric patients and their caregivers should include experienced nutrition clinicians and support staff who are in regular contact with the family to monitor patient progress. They should be proactive in problem solving to avoid interruptions in therapy and should function as partners in addressing patient concerns and educational needs. The home care team should encourage regular clinic visits and follow-up care with their primary healthcare providers. They are the first line of communication between the patient/caregivers and the physician and often alert the physician when problems arise.

MONITORING GROWTH

Until the child reaches the age of 20 years, regular monitoring of height, weight, head circumference (≤3–5 years), weight for height (<2 years), and BMI (≥2 years) on the revised 2000 growth charts published by the NCHS (National Center for Health Statistics) of the CDC is imperative to ensure that the pediatric patient's established goals for optimal growth and nutritional status are continually being met.

In clinical practice, patients who are nutritionally wasted will show the greatest sensitivity to weight gain. Height improvement may lag behind improvements in weight in stunted patients and it may take up to one year to reverse linear growth failure.[80] Not all children on HEN will have improved growth as an outcome measure. This does not necessarily imply treatment failure. For instance, children with conditions such as terminal cancer, severe cerebral palsy, congenital human immunodeficiency virus, and certain metabolic disorders will have impaired linear growth no matter how much their intake improves.[77] Adequacy of growth is best interpreted through assessment of serial measurements. Significant changes in an individual's usual growth percentile should signal the need to evaluate the cause and to adjust treatment and nutrition support as needed. Weight-for-height (children 0–3 years) and Body Mass Index (children ≥3 years) evaluate current nutritional status, acute changes (loss or gain), or degree of wasting specific to the individual's body size. One week between measurements should be allowed before concluding that the weight change is accurate.[81] Length/height-for-age compared with the standard is an index of past nutritional and growth status and degree of stunting.

The clinical growth charts have the grids scaled to metric units (kg, cm), with English units (lb, in) as the secondary scale. Clinical charts are available for boys and for girls.

Clinical charts are available in English, French, or Spanish. Anthropometric measurements can be plotted on these growth charts as follows:

Infants, birth to 36 months:

- Length-for-age and weight-for-age
- Head circumference-for-age and weight-for-length

Children and adolescents, 2 to 20 years:

- Stature-for-age and weight-for-age
- BMI-for-age

Preschoolers, 2 to 5 years:

- Weight-for-stature

Growth charts for length and weight are available elsewhere for males and females with:

- Prematurity based on gestational age[82]
- Myelomeningocele (spina bifida) for males and females aged 2–18 years[83] cerebral palsy-quadraplegia for males and females aged 0–10 years[84,85]
- Down Syndrome for males and females from birth to 36 months and 2–18 years[85,86]
- Achondroplasia for males and females from birth to 18 years[87,88]

Growth charts for height are available for males and females with:

- Noonan Syndrome[85]
- Prader-Willi Syndrome[85,87]
- Turner Syndrome[85]

These specialized growth charts provide useful growth references, but are limited in that they are developed from relatively small samples. One option suggested by the NCHS is to plot the growth patterns of these children on the specialized charts and the CDC charts. This will allow comparisons of growth to the general population and to the references for children with a given condition. The CDC growth charts can also be used to monitor weight in relation to stature in those instances where weight curves do not exist for that condition (www.cdc.gov/growthcharts).[88] Anthropometric monitoring of stable pediatric HEN patients should be performed at least monthly in infants and young children and plotted on their curves. Once stable, older children and adolescents can be monitored approximately every 6–12 months.[81,38] Goals must be reevaluated and HEN therapy must be adjusted as indicated based upon the patient's tolerance to the regimen and response to therapy, and as clinical status, nutritional needs, and stress factors change.

GROWTH VELOCITY

Knowledge of average growth velocities are useful for monitoring the adequacy, safety, and effectiveness of nutrition support more quickly than can be detected through use of standard growth charts. Table 9–27 lists growth velocity data based on the 50th percentile of weight-for-age[89] and height-for-age[81] from the National Center for Health Statistics growth charts. It should be remembered that growth suppression can occur from illness or injury. During recovery growth velocity may increase above average rates. Rates should not exceed ½ normal velocities, or 5–6 cm/month in height and 6–7 kg in weight every 6 months.[81]

SUMMARY

Treatment of feeding disorders or chronic undernutrition in infants and children includes the administration of enteral nutrition. The efficacy of the HEN plan is especially important in light of the significant expense and growing popularity of enteral nutrition support. Many studies of children on long-term HEN have demonstrated that effective therapy can promote catch-up growth or maintain growth along appropriate percentiles in the majority of children in a variety of conditions.[90–99] With proper diligence to safe practices, serious complications can be minimized.[90] The clinician caring for the pediatric HEN patient must have special skills to effectively treat and monitor these patients at home. Nutrition evaluation, HEN (and/or HPN) therapy, and education can be beneficial and cost-effective for children with special health care needs at home.[99]

HEN RESOURCES

Oley Foundation
www.oley.org
800-776-OLEY
Large patient network that allows parents to communicate with other patients in similar situations
Provides online Web site information
Free newsletter for patients
Toll free network

TABLE 9–27: Troubleshooting chart for enteral feeding tube occlusions[1,65]

Cause	Prevention
1. Inadequate flushing	**Always** flush the tube with at least 30 ml of warm water before and after any administration of medications **and** formula.
	Always provide water flushes between meds and formula.
2. Administration of medications	Evaluate all meds to determine whether they are needed and whether they are appropriate to administer through a tube. All enteric coated and time-released meds cannot be crushed and should be changed to an alternative.
	If a med comes in liquid form evaluate whether this can be substituted. Determine whether the liquid contains sorbitol and whether this could cause or exacerbate diarrhea.
	If there is no liquid form or the liquid form is undesirable then most pharmacies can provide pill crushers to efficiently pulverize the drug into small particles. Use glass or plastic (not wood) pill crushers.
3. Administration of formula additives	Evaluate all formula additives—protein powders or other modular components—and determine whether they are still needed or whether another enteral formula can be tried that provides the extra nutrients or additive.
	If a modular component must be used it must be carefully mixed with warm water to avoid clumping and clotting.
	Use of a larger bore feeding tube may be necessary if multiple medications or additives are necessary.
4. Formula viscosity	Check appropriateness of tube diameter for high caloric density, powdered formulas, or fiber-containing formulas.
	Mix powdered formulas well, ensure no clumps remain before infusing.
	Consider post-pylorus feeds or continuous infusion.

Equipment exchange list specified in the newsletter
Strong parental support group
Annual national conference for patients, families/caregivers

American Society of Parenteral and Enteral Nutrition (ASPEN)

www.nutritoncare.org
800-727-4567
Established Standards of Practice and Clinical Guidelines for Enteral

TABLE 9–28   Growth Velocities for Healthy Children[89,81]

Weight:	age	g/day	head circumference_(cm/wk)
	0–3 mo	25–35	0.5
	3–6 mo	15–21	0.5
	6–12 mo	10–13	0.5
	1–3 yr	4–10	
	4–6 yr	5–8	
	7–10 yr	5–12	
	12–18	8	
Height:	age(yr)	cm/yr	
	0–1 yr	25cm/yr	
	2–3 yr	11cm/yr	
	4–12 yr	6cm/yr	
males,	12–18yr	4cm/6mo	
females,	12–18yr	3cm/6mo	

Nutrition Therapy and Home Nutrition Support For Adult and Pediatric populations

REFERENCES

1. Barnadas, G. Navigating Home Care: Enteral Nutrition-Part One. Nutrition Issues in Gastroenterology, October 2003; Series #10: p.13. Available at http://www.healthsystem.virginia.edu/internet/digestive-health/nutrition.cfm.
2. Howard L, Malone, M. Clinical outcome of geriatric patients in the United States receiving home parenteral and enteral nutrition. *Am J Clin Nutr.* 1997; 66(6):1364–1370.
3. Heird WC, Greene HL. Panel report on nutritional support of pediatric patients. *Am J Clin Nutr.* 1981;34(suppl 6):1223–1234.
4. Heird WC, Driscoll JM Jr, Schullinger JN, Grebin B, Winters RW. Intravenous alimentation in pediatric patients. *J Pediatr.* 1972;80(3):351–372.
5. Groh-Wargo, S. Recommended enteral nutrient intakes. In: Groh-Wargo S, Thompson M, Cox J, eds. *Nutritional Care of High-Risk Newborns.* Chicago, Ill: Precept Press, Inc; 2000:232.
6. Schwenk WF 2nd. Specialized nutrition support: the pediatric perspective. *JPEN.* 2003;27(3):160–167.
7. Position Paper: American Dietetic Association: Nutrition monitoring of the home parenteral and enteral patient. Available at: http://www.penpages.psu. edu/penpages-reference/12101/12101506.HTML. Accessed September 27, 2004.

8. Klotz KA, Wessel JJ. Hennies GA. Goals of pediatric nutrition support and nutrition assessment. In: *The ASPEN Nutrition Support Manual.* Silver Spring, Md. 1998: 23–1-9.

9. Davis A. Indications and techniques for enteral feeds. In: Baker SB, Baker RD, Davis A. eds. *Pediatric Enteral Nutrition.* New York: Chapman and Hall; 1994: 67–94.

10. Marian, M. Pediatric nutrition support. *Nutr Clin Pract.* 1993;8(5): 199–209.

11. Bentley D, Lifschitz C, Lawson M. Enteral and parenteral nutrition. In: Eds. *Pediatric Gastroenterology and Clinical Nutrition.* London, UK: ReMedica Publishing; 2001.

12. Abad-Sinden A, Stuphen, J. Nutritional management of pediatric short bowel syndrome. nutrition issues. *Gastroenterology.* 2003;12:28–48.

13. ASPEN Board of Directors and The Clinical Guidelines Task Force. Section XII: "Administration of specialized nutrition support—issues unique to pediatrics." In: eds. Guidelines for the use of parenteral and enteral nutrition in adult and pediatric patients. *JPEN.* 2002;26(suppl 1):97SA-100SA.

14. Jenkins AP, Thompson RP. Enteral nutrition and the small intestine. *Gut.* 1994;35:1765–1769.

15. Lucas A, Bloom SR, Aynsley-Green A. Postnatal surges in plasma gut hormones in term and preterm infants. *Biol Neonate.* 1982;41:63–67.

16. Zenel JA Jr. Failure to thrive: a general pediatrician's perspective. *Pediatr Rev.* 1997;18(11):371–378.

17. Bithoney W, Dubowitz H, Egan H. Failure to thrive/growth deficiency. *Pediatr Rev.* 1992;13:453–460.

18. Skuse D, Pickles A, Wolke D, Reilly S. Postnatal growth and mental development: evidence for a "sensitive period." *J Child Psychol Psychiatry.* 1994; 35:521–545.

19. Hovasi Cox J. Bronchopulmonary dysplasia. In: Groh-Wargo S, Thompson M, Cox J, eds. *Nutritional Care for High-Risk Newborns.* Chicago, Ill: Precept Press, Inc; 2000:379.

20. Davis A. Pediatrics. In: Matarese LE, Gottsclich MM, eds. *Contemporary Nutrition Support Practice: A Clinical Guide.* Philadelphia, Pa: WB Saunders, Co; 1998:347–364.

21. Food and Nutrition Board, Institute of Medicine: Dietary Reference Intakes for Energy, Carbohydrate, Fiber, Fat, Fatty Acids, Cholesterol, Protein, and Amino Acids (Macronutrients). National Academies Press, Washington, DC. 2002:93–206.

22. Nevin-Folino NL. Neurological impairment. In: Groh-Wargo S, Thompson M, Hovasi Cox J, eds. *Nutritional Care for High-Risk Newborns.* Chicago, Ill: Precept Press, Inc; 2000:521.

23. Nutritional status assessment and feeding guidelines. In: *The Baylor Pediatric Nutrition Handbook for Residents.* Baylor College of Medicine, Nestle Nutrition Institute; 2003:15–33.

24. Nutrition Committee, Canadian Paediatric Society. Nutrient needs and feeding of premature infants. *CMAJ.* 1995;152(11):1765–1785.
25. Sapsford A. Human milk and enteral nutrition products. In: Groh-Wargo S, Thompson M, Hovasi Cox J, eds. *Nutritional Care for High-Risk Newborns.* Chicago, Ill: Precept Press, Inc; 2000:266.
26. National Research Council, Food and Nutrition Board. Recommended Dietary Allowances. 10th Edition. Washington, DC. National Academy of Sciences. 1989.
27. Foulkes D. Fluids and electrolytes. In: Gunn VL, Nechyba C eds. *The Harriet Lane Handbook,* 16th ed. Philadelphia, Pa: Mosby; 2002:233–235.
28. Holliday MA, Segar WE. The maintenance need for water in parenteral fluid therapy. *Pediatrics.* 1957;19:823–832.
29. CeraProducts, Inc. Columbia, Md, 210451999-2006. Available at http://www.ceraproductsinc.com 1-888-Ceralyte. http://www.ceraproductsinc.com/productline/ceralyte.cfm. Accessed 11/12/06.
30. Position of the American Dietetic Association: promotion of breast feeding. *J Am Diet Assoc.* 1997;97:662–666.
31. Hurst HM, Myatt A, Schanler RJ. Growth and development of a hospital-based lactation program and mother's own milk bank. *J Obstet Gynecol Neonatal Nurs.* 1998;27:503–510.
32. Reis BB, Hall RT, Schanler RJ, Berseth CL, Chan G, Ernst JA, et al. Enhanced growth of preterm infants fed a new powdered human milk fortifier: A randomized, controlled trial. *Pediatrics.* 2000;106(3):581–588.
33. American Academy of Pediatrics Committee on Nutrition: Pediatric Nutrition Handbook, 4th ed. AAP, Elk Grove Village, Ill: 1998.
34. Lozoff B, Jimenez E, Hagen J, Mollen E, Wolf AW. Poorer behavioral and developmental outcome more than 10 years after treatment for iron deficiency in infancy. *Pediatrics.* 2000;105(4):E51.
35. American Academy of Pediatrics Committee on Nutrition. Iron fortification of infant formulas. *Pediatrics.* 1999;104:119–123.
36. Bowen PE, Mobarhan S, Henderson C, et al. Hypocarotenemia in patients fed enterally with commercial liquid diets. *JPEN.* 1988;12:484–489.
37. Weckwerth JA. Monitoring enteral nutrition support tolerance in infants and children. *Nutr Clin Pract.* 2004;19:496–503.
38. Position Paper: American Dietetic Association: Nutrition monitoring of the home parenteral and enteral patient. September 27, 2004. Available at eds. http://www.penpages.psu.edu/penpages-reference/12101/12101506.html.
39. Schwenk WF, Olson D. Pediatrics. In: eds. *The Science and Practice of Nutrition Support: A Core-Based Curriculum.* American Society for Parenteral and Enteral Nutrition. Dubuque, Iowa: Kendall/Hunt Publishing Co; 2001:347–372.
40. "FARRELL Valve," CORPAK MedSystems, http://www.corpakmedsystems.com/products/enteral/farrell.htm). Accessed 11/17/06.

41. Innis SM, Adamkin DH, Hall RT, et al. Docosahexaenoic acid and arachidonic acid enhance growth with no adverse effects in preterm infants fed formula. *J Pediatr.* 2002;140(5):547–554.

42. Brenna T. Infant formulas containing DHA & ARA. Cornell Cooperative Extension. Ithica, NY: Cornell University; April 4, 2003.

43. Pediatric Products Handbook (2004) Mead Johnson & Company, Evansville, Ind. 47721.

44. Lucas A, Morley R, Cole TJ, Gore SM. A randomised multicentre study of human milk versus formula and later development in preterm infants. *Arch Dis Child Fetal Neonatal Ed.* 1994;70:F141-F146.

45. Lucas A, Morley R, Cole TJ. Randomised trial of early diet in preterm babies and later intelligence quotient. *BMJ.* 1998;317(7171):1481–1487.

46. Sampson HA, Bernhisel-Broadbent J, Yang E, Scanlon SM. Safety of casein hydrolysate formula in children with cow milk allergy. *J Pediatr.* 1991; 118:520–525.

47. Hill DJ, Heine RG, Cameron DJ, Francis DE, Bines JE. The natural history of intolerance to soy and extensively hydrolyzed formula in infants with multiple food protein intolerance. *J Pediatr.* 1999;135:118–121.

48. Corrales KM. Enteral nutrition. In: Hendricks KM, Duggan C, Walker WA., eds. *Manual of Pediatric Nutrition,* 3rd ed. London: BC Decker; 2000:186–241.

49. Kraft D, Btaiche IF, Sacks GS. Review of the refeeding syndrome. *Nutr Clin Pract.* 2005;20(6):625–633.

50. Frederick A. Practical tips for tube feeding. Nutrition Focus. January/February 2003;16(1):1–8.

51. Sapsford AL, Grog-Wargo S. Potential renal solute load and osmolality. In: Groh-Wargo S, Thompson M, Cox J, eds. *Nutritional Care for High-Risk Newborns.* Chicago, Ill: Precept Press, Inc; 2000:643.

52. Kuzma-O'Reilly B. Preparing formulas with various caloric densities. In: Groh-Wargo S, Thompson M, Cox J, eds. *Nutritional Care for High-Risk Newborns.* Chicago, Ill: Precept Press, Inc; 2000:651.

53. Breedon, C. Increasing the Caloric Density of Infant Formulas. Nutrition Focus: for children with special health care needs. Child Development and Mental Retardation Center, University of Washington, Seattle, Wash. Nov/Dec. 1993;8(6):1–6.

54. Ziegler EE, Fomon SJ. Fluid intake, renal solute load, and water balance in infancy. *J Pediatr.* 1971;78:561–568.

55. Puangco MA, Schanler RJ. Clinical experience in enteral nutrition support for premature infants with bronchopulmonary dysplasia. *J Perinatol.* 2000; 20:87–91.

56. A.S.P.E.N. Board of Directors. Definition of terms used in A.S.P.E.N. guidelines and standards. *Nutr Clin Pract.* 1995;10(1):1–3.

57. "Enteral Nutrition" In: Eds. The Baylor Pediatric Nutrition Handbook for Residents, 3rd ed, Conkin Calif, Gilger MA, Klish WJ, Motil KJ, Philips SM, Shulman RJ. Baylor College of Medicine, 2003:72–106.

58. Pederson AL. Tube feeding update. *Nutrition Focus.* November/December 2002;17(6):4.

59. Food and Drug Administration: Available at: http://www.cfsan.fida.gov/%7Edms/inf-ltr3.html. Accessed 11/17/06.

60. Anderson D. Nutrition support for neonates. In: Matarese LE, Gottsclich MM, eds. *Contemporary Nutrition Support Practice: A Clinical Guide.* Philadelphia, Pa: WB Saunders, Co; 1998:335–346.

61. Glass RP, Nowak-Cooperman KM. Helping children who are tube-fed learn to eat. *Nutrition Focus.* March/April 2003;18(2):1–6.

62. Pediatric enteral nutrition support. *The American Dietetic Association: Manual of Clinical Dietetics.* Chicago, Ill; 2000:358.

63. Duperret E, Trautlein J, Klein MD. Homemade blenderized tube feedings. *Nutrition Focus.* September/October 2004;19(5):1–8.

64. Guenter, Jones, Sweed, and Ericson. Delivery systems and administration of enteral nutrition. In: Clinical Nutrition, Enteral and Tube Feeding, 3rd ed. Rombeau and Rolandelli, Philadelphia, PA: WB Saunders Co; 1997:254–255.

65. Lysen LK, Samour PQ. Enteral equipment. In: Matarese LE, Gottsclich MM, eds. *Contemporary Nutrition Support Practice: A Clinical Guide.* Philadelphia, Pa: WB Saunders, Co; 1998:202–215.

66. Choices In Low Profile Gastrostomy Tubes (2002). Ross Products Division Abbott Laboratories Inc, Columbus, Ohio, 43215.

67. Minard G, Lysen LK. Enteral access devices. In: Gottsclich, Michele M., ed. *The Science and Practice of Nutrition Support: A Case-Based Core Curriculum.* Dubuque, Iowa: Kendall/Hunt Publishing Company; 2001.

68. Kimberly Clark Interventional Catalog, 2003, Kimberly-Clark Corporation, Draper, Utah, 84020.

69. PVC and DEHP. Healthcare Without Harm. Dec 10 2004 Available at http://www.noharm.org/pvcDehp/pvcFree. Accessed 11/17/06.

70. Feigal Jr, David W. Public Health Notification: PVC Devices Containing Plasticizer DEHP. Food and Drug Administration, July 12 2002.

71. Bowers S. Tubes: a nurse's guide to enteral feeding devices. *Medsurg Nurs.* 1996;5:313–324.

72. Fuchs GJ. Enteral support of the hospitalized child. In: Suskind RM, Lewinter-Suskind L, eds. *Textbook of Pediatric Nutrition,* 2nd ed. New York, NY: Raven Press; 1993:243.

73. Horn D, Chaboyer W. Gastric feeding in critically ill children: a randomized controlled trial. *Am J Crit Care.* 2003;12:461–468.

74. Rees Parrish C, McCray S. Enteral feeding: dispelling myths, nutrition issues in Gastroenterology, Series #9, Practical Gastroenterology, September

2003:33–50. Available at: http://www.healthsystem.virginia.edu/internet/digestive-health/nutrition.cfm. Accessed 11/10/06.

75. Tween 80, UniQema, Inc. 800-424-2024.

76. Bliss DZ, Johnson S, Savik K, et al. Acquisition of Clostridium difficile and Clostridium difficile-diarrhea in hospitalized patients receiving tube feeding. *Ann Intern Med.* 1998; 129:1012–1019.

77. Kang A, Zamora SA, Scott RB, Parsons HG. Catch-up growth in children treated with home enteral nutrition. *Pediatrics.* 1998;102(4):951–955.

78. Lifeline Letter, The Oley Foundation, May/June 2004; XXV(3):3.

79. Fish J. Tube Feeding in the ICU: Overcoming the Obstacles. Columbus, Ohio: Ross Products Division, Abbott Laboratories, Inc; 2002:12.

80. Walker SP, Golden MH. Growth in length of children recovering from severe malnutrition. *Eur J Clin Nutr.* 1988;42:395–404.

81. Assessment of growth. In: Conkin CA, Gilger MA, Klish WJ, Motil KJ, Philips SM, Shulman RJ. *The Baylor Pediatric Nutrition Handbook for Residents, 3rd ed.* Baylor College of Medicine; 2003:6–14.

82. Growth charts: appendix D. In: Groh-Wargo S, Thompson M, Cox J., ed. *Nutritional Care of High-Risk Newborns.* Chicago, Ill: Precept Press, Inc; 2000:611.

83. Ekvall SW, Bandini L, Ekvall V. Obesity. In: Evall SW, ed. *Pediatric Nutrition in Chronic Diseases and Developmental Disorders.* New York: Oxford University Press; 1993:168.

84. Krick J, Murphy-Miller P, Zeger S, Wright E. Pattern of growth in children with cerebral palsy. *J Am Diet Assoc.* 1996;96:680–685.

85. Appendix: growth charts. In: Conkin CA, Gilger MA, Klish WJ, Motil KJ, Philips SM, Shulman RJ. *The Baylor Pediatric Nutrition Handbook for Residents,* 3rd ed. Baylor College of Medicine; 2003:143–167.

86. Cox J, Jordan LC. Nutrition and growth. In: Gunn VL, Nechyba C, eds. *The Harriet Lane Handbook,* 16th ed. Philadelphia, Pa: Mosby; 2002:436–459.

87. Quinn H. Appendix E. In: Hendricks KM, Duggan C, Walker WA, eds. *Manual of Pediatric Nutrition,* 3rd ed. London: BC Decker;2000:574–585.

88. Kuczmarski RJ, Ogden CL, Guo SS, et al. 2000 CDC Growth Charts for the United States: methods and development. *Vital Health Stat 11.* 2002; 246:1–190.

89. Fomon SJ, Haschke F, Zeigler EE, Nelson SE. Body composition of reference children from birth to 10 years. *Am J Clin Nutr.* 1982;35:1169–1175.

90. Rees Parrish, C. The Clinician's Guide to Short Bowel Syndrome. Nutrition Issues in Gastroenterology, Series #31, September 2005;67–106. Available at: http://www.healthsystem.virginia.edu/internet/digestive-health/nutrition.cfm.

91. Moreno LA, Gottrand F, Hoden S, et al. Improvement of nutritional status in cholestatic children with supplemental nocturnal enteral nutrition. *J Pediatr Gastroenterol Nutr.* 1991;12:213–216.

92. Brewer E. Growth of small children managed with chronic peritoneal dialysis and nasogastric tube feedings: 203-month experience in 14 patients. *Adv Perit Dial.* 1990;6:269–272.

93. Heine RG, Reddihough DS, Catto-Smith AG. Gastro-eosophageal reflux and feeding problems after gastrostomy in children with severe neurological impairment. *Dev Med Child Neurol.* 1995;37:320–329.

94. Papadopoulou A, Holden CE, Paul L, et al. The nutritional response to home enteral nutrition in childhood. *Acta Paediatr.* 1995;84:528–531.

95. Howard L, Ament M, Fleming CR, Shike M, Steiger E. Current use and clinical outcome of home enteral nutrition therapies in the United States. *Gastroenterology.* 1995;109:355–365.

96. Guimber D, Michaud L, Storme L, et al. Gastrostomy in infants with neonatal pulmonary disease. *J Pediatr Gastroenterol Nutr.* 2003;36(4):459–463.

97. Reed EE, Roy LP, Gaskin KJ, Knight JF. Nutritional intervention and growth in children with chronic renal failure. *J Ren Nutr.* 1998;8(3):122–126.

98. Corwin DS, Isaacs JS, Georgeson KE, et al. Weight and length increases in children after gastrostomy placement. *J Am Diet Assoc.* 1996;96(9):874–879.

99. Johnson DB, Cheney C, Monsen ER. Nutrition and feeding in infants with bronchopulmonary dysplasia after initial hospital discharge: risk factors for growth failure. *J Am Diet Assoc.* 1998;98:649–656.

READINGS

Savy, GK. Enteral Glutamine Supplementation: Clinical review and practical guidelines. *Nutrition in Clinical Practice.* December 1997;12(6):259–262.

Pennington, J. Bowes and Church's Food Values of Portions Commonly Used, 16th ed. Philadelphia, Pa: Lippincott Co; 1994:127.

Institute of Medicine of the National Academies. Dietary reference intakes for energy, carbohydrate, fiber, fat, fatty acids, cholesterol, protein and amino acids. *J Am Diet Assoc.* 2002;102:1621–1630.

CHAPTER 10

Home Parenteral Nutrition Support in Pediatrics

Phuong Christine Nguyen, MD
John A. Kerner, Jr., MD

INTRODUCTION

Home parenteral nutrition (HPN) delivers the patient's nutrient and fluid requirements intravenously outside of the hospital setting. It decreases the length of the patient's hospital stay, reduces patient readmissions, reduces health-care costs, and promotes an environment that is more appropriate for growth and development in the pediatric patient.

INDICATIONS

The clinical conditions requiring HPN for pediatric patients are the same as those for parenteral nutrition in the hospital, except that the patient no longer requires acute hospital care (see Table 10–1). The child needs intravenous fluid and nutrition because he or she is unable either to sustain or to maintain his or her weight.

Initiating HPN is time-consuming and expensive, requiring intensive work from the physician, hospital nutrition support team, home infusion provider, and family members. Some centers do not initiate HPN unless it is clear the patient will need at least 30 days of therapy.[1,2] How-

TABLE 10–1   Indications and Contraindications for Home
Parenteral Nutrition[3]

Indications
- Nutritional requirements cannot be met by enteral means
  - renal failure
  - cardiac cachexia
  - cystic fibrosis
  - prior to orthotopic liver transplantation
- Short-bowel syndrome
  - necrotizing enterocolitis
  - surgical resection (e.g., secondary to Crohn's disease)
- Surgical gastrointestinal disorders (leading to short-bowel syndrome)
  - gastroschisis
  - midgut volvulus
  - intestinal atresias
- Motility disorders: pseudo-obstruction
- Intractable diarrhea
  - intestinal lymphangiectasia
  - microvillus inclusion disease
- Inflammatory bowel disease
- Gastrointestinal fistulas
- AIDS
- Cancer-related
  - post-bone marrow transplantation
  - graft-versus-host disease
  - radiation
  - nausea
- Chylothorax or chylous ascites

Contraindications
- A functional gastrointestinal tract
- Lack of vascular access
- Home caretakers do not have psychological or cognitive ability to provide home therapy
- Unstable home environment

ever, discharging a patient on HPN may be cost saving to all parties. In addition, it often provides a quality of life improvement for both the patients and their families.

HPN does not preclude a pediatric patient from receiving oral nutrients, if possible. Home parenteral nutrition patients should take some oral nutrients to ensure maximal stimulation of the gastrointestinal tract, for gastrointestinal tract adaptation, and to diminish bacterial translocation. Oral intake also stimulates bile flow and decreases the likelihood of developing sludge or forming gallstones. Speech therapy and occupational therapy should be offered to infants and toddlers to prevent oral aversion.

PREPARATION FOR HOME PARENTERAL NUTRITION

Caretakers and Discharge Requirements

Home parenteral nutrition requires a multidisciplinary team including medical specialists, nurses, pharmacists, dietitians, social workers, and child psychiatrists. Expect at least a week for family caretakers to become familiar and competent in the basics of HPN. Family members need to be taught aseptic technique and central line care. They need to know how to add medications to the solution, how to operate an infusion pump, how to identify potential complications, and the expected outcome of therapy. To ensure that caregivers are competent, it is recommended that they room-in with the patient prior to discharge and demonstrate competency in giving care. Two home caretakers are preferable to one. Prior to discharge, a home visit should confirm that there is a phone, adequate space for HPN supplies, and a refrigerator to store HPN solutions. Cleanliness of the home is also critical. Equipment should be delivered to the home prior to discharge from the hospital. A nurse should visit the home in the first 24 hours after beginning HPN to evaluate competency and the need for ongoing visits.

Home Infusion Provider Requirements

The home infusion provider (homecare company) should be experienced in providing care for pediatric HPN patients (see Table 10–2) and licensed and accredited by the Joint Commission on Accreditation of Healthcare Organizations (JCAHO) or another accrediting organization specific to homecare such as the Accreditation Commission for Health Care, Inc (ACHC). The home infusion provider should employ nursing staff with pediatric experience and have 24-hour on-call support staff. The pharmacy providing the HPN should be experienced in pediatric needs for HPN and be licensed by a state board of pharmacy.

TABLE 10–2   Evaluation of a Home Infusion Provider

Background
- Size of company
- Years in operation
- Number of pediatric patients served
- Other groups using the company

Geography
- Area served
- Location of company headquarters
- Location of pharmacy

Pharmacy
- Frequency of solution mixing
- Frequency of deliveries
- Ability to respond to emergencies

Personnel
- Pharmacist
- Pediatric nurse
- Dietitian
- 24-hour nurse and pharmacist availability
- Blood drawing capabilities

Patient Education
- Availability of in-hospital teaching
- Home teaching

Financial
- Insurance contracts
- Governmental coverage — Medicaid/Medicare
- State-sponsored programs [e.g., California Children's Services (CCS)]
- Indigent care policy

Equipment and Supplies

Regardless of the types of technology used, pediatric HPN patients require an individualized list of supplies that needs periodic updating (see Table 10–3). For safety, the pump should have a lockout and the company should be able to supply replacement equipment quickly in the event of equipment malfunction. A back-up pump may be helpful.

TABLE 10–3   Sample Supply List for Pediatric HPN[4]

- HPN solution
- Lipid solution
- Multivitamin injection
- Medication additives?
- Infusion pumps — two or multi-channel
- IV pole
- Tubing for infusion of HPN and lipids
- Extension sets
- Alcohol wipes
- Heparin flush syringes
- Normal saline flush syringes
- Injection connectors without needles
- Hypodermic syringes/needles for additives
- Site dressing supplies
- Dextrose 10% for emergency use
- Sharps container
- Adequate refrigerator space for HPN and medication storage
- Portable backpack for HPN solutions with an appropriate pump

---

ADMINISTRATION OF HPN

Access

The type of access depends on the duration of therapy, the child's other needs, the child's lifestyle, family preference, and the physician and healthcare team's experience and knowledge of available products (see Table 10–4). Choices include:

- Peripherally inserted central venous catheters (PICCs)
- Tunneled venous catheters: Hickman-Broviac®
- Totally implantable venous access systems: Infuse-A-Port®, Port-A-Cath®, MediPort®

Special catheters

- Catheters impregnated with chlorhexadine and silver sulfadiazine may reduce the incidence of catheter sepsis.[8,9]
- Silicone (Silastic) catheters can lower the incidence of thrombosis and vein perforation.

TABLE 10–4   Access for Parenteral Nutrition[5]

Type	Duration of HPN	Advantages	Disadvantages
Peripheral IV	<2 weeks	—Can maintain existing weight for normally nourished patient	—Can only tolerate osmolarity of 300–900 mOsm/L —High risk of losing IV, sclerosis, phlebitis
PICC	1 month	—Single or double lumens available	
Non-implanted catheters	>1 month	—Single, double, or triple lumens available	—Not recommended for home use
Implanted (tunneled catheters)	>1 month	—Single, double, or triple lumen	
Totally implanted venous system ("Port")	>1 month	—Single or double lumen —No external portion allows free mobility when not using an access needle —Best for intermittent access —More difficult to clear catheter infections than with tunneled catheters[6,7]	—Needle access may be painful —Daily need for needle access makes it less desirable for HPN —Mobility may be limited during port access due to risk of needle dislodgement

Evaluating Placement

A physician is often required to evaluate or re-evaluate proper placement of the tip of a central venous catheter. Parenteral nutrition solutions infused in a noncentral catheter should be limited to an osmolarity ≤ 900 mOsm/L. Clinicians should consult their pharmacy for an estimation of solution osmolarity if solutions of high osmolarity are desired (see Table 10–5). The location of the catheter tip, central or noncentral, must be confirmed by X-ray and must be documented in the medical record.

- **"Central"** The tip is in the superior vena cava (SVC) (including the brachiocephalic-SVC junction, right atrium (RA) or inferior

TABLE 10–5 Osmolarity of Selected Parenteral Nutrition Preparations

Dextrose %	Amino acid %	Additives	Osmolarity
10	2	Standard	830
10	2	Standard, 40 mEq KCl/L	870
10	2	Standard, 60 mEq KCl/L	910
12.5	2	Standard	956

vena cava (IVC). The tip of the catheter should be in the SVC, near but not in the right atrium. Ideally, the catheter should be at the junction of the SVC and right atrium.

- **"Non-central"** The tip is in the internal jugular, external jugular, subclavian, axillary, and saphenous veins.

Cycling Parenteral Nutrition

Cycling PN (parenteral nutrition) is defined as providing PN over a time less than 24 hours a day. It allows patients to have increased mobility to perform tasks of daily living and to achieve motor developmental milestones, because they are not connected to the infusion pump for the entire day. Most patients can receive a cyclic HPN cycle. A prerequisite is a stable HPN regimen. Duration of infusion time may vary from 8 to 17 hours, depending on the patient's age, nutritional requirements, medications, and enteral intake. In general, infants less than 6 months old should be cycled over at least 16 hours. Many centers have successfully tapered such patients to 4 to 6 hours off PN. Infants between 6 and 12 months can tolerate cycles of 12 hours, and older children may tolerate times as short as 8 hours. Regardless of the total time, the infusion should not be stopped abruptly. Daily HPN administration should be initiated gradually, increasing usually over the first hour to goal rate and gradually decreased over the last hour or so of the infusion. This will help avoid the metabolic complications of hyperglycemia and hypoglycemia.

An HPN cycling calculator is available at http://peds.stanford.edu/tpn.html.[10] Some pumps can be programmed to automatically ramp up and down on cycled HPN.

PARENTERAL NUTRITION REQUIREMENTS

Calories

There are many different recommendations and methods to calculate the caloric needs of children (see Table 10–6 and Table 10–7). The Harris-Benedict equations were developed for use with normal adults and have been applied empirically to children.[11] The World Health Organization (WHO) recommendations provide an estimated resting energy expenditure (REE), which may then be multiplied by a factor to adjust for catch-up growth, activity, and medical status.[12] In obese patients (>120% ideal body weight), the Schofield height/weight equation has been used to more accurately predict energy needs.[13]

Predictive equations often do not accurately reflect the patients' needs.[14] Earlier studies of adults suggested that stresses, such as sepsis, increased caloric requirements by as much as 40%. These conclusions have since been questioned. Severe stress in children probably does not increase requirements by any more than 15%. Decreased physical activity may reduce demands and balance the increased needs due to the stress of underlying disorders. If extremely accurate measurements are needed, then energy expenditure can be measured using indirect calorimetry.[15,16] Indirect calorimetry can be helpful in assessing the patient with increased needs and for those not responding appropriately to nutritional therapy. Indirect calorimeters can measure resting energy expenditure in infants as small as 3 kg as well as children and adolescents.

Protein

Adequate protein intake must be provided for optimal caloric utilization and growth (see Table 10–8). Infants and children have better weight gain and positive nitrogen balance when receiving "pediatric formulations" than when receiving adult formulations. Children with catabolic states or with a protein-losing enteropathy may require more protein than standard recommendations. The following are available types of amino acid solutions:

TABLE 10–6   Equations Used for Estimation of Basal Energy Expenditure

Harris-Benedict (kcal/day)[11]
   Boys: REE = 66.437 + (13.752 x wt) + (5.003 x ht) − (6.755 x age)
   Girls: REE = 655.096 + (9.563 x wt) + (1.85 x ht) − (4.676 x age)
 (wt = kg, ht= cm, age = years)

Schofield weight and height (MJ/day)[13]
   Children less than 3 years of age
      Boys: REE = 0.0007 x weight (kg) + 6.349 x height (m) − 2.584.
      Girls: REE = 0.068 x weight (kg) + 4.281 x height (m) − 1 730
   Children 3 to 10 years of age
      Boys: REE = [0.082 x weight (kg)] + [0.545 x (height /100)] + 1.736
      Girls: REE = (0.071 x wt) + [0.677 x (ht/100)] + 1.553
   Children 10 to 18 years of age
      Boys: REE = (0.068 x wt) + [0.574 x (ht/100)] + 2.157
      Girls: REE = (0.035 x wt) + [1.948 x (ht/100)] + 0.837
 (1 kcal = 4.186 x 10^3 joules (J)[1] 1 mega joule (MJ) = 10^6 joules)

World Health Organization (kcal/day) for children less than 3 years of age[12]
   Children less than 3 years of age
      Boys: REE = 60.9 x weight (kg) − 54
      Girls: REE = 61.0 x weight (kg) − 51
   Older Children
      Boys: REE = (16.6 x wt) + (77 x ht) + 572
      Girls: REE = (7.4 x wt) + (482 x ht) +217

TABLE 10–7   Recommended Energy Intake for Age

Age (years)	Females (kcal/kg/day)	Males (kcal/kg/day)
0–0.5	90–110	90–110
0.5–1	80–100	80–100
1–3	90	90
4–6	80–90	80–90
7–10	70–80	70–80
11–14	45	55
15–18	40	45

For patients who are normally nourished, use actual weight; for those who are malnourished, use the ideal.

TABLE 10–8   Protein Requirements

Age (yr)	Protein (g/kg/day)
0–0.5	2.5–3 (occasionally 3.5–4)
0.5–1	2–2.5
1–14	1–2
15–18 (boys)	0.9–2
15–18 (girls)	0.8–2

- **Adult amino acid solutions** can lead to high plasma concentrations of some amino acids such as methionine, glycine, and phenylalanine and low plasma concentrations of branched-chain amino acids (leucine, isoleucine, and valine). They can also be deficient in histidine, aspartic acid, glutamic acid, tyrosine, and cysteine. Adult formulas lack taurine.
- **TrophAmine®** (B Braun, Irvine, CA) is a pediatric solution that normalizes plasma amino acid levels within the range for 2-hour postprandial levels in healthy 30-day-old infants that are breast-fed.[17] Studies of this product have been conducted in preterm and term infants and older children.
- **Aminosyn-PF®** (Abbott Laboratories) is a pediatric product marketed as comparable to TrophAmine. However, two studies have shown lower incidence of cholestasis with TrophAmine than Aminosyn-PF.[18–20]

Carbohydrate

The major source of nonprotein calories in parenteral nutrition is D-glucose, provided in monohydrate form.

- D-glucose yields 3.4 kcal/g (rather than 4 kcal/g of enteral glucose) and provides most of the osmolality in the HPN solution.
- Glucose should be increased incrementally to allow an appropriate response of endogenous insulin.
- Keeping volume constant, glucose concentration can be increased in increments of 2.5% to 5% dextrose per day.
- Signs and symptoms of excessive glucose load include: hyperglycemia, glucosuria and osmotic diuresis, water retention, increased car-

TABLE 10–9 Dosing for Intravenous Fat

Age (yr)	Starting Dose (g/kg/day)	Daily Dose Increase (g/kg/day)	Maximum Dose (g/kg/day)
0–0.5	1–1.5	1–1.5	3.5
0.5–1	1–1.5	1–1.5	3
1–10	1	1–1.5	3
11–18	1	1	2–3

bon dioxide production with respiratory compromise, and hepatic steatosis.

Fat

Intravenous fat provides a concentrated source of isotonic calories and prevents or reverses essential fatty acid deficiency (see Table 10–9).

- Infuse fat separately from the dextrose/amino acid solution.
- Administer at least 2–4% of calories from fat (0.5 to 1 g/kg/day) to avoid essential fatty acid deficiency.
- Do not administer more than 60% of calories as fat to avoid ketosis.
- Use a 20% solution (2 kcal/mL), which is cleared more effectively than a 10% solution.
- Infuse over 24 hours whenever possible to avoid large fluctuations in plasma lipids.
- Do not use an infusion rate exceeding 0.15 g/kg/hour.
- Current solutions do not contain eicosapentaenoic and docosahexaenoic acid (EPA, DHA).

Fluids and Electrolytes

- Fluid requirements depend on size, age, environmental factors, and underlying disease (see Table 10–10).
- It may be necessary to give fluids in excess of maintenance to provide adequate calories.
- Do not use PN to replace ongoing losses, because PN contains not only electrolytes, but also protein, vitamins, and minerals.

TABLE 10–10   Fluid Recommendations for Parenteral Nutrition

Initial volume for patients free of cardiovascular or renal disease:

- < 10 kg = 100 ml/kg/day
- 10–30 kg = 2,000 ml/m²/day
- 30–50 kg = 100 mL/hour (2.4 L/day)
- > 50 kg = 124 mL/hour (3 L/day)

Increase in volume to reach desired caloric intake:

- In infants, by 10 ml/kg/day (maximum 200 mL/kg/day, if tolerated)
- Patients > 10 kg by 10% of initial volume per day (maximum 4,000 mL/m²/day, if tolerated)

- Specifically designed replacement fluids should be used for ongoing losses.
- Electrolyte provision and supplementation is done based on individual and patient-specific needs and based on published expert guidelines.[21] If a patient receives PN for more than 30 days without significant enteral intake, then trace elements should be added. (see Table 10–11, Table 10–12, and Table 10–13).

Trace Elements

- Omit copper and manganese in cases of significant cholestasis. Omit selenium, chromium, and molybdenum in patients with significant renal dysfunction.
- Many centers do not routinely add molybdenum due to rare evidence for deficiency states. One source recommends 1 μg/kg/day for the low birth weight infant.[22]

Calcium and Phosphorus

- Serum calcium can be normal despite bone demineralization.
- Serum phosphorus is a better indicator of total body stores.
- Plasma alkaline phosphatase levels six times the adult upper limit of normal should prompt investigation for rickets.
- The ideal calcium to phosphorus ratio is 1.3:1 to 1.7:1.
- Calcium and phosphorus may precipitate in solution. Solubility is dependent on
  - Concentration
  - Calcium to phosphorus ratio

TABLE 10–11 Electrolyte, Mineral, Trace Element Requirements[23]

Additive	Infants and Toddlers	Children	Adolescents
Sodium	2–4 mEq/kg	2–4 mEq/kg	60–150 mEq
Potassium	2–4 mEq/kg	2–4 mEq/kg	70–180 mEq
Chloride	2–4 mEq/kg	2–4 mEq/kg	60–150 mEq
Magnesium (125 mg/mEq)	0.25–1 mEq/kg	0.25–1 mEq/kg	8–32 mEq
Trace elements	0.2 mL/kg, max 5 mL (Pediatric trace elements)	0.2 mL/kg, max 5 mL (Pediatric trace elements)	5 mL (Adult trace elements)
Selenium (maximum 60 μg/day)[40]	2 μg/kg	2 μg/kg	2 μg/kg
Molybdenum (maximum 5 μg/day)	0.25 μg/kg/day	0.25 μg/kg/day	0.25 μg/kg/day

TABLE 10–12 Composition of Parenteral Trace Element Solutions

Ingredient	Adult Trace Elements/mL	Pediatric Trace Elements/mL
Zinc	1 mg	1 mg
Copper	0.4 mg	0.1 mg
Manganese	100 μg	25 μg
Chromium	4 μg	1 μg

- ○ Temperature
- ○ pH
- The pH determined primarily by the amino acid solution.
- Aminosyn-PF and TrophAmine have a lower pH than adult formulations.
- Calcium phosphate is more soluble at cooler temperatures.
- Avoid three-in-one (amino acid, carbohydrate, and lipid) solutions.
  - ○ Maximal calcium and phosphorus levels cannot be achieved in three-in-one solutions.

TABLE 10–13   Individual Trace Elements Supplementation if Parenteral Trace Elements are Unavailable or Omitted[24]

Trace Element	<5 years old	>5 years to adolescent
Zinc	50–125 µg/kg	2–5 mg
Copper	5–20 µg/kg	200–500 µg
Chromium	0.14–0.2 µg/kg	5–15 µg
Manganese	1 µg/kg	50–150 µg
Selenium (maximum 60 µg)	1–2 µg/kg	40–60 µg

TABLE 10–14   Recommended Amounts of Calcium and Phosphorus

Age Group	Calcium Gluconate (mg/kg/day)*	Phosphate (mM/kg/day)**
Full-term infants	300–500	1–1.5
Older infants and children	100–200	1
Adolescents	50–100	0.5–1

*20 mg Ca to each mEq Ca; 1 mL of a 10% solution of calcium gluconate gives 9.3 mg of elemental calcium.

**31 mg PO4 to each mMole PO4.

- o Three-in-one solutions may disguise calcium-phosphorus precipitates.

Vitamins

(see Table 10–15)

- There are multivitamin preparations for IV administration with PN designed for children older than 11 years old and for children older than 11 years old to adult. Appropriate dosage amounts should be based on weight and/or age in children.
- Previously, Vitamin K was not supplied in multivitamin preparations. Intravaneous multivitamins are currently available with and without Vitamin K.
- Patients receiving oral supplements may need adjustments of their parenteral multivitamin dose.

TABLE 10–15   Parenteral Vitamin Solutions Currently Available

Ingredient	MVI®* Adult/10 mL	MVI® Pediatric/5 mol
Vitamin A	1 mg (3300 IU)	0.7 mg (2300 IU)
Vitamin C	200 mg	80 mg
Vitamin D	5 μg (200 IU)	10 μg (400 IU)
Vitamin E	10 mg (10 IU)	7 mg (7 IU)
Vitamin B₁ (thiamine)	6 mg	1.2 mg
Vitamin B₂ (riboflavin)	3.6 mg	1.4 mg
Vitamin B₆ (pyridoxine)	6 mg	1 mg
Vitamin B₁₂ (cyanocobalamin)	5 μg	1 μg
Vitamin K	150 μg**	200 μg***
Niacin	40 mg	17 mg
Dexpanthenol	15 mg	5 mg
Folic acid	600 μg	140 μg
Biotin	60 μg	20 μg

*MVI is a registered trademark of Mayne Pharmaceuticals.

Infuvite® is a registered trademark of Baxter. Infuvite Pediatric is an acceptable alternative (also in 5 ml vials).

**As phylloquinone.

***As phytonadione.

- Failure to provide parenteral vitamins may lead to clinical deficiency states, especially thiamine deficiency.
- Vitamins may be lost through adsorption to plastic PN bags and tubing.
- Light may cause biodegradation.

PARENTERAL IRON

Pediatric patients have received iron dextran (INFeD®) in their infusates at a daily dose of 0.5 mg to 1 mg of elemental iron per day. Adults have received 2 mg of elemental iron per day. There have been no published adverse physiochemical or clinical effects. Such use is only with non-IV fat emulsions. INFeD® is not compatible with 3-in-1 PN solutions. Even then, this use of INFeD® requires caution because of compatibility issues. The INFeD® package insert states, "Do not mix INFeD® with other medications or add to parenteral nutrition solutions for intravenous infusion."

Iron infusions should be administered separate from the HPN. Iron can be provided as sodium ferric gluconate complex in sucrose (Ferrlecit®) or as iron dextran. There are standard equations for iron supplementation.[25]

INSULIN

- Insulin may be required to improve caloric intake in the face of hyperglycemia.
- Typical dosage is 1 unit of regular insulin per 10 g of glucose; check serum glucose. (See Chapter 12 for more information on glucose management.)

OTHER ADDITIVES

H_2-receptor antagonists such as famotidine or ranitidine can reduce amino acid-associated gastric acid secretion and ostomy output in children with short-bowel syndrome and hypersecretion.

MONITORING

The frequency and breadth of monitoring depends on the stability of the patient and the patient's underlying condition. Initially, anthropometrics and laboratory draws are frequent, but as the patient reaches a stable HPN regimen, both anthropometrics and laboratory draws can be spaced out over longer periods of time. Guidelines for patients on long-term HPN monitoring in children is found in Table 10–16.

COMPLICATIONS

An experienced team minimizes the incidence of complications. In large studies of catheter-related complications,[26,27] deaths were rare, and few were related to HPN. Of the HPN-related deaths, the most common causes were catheter-related and cirrhosis. As experience is increasing with minimizing the risk for hepatic complications, catheter complica-

TABLE 10–16 Clinical and Laboratory Monitoring for Home PN

Clinical or laboratory parameter	Initial monitoring	Long-term monitoring
Anthropometrics[1]	Baseline Daily weight check	<2 years old: every 2–4 weeks >2 years old: every month
Complete blood count	Baseline then weekly	Weekly to monthly
Electrolytes[2]	Baseline then daily	Weekly to monthly
BUN and creatinine	Baseline then daily	Weekly to monthly
Calcium, magnesium, phosphorus	Baseline then daily	Weekly to monthly
Serum or finger-stick glucose[3]	Daily	Weekly to monthly
Serum triglycerides[4]	Baseline then daily	Weekly to monthly
Serum cholesterol	Baseline then weekly	Weekly to monthly
Alkaline phosphatase	Baseline then weekly	Weekly to monthly
Total protein and albumin	Baseline then weekly	Weekly to monthly
Prealbumin	Baseline then weekly	Weekly to monthly
Liver function studies[5]	Baseline then weekly	Weekly to monthly
Iron studies[6]	Baseline	Every 3 months
Vitamin A, Vitamin E, 25-OH Vitamin D		Every 6 months
Prothrombin time		Every 6 months
Serum selenium, zinc, copper, chromium, and whole blood manganese		Every 6 months
Bone mineral density		Yearly

[1] Anthropometrics include baseline weight, length, mid-arm circumference, and if applicable, head circumference.

[2] Sodium, potassium, chloride, carbon dioxide.

[3] Serum glucose should be closely monitored during 1) periods of glucosuria, 2) for 2 to 3 days after cessation of PN.

[4] Triglycerides should be measured fasting or 4 hours after an increase in cose.

[5] ALT (SGPT), AST (SGOT), total and conjugated bilirubin, GGT.

[6] Serum ferritin, TIBC, serum iron.

tions have become the most significant. Nonfatal complications can include, in order of frequency, mechanical complications (obstruction, dislodgement, rupture, and superior vena cava syndrome), sepsis, hepatic complications, and metabolic complications.[27]

CATHETER SEPSIS

Children have a higher incidence of catheter infection than do adults.[28] However, catheter sepsis is less frequent among patients on HPN than among hospitalized patients receiving PN.[1] Catheter infections are usually caused by a known or unsuspected break in standard technique for HPN. The lower incidence of catheter infection at home reflects the positive impact of one dedicated caregiver who is well trained in meticulous catheter care. There is a longer lifespan of the second catheter as well as a higher incidence of catheter-related complications of HPN in the first 2 years versus later years. This decreasing incidence of infections reflects increased experience and vigilance. The most effective ways to prevent catheter sepsis are to educate and train healthcare providers who maintain the catheters, to use maximal sterile barrier precautions, and to use 2% chlorhexadine preparation for skin antisepsis.[29] Scrubbing the catheter hub and the area surrounding the catheter is important. Catheters should not be routinely replaced to prevent infection.[30]

With each fever, HPN patients should be evaluated with a careful history and physical examination. If there is no identifiable source of infection, then the differential is most likely a catheter infection or intercurrent viral infection.

Evaluation of a fever in a patient on HPN should include the following:[31]

- Complete blood count (CBC)
- Central and peripheral blood culture: aerobic, anaerobic, fungal; culture all ports
- Urinalysis, urine culture
- Chest X-ray
- If suspected, the HPN solution should be cultured for possible contamination; there are reports of contaminated HPN solution leading to sepsis[23]

Treatment may be started empirically or the clinician may await test results. Usually, the patient should be admitted for initial treatment. Once the patient is afebrile and clinically stable for 24 hours, the physician can consider continuing treatment at home, provided the family is adequately trained to administer IV antibiotics and is competent in recognizing signs of deterioration. The empiric antibiotics should cover staphylococcal and gram-negative organisms. The patient should receive intravenous antibiotics because most HPN patients cannot absorb oral antibiotics. Bloodstream infections should be treated "through the line," and antibiotics should be alternated through all lumens of the catheter. Antibiotic locks can be used when the identity of an organism and sensitivity are known.[32] The use of antibiotic locks is not in the scope of this chapter; consultation with pediatric infectious disease is recommended. In general, preserving the line is important because of the long-term need for vascular access. Fever alone is not an indication for removal of a catheter. Typically, infections with gram-negative organisms are more difficult to treat than infections with gram-positive organisms. In a large series, 87% of gram-positive and 53% of gram-negative infections were treated successfully without catheter removal.[24]

Catheter removal is required for the following reasons:

- Fungal infections (uncomplicated fungal infections may have exceptions)
- Septic shock
- Endocarditis
- Embolism
- Persistent fever with positive blood culture growth
- Disseminated intravascular coagulation (DIC)
- Peristent positive blood cultures after 72 hours of appropriate intravenous antibiotic treatment

After the catheter is removed, antimicrobial or antifungal therapy is continued for 5 to 7 days, and a new catheter is inserted after the patient is afebrile for 72 hours and blood cultures no longer contain the infectious organism. If the patient requires fluids, medications, or PN then a peripheral line may be placed with care taken to ensure osmolality of the formula is within the acceptable range for the peripheral venous system.

TABLE 10–17 Causes and Management of Catheter Occlusion

Cause	Management
Clot or thrombus	t-PA (Alteplase)
Fat deposition	70% ethanol
Calcium-phosphorus deposition	0.1 N Hydrochloric acid
Drug precipitation	0.1 N Hydrochloric acid or 0.1 N NaOH

TUNNEL TRACT INFECTIONS

Tunnel tract infections usually require catheter removal. Fifty percent of exit-site infections were successfully treated without catheter removal.[33–35] Fifty percent is not an excellent success rate. Most pediatric infectious physicians would recommend removal.

CATHETER OCCLUSION

Flushing with saline helps prevent fibrin sheath formation and clot development, which can occlude a line. The saline flush should be five times the catheter volume, and the catheter should be locked off with heparin. Nevertheless, occlusions can occur, and management depends on the type of occlusion (see Table 10–17). Causes of catheter occlusion include:

- Clot or thrombus
- Fibrin deposition
- Fat deposition
- Calcium-phosphorus precipitation
- Drug precipitation
- Kinking of the catheter
- Catheter tip against venous wall
- Excessively tight suture

Preventing occlusion should be a goal of HPN. Sola and associates[6] recommended administering low-dose aspirin therapy (80 mg/day) to all patients who did not have liver disease or other risks of bleeding. Acid-suppressing agents, such as H2 blockers, can decrease the gastric and duodenal irritation associated with long-term aspirin therapy. Treatment of catheter occlusion can include warfarin or low molecular weight heparin. The use of these drugs has been studied most extensively in cancer patients.[36,37] Ultrasonography can be helpful to identify a clot or to demonstrate catheter kinking or impingement against the vessel wall.

CATHETER MALPOSITION OR DISLODGEMENT

- Malposition of catheter can occur outside the vein, and hypertonic solutions can infuse into pleural or pericardial space.
- Symptoms are rapid hypoglycemia, circulatory or respiratory compromise, and hemorrhage.

CATHETER EMBOLI

- Silicone elastomer catheters perfused under high pressure can rupture.
- Tips of polyethylene catheters can shear during needle access.

CATHETER BREAKS OR LEAKS

Trauma, accidents, or repeated clamping can cause the external catheter tubing to break. Breaks require immediate repair, because there is a high risk of subsequent line sepsis. Repair kits are available, but if the damage is close to the catheter exit site, then the entire catheter will need to be replaced.

THOMBOPHLEBITIS

- Usually caused by hypertonic solutions infused through peripheral veins.
- Skin slough can result.
- Hyaluronidase (Wydase) can be helpful if given subcutaneously or intradermal within 1 hour after the event.

TABLE 10–18   Strategies to Prevent Hepatobiliary Complications

- Avoid overfeeding
- Avoid excessive lipid or glucose infusions
- Use pediatric amino acid formulations
- Cycle TPN
- Provide enteral stimulation
- Use strict catheter-care protocols to avoid sepsis

HEPATOBILIARY DISEASE

Cholestasis in children on long-term HPN has been associated with many factors (see Table 10–18). These include the patient's length of time on PN, length of time without gut stimulation, underlying disease (i.e., Crohn's disease), infection, and bacterial overgrowth. Deficiencies in some amino acids and excess in some elements (i.e., manganese) or nutrients such as phytosterols in lipid solutions are associated with cholestasis. (Length of remaining small bowel?) A lack of gut stimulation leads to bile stasis and chemical changes that can predispose patients on HPN to cholelithiasis or biliary sludge. Enteral feeding can reduce the incidence of these complications as well as chronic liver disease. Using pediatric amino acid formulations can decrease the incidence of chronic liver disease.[38]

Before attributing elevated transaminases to HPN, the clinician should evaluate the patient for viral hepatitis, drug reaction, or evidence of ischemic injury. Patients may have mildly elevated transaminases due to their preexisting disease.

When patients receiving HPN develop cholestasis, it is routine to remove copper and manganese from the HPN solution. Both of these trace elements are hepatotoxic and cleared by the liver. Because many centers use a solution of four trace elements (zinc, copper, manganese, and chromium), the trace element solution is held and zinc is added back separately. Severe copper deficiency has been reported in cholestatic patients who have had their trace elements withheld. Symptoms of copper deficiency include pancytopenia, depigmentation of the hair, and pseudoscurvy. Therefore, when withholding trace elements, it is wise to monitor serum copper at least monthly. Copper should be replaced if values are low.[39]

HEMATOLOGIC DISORDERS

There is a series report in the literature of thrombocytopenia in seven children on long-term HPN, all of whom were receiving only 1 to 2 g/day of fat emulsion;[40] however, the overall risk is low. The group at the University of California at Los Angeles, reporting their 18-year HPN experience, had no patients on long-term daily HPN with significant thrombocytopenia.[24]

NEUROLOGIC DISORDERS

There is also a report in the literature of two children on PN who experienced neurological complications of fat emulsion therapy without other systemic signs.[41] These children had seizures, weakness, and altered mental status. Biopsy revealed endothelial and intravascular lipid deposition.

Manganese toxicity can also lead to neurological disorders such as seizures and dystonia.[42] There are reports of manganese toxicity in patients on long-term HPN. Symptoms have included disturbed thought processes, gait abnormalities, hallucinations, and Parkinsonian symptoms. Because manganese is excreted in bile, it may be especially hazardous in patients with existing liver disease. Cholestatic patients should definitely have manganese removed from their HPN. Magnetic resonance imaging (MRI) of the brain in patients with manganese toxicity shows bilateral, symmetrical signal changes in the basal ganglia. These changes can be reversed, but the long-term neurological outcome in children with developing nervous systems is unknown. Until more data are available, it may be prudent to measure serial whole blood manganese levels, which is the most sensitive noninvasive monitoring technique. Clinicians should consider periodic brain MRIs. There have been no reports of manganese deficiency on long-term HPN.

METABOLIC DISORDERS

Electrolyte abnormalities may occur as a complication of HPN. These are usually avoidable if there is appropriate monitoring and follow-up.

Fluid imbalances are another avoidable complication. When initiating and weaning HPN, patients should keep strict input and output records, and practitioners should carefully monitor the patient for electrolyte disorders and hyperglycemia.

Low magnesium is a special concern among patients with short-bowel syndrome. Magnesium status is best measured with a 24-hour urine collection (some centers are capable of administering the sensitive "magnesium load" test).

NUTRIENT DEFICIENCIES AND EXCESSES

Since the guidelines for trace elements and vitamins (copper, zinc, manganese, chromium, selenium, biotin) have been developed, deficiency states previously described rarely occur on long-term HPN.[21] Serum zinc and selenium supplementation may be required in patients who have massive diarrhea and malabsorption.

Evidence suggests that chromium supplementation may lead to elevated chromium levels.[43] Chromium deficiencies can lead to diabetic symptoms,[44] and chromium excesses can lead to decreased glomerular filtration rates.[45] Iodide is a contaminant in water used in PN and is also a natural contaminant of a number of PN salts. Additionally, if iodide aseptic solutions are used in central venous line care, then this iodide is absorbed through the skin and contributes to normal iodide levels. Therefore, adding supplemental iodine to PN solutions is not necessary.

OUTCOMES

When initiating HPN, the physician should follow the family closely for the first few weeks. An appropriate follow-up plan for infants starting HPN should be weekly for the first month, then every 2 to 4 weeks. Older children can be seen every 1 to 3 months.

Physicians should emphasize enteral feedings at all visits. In children with extreme short-bowel syndrome, even small amounts of an oral diet facilitate socialization. When a child tolerates 50–75% of his or her calories from oral or enteral feeds, HPN can be gradually reduced. The physician can begin with decreasing calories from HPN by 10%. Commonly, children lose some weight immediately after stopping HPN. A study of children who received an average of over 1 year of HPN showed that long-term HPN, early in life, increased the risk for growth and nutritional abnormalities. The child's underlying primary gastrointestinal disorder can contribute to malabsorption. A significant proportion of patients will have abnormal bone density.[46]

The physician should perform a developmental evaluation at each visit. Frequent hospitalizations can lead to developmental delay. Home parenteral nutrition patients, appropriately managed, can have normal intelligence and motor function. A study of long-term HPN patients evaluating expressive language, perceptual motor function, visuomotor skills, and oromotor skills showed that long-term HPN patients are at risk for lower perceptual motor performance. Strength, range, and accuracy of oral movements in a group of long-term HPN patients were normal.[46]

RESOURCES FOR PRACTITIONERS

The following resources are helpful resources for medical providers:

- *Pediatric Nutrition Handbook*, from the American Academy of Pediatrics[21]
- "Parenteral Nutrition," by John Kerner, Jr. In: *Nutrition in Pediatrics: Basic Science and Clinical Applications*[47]
- "Parenteral Nutrition," by Susan Baker. In: *Pediatric Gastrointestinal Disease*[48]
- "Overview of Considerations for the Pediatric Patient Receiving Home Parenteral and Enteral Nutrition," by Jon A. Vanderhoof and Rosemary J. Young. In *Nutrition in Clinical Practice*, June 2003.[49]

RESOURCES FOR PATIENTS

The Oley Foundation is a national, independent, nonprofit organization that distributes information, organizes conference activities, and provides emotional support for families and caregivers. Families can access the Foundation's many resources including:

- Lifeline Letter, a bi-monthly newsletter for consumers
- "Choices in Nutrition: Understanding HPN Therapy Options" video available for rent or purchase. To obtain a copy, go to the

website at http://www.oley.org or call 800-776-OLEY or 518-262-5079.

- Regional coordinators to provide speakers and coordinate meetings
- Information Clearinghouse, which provides reputable information and access to similar families to discuss insurance issues, traveling, catheter care, and medical and research updates.

The Oley Foundation
214 Hun Memorial, A-28
Albany Medical Center
Albany, NY 12208-3478
1-800-776-OLEY (toll free in the USA and Canada)
1-518-262-5528 (outside the USA)
fax: 1-518-262-5528
e-mail: bishopj@mail.amc.edu

REFERENCES

1. Moukarzel AA, Ament, MA. Home parenteral nutrition in infants and children. In: Rombeau JL, Caldwell MD, eds. *Clinical Nutrition: Parenteral Nutrition. 2nd ed.* Philadelphia: W.B. Saunders;1993.
2. Misra S, Ament M, Reyen L. Home Parenteral Nutrition. In: Baker R, Jr, Baker S, Davis A, eds. *Pediatric Parenteral Nutrition.* New York: Chapman and Hall;1997:354–369.
3. American Society for Parenteral and Enteral Nutrition. Standards for nutrition support physicians. A.S.P.E.N. Board of Directors. *Nutr Clin Pract.* 1996;11:235–240.
4. Poole RL, Nishioka FY, Kerner J, Jr. Selecting a home infusion company. In: McConnell M, ed. *Guidelines for Pediatric Home Health Care.* Elk Grove Village, Ill: American Academy of Pediatrics;2002:97–103.
5. Maki DG, Stolz SM, Wheeler S, et al. Prevention of central venous catheter-related bloodstream infection by use of an antiseptic-impregnated catheter. A randomized, controlled trial. *Ann Intern Med.* 1997;127:257–266.
6. Veenestra DL, Saint S, Somnath S, et al. Efficacy of antiseptic-impregnated central venous catheters in preventing catheter-related bloodstream infection: a meta-analysis. *JAMA.* 1999;281:261–267.
7. Ament ME, Reyen L. The physician's perspective on home infusion therapy. In: McConnell M, ed. *Guidelines for Pediatric Home Health Care.* Elk Grove Village, Ill: American Academy of Pediatrics;2002:105–111.
8. Sola JE, Stone MM, Wise B, et al. Atypical thrombotic and septic complications of totally implantable venous access devices in patients with cystic fibrosis. *Pediatr Pulmonol.* 1992;14:239–242.

9. Flynn PM, Willis B, Gaur AH, Shenep JL. Catheter design influences recurrence of catheter-related bloodstream infection in children with cancer. *J Clin Oncol.* 2003;21(18):3520–3525.

10. Longhurst C, Naumovski L, Garcia-Careaga M, Kerner J. A practical guideline for calculating parenteral nutrition cycles. *Nutr Clin Pract.* 2003; 18:517–520.

11. World Health Organization. Energy and protein requirements: report of a joint FAO/WHO/UNU expert consultation. Geneva: World Health Organization; 1985.

12. Pencharz PB, Azcue MP. Measuring resting energy expenditure in clinical practice. *J Pediatr.* 1995;127:269–271.

13. Schofield WN. Predicting basal metabolic rate, new standards and review of previous work. *Hum Nutr Clin Nutr.* 1985;39(suppl 1):5–41.

14. Thomson MA, Bucolo S, Quirk P, Shepherd RW. Measured versus predicted resting energy expenditure in infants: a need for reappraisal. *J Pediatr.* 1995; 126(1):21–27.

15. Harris J, Benedict F. (Carnegie Institute of Washington). A biometric study of basal metabolism in man. 1919. Report No. 279.

16. Kaplan AS, Zemel BS, Neiswender KM, Stallings VA. Resting energy expenditure in clinical pediatrics: measured versus prediction equations. *J Pediatr.* 1995;127:200–205.

17. Wu PY, Edwards N, Storm MC. Plasma amino acid pattern in normal term breast-fed infants. *J Pediatr.* 1986;109:347–349.

18. Cloney DB, Bouthillier MJ, Staublin SA, et al. Total parenteral nutrition-associated cholestasis in neonates receiving two different pediatric amino acid formulation (Abstract). *Pharmacotherapy.* 1996;16:66.

19. Ernst K, Gaylord M, Burnette T, et al. Aminosyn PF associated with doubled incidence of neonatal cholestasis (Abstract). *Pediatr Res.* 2000;47:286A.

20. Wright K, Ernst KD, Gaylord MS, et al. Increased incidence of parenteral nutrition-associated cholestasis with aminosyn PF compared to trophamine. *J Perinatol.* 2003;23:444–450.

21. Greene HL, Hambidge KM, Schalner R, et al. Guidelines for the use of vitamins, trace elements, calcium, magnesium, and phosphorus in infants and children receiving total parenteral nutrition: report of the Subcommittee on Pediatric Parenteral Nutrient Requirements from the Committee on Clinical Practice Issues of the American Society for Clinical Nutrition. *Am J Clin Nutr.* 1988;48:1324–1342.

22. Friel JK, MacDonald AC, Mercer CN, et al. Molybdenum requirements for low-birth-weight infants receiving parenteral and enteral nutrition. *J Parenter Enteral Nutr.* 1999;23(3):155–159.

23. Kleinman RE, ed. *Pediatric Nutrition Handbook.* 5th edition: American Academy of Pediatrics, Committee on Nutrition; 2004.

24. Safe practices for parenteral nutrition formulations. National Advisory Group on Standards and Practice Guidelines for Parenteral Nutrition. *J Parenter Enteral Nutr.* 1998;22(2):49–66.

25. Kumpf VJ. Update on parenteral iron therapy. *Nutr Clin Pract.* 2003; 18:318–326.

26. De Potter S, Goulet O, Lamor M, et al. 263 patient-years of home parenteral nutrition in children. *Transplant Proc.* 1992;24:1056–1057.

27. Knafelz D, Gambarara A, Diamanti A, et al. Complications of home parenteral nutrition in a large pediatric series. *Transplant Proc.* 2003;35: 3050–3051.

28. National Nosocomial Infections Surveillance (NNIS) System Report. Data Summary from January 1992 through June 2004, issued October 2004. *AMJ Infect Control.* 2004 Dec;32(8):470–485.

29. Chaiyakunapruk N, Veenstra DL, Lipsky BA, Sullivan SD, Saint S. Vascular catheter site care: the clinical and economic benefits of chlorhexidine gluconate compared with povidone iodine. *Clin Infect Dis.* 2004 Sep 15;37(6): 764–771.

30. O'Grady NP, Alexander M, Dellinger EP, et al. Guidelines for the prevention of intravascular catheter-related infections. *Infect Control Hosp Epidemiol.* 2002;23(12):759–769.

31. Hodge D, Puntis JW. Diagnosis, prevention, and management of catheter related bloodstream infection during long term parenteral nutrition. *Arch Dis Child Fetal Neonatal Ed.* 2002;87(1):F21–F24.

32. Messing B, Peitra-Cohen S, Debure A, Beliah M, Bernier JJ. Antibiotic-lock technique: a new approach to optimal therapy for catheter-related sepsis in home-parenteral nutrition patients. *J Parenter Enteral Nutr.* 1988; 12:185–189.

33. Buchman AL, Moukarzel A, Goodson B, Herzog F, et al. Catheter-related infections associated with home parenteral nutrition and predictive factors for the need for catheter removal in their treatment. *J Parenter Enteral Nutr.* 1994;18:297–302.

34. Severien C, Nelson JD. Frequency of infections associated with implanted systems vs cuffed, tunneled Silastic venous catheters in patients with acute leukemia. *Am J Dis Child.* 1991;45:1433–1438.

35. Mermel LA, Farr BM, Sherertz RJ, et al. Guidelines for the management of intravascular catheter-related infections. *Clin Infect Dis.* 2001;32(9): 1249–1272.

36. Mismetti P, Mille D, LaPorte S, et al. Low-molecular-weight heparin (nadroparin) and very low doses of warfarin in the prevention of upper extremity thrombosis in cancer patients with indwelling long-term central venous catheters: a pilot randomized trial. *Haematologica.* 2003;88:67–73.

37. Bern MM, Lokich JJ, Wallach SR, et al. Very low doses of warfarin can prevent thrombosis in central venous catheters. A randomized prospective trial. *Ann Intern Med.* 1990;112:423–428.

38. Adamkin DH, McClead RE, Desai NS. Comparison of two neonatal intravenous amino acid formulations in preterm infants: a multicenter study. *J Perinatology.* 1991;11(4):375–382.

39. Hurwitz M, Garcia MG, Poole RL, Kerner JA. Copper deficiency during parenteral nutrition: a report of four pediatric cases. *Nutr Clin Pract.* 2004; 19:305–308.

40. Goulet O, Girot R, Maier-Redelsperger M, et al. Hematologic disorders following prolonged use of intravenous fat emulsions in children. *J Parenter Enteral Nutr.* 1986;10:284–288.

41. Colomb V, Jober-Giraud A, Lacaille F, et al. Role of lipid emulsions in cholestasis associated with long-term parenteral nutrition in children. *J Parenter Enteral Nutr.* 2000;24(6):345–350.

42. Fell JM, Reynolds AP, Meadows N, et al. Manganese toxicity in children receiving long-term parenteral nutrition. *Lancet.* 1996;347:1218–1221.

43. Hak EB, Storm MC, Helms RA. Chromium and zinc contamination of parenteral nutrient solution components commonly used in infants and children. *Am J Health Syst Pharm.* 1998;55(2):150–154.

44. Anderson RA. Chromium and parenteral nutrition. *Nutrition.* 1995;11(suppl 1):83–86.

45. Moukarzel AA, Song MK, Buchman AL, et al. Excessive chromium intake in children receiving total parenteral nutrition. *Lancet.* 1992;339:385–388.

46. Leonberg BL, Chuang E, Eicher P, et al. Long-term growth and development in children after home parenteral nutrition. *J Pediatr.* 1998;132(3):461–466.

47. Kerner J, Jr. Parenteral nutrition. In: Walker WA, Watkins JB, Duggan C, eds. *Nutrition in Pediatrics.* 3rd ed. Hamilton, Ontario, Canada: B.C. Decker;2003:957–985.

48. Baker SS, Baker RD. Parenteral nutrition. In: Walker WA, Goulet O, Kleinman RE, Sherman PS, Schneider BL, Sanderson IR, eds. *Pediatric Gastrointestinal Disease.* 4th edition, Vol. II. Hamilton, Ontario, Canada: B.C. Decker;2004:1958–1980.

49. Vanderhoof JA, Young RJ. Overview of considerations for the pediatric patient receiving home parenteral and enteral nutrition. *Nutr Clin Pract.* 2003; 18:221–226.

CHAPTER 11

Nursing Considerations in Home Parenteral and Enteral Nutrition

Sharon Woods, RN, MSN, CNSN
Marcia Boatwright, RN, CRNI

INTRODUCTION

Nutrition therapy based nursing care has changed dramatically over the years since nutrition support was first applied in the home in the 1970s. Early on, patients going home on parenteral nutrition (PN) received most of their instruction for their home care while in the hospital. Often this training period lasted 2 to 3 weeks. Home care technology has advanced and education techniques have also advanced to the point that some patients are initiated on parenteral and enteral nutrition in the home without hospital admission.

There are many components of nursing care for home parenteral and enteral nutrition (HPEN) patients. These include evaluation and preparation of the patient for home nutrition support, education, clinical monitoring, and psychosocial considerations. Many excellent resources are available that outline the care of the HPEN patient. In addition to providing an overview of the components of nursing care in the home, this chapter will include information gleaned from years of providing nursing care for HPEN patients, specifically, home parenteral nutrition (HPN) patients.

PREDISCHARGE PLANNING

Many patients today experience shorter hospitalization periods, are discharged more acutely ill, and have had minimal or no instruction regarding HPEN therapy during their hospital admission. These patients are not in a "readiness to learn" state because of their heightened anxiety level, having received medical determination that an invasive therapy, HPN, is required for restitution of their health. They experience an apprehension of what HPN therapy entails as well as the impact on their lifestyle and quality of life. The nurse clinician must consider that these patients are struggling through a grieving process for what they may consider as their "failing body" and recent disease diagnosis.

Many times, patients have some limited knowledge and understanding of others who have received HPN therapy, or they have been provided with sketchy information from friends. Anxiety and fear may compound as the anticipated discharge date approaches. A predischarge hospital visit to the patient and care partner by the nurse who will be providing the HPN in the home can aid in alleviation of their anxiety. During the initial visit, the nurse clinician has the opportunity to introduce himself/herself, to introduce the nutrition support team, and to provide an overview of the infusion provider, the purpose and principles of HPEN therapy, therapy requirements, patient rights and responsibilities, and a customized plan of care.

Patient and care-partner teaching within the hospital setting prior to discharge can be challenging for all involved parties. Routine hospital nursing care can create frequent interruptions. Placing a "teaching in progress" sign on the patient's door can help to eliminate a portion of the interruptions. A care partner may not have the ability to take time away from work or other family responsibilities for scheduled predischarge teaching sessions. This can cause additional stress in an already stressed patient, if he or she feels that he or she must understand and remember a significant amount of new information. Assuring the patient and care partner that HPN therapy teaching can be done safely within the home setting can help to minimize that concern.

Similarly, patients who will receive home enteral nutrition (HEN) can benefit from a predischarge visit from the clinician (nurse or dietitian) working with the HEN provider. This visit may not be a part of the discharge planning, and the patient/caregiver must rely on the hospital staff or nutrition support team for instructions. An initial nursing visit can usually be arranged after discharge to teach HEN administration. If the patient is receiving his or her HEN via a pump, then there are video programs that the patient can obtain (from the home care provider or the pump manufacturer) that can teach them how to operate the equipment. Detailed booklets on HEN therapy are also available from the home care provider or the manufacturer of the enteral formula (see Chapter 6).

Keeping the patient and care partner informed of care coordination and discharge planning also empowers their active participation in their plan of care. With predischarge visits, the nurse clinician is able to establish a strong, ongoing relationship with the patient and care partner that serves as a positive introduction to the multidisciplinary home nutrition support team (HNST).

With subsequent predischarge visits, the nurse clinician has the opportunity to provide a basic overview of the following topics: HPN services, safety and infection control, supply management, HPN solution storage and preparation, administrative procedures, catheter care, self monitoring, management of potential complications, and medical care coordination. This basic overview provides the patient and care partner the opportunity to identify questions of concern. It also allows the nurse clinician the opportunity to clarify any misconceptions or unnecessary fears. A visit from another experienced HPN client to the patient and care partner to discuss his or her HPN experience prior to discharge can assist in decreasing the patient's anxiety and fear.

PSYCHOSOCIAL IMPLICATIONS WITH HPEN

Patients experience many psychological stressors when dealing with their underlying disease states that necessitate the need for HPEN therapy. This may include the effects of body image changes due to central vascular device placement, incisions, wounds, stomas, gastrointestinal (GI) tubes and/or drains, and the knowledge that HPEN will be necessary for a period of time or for a lifetime. Patients may have a previous history of pain, depression, substance abuse, or ineffective coping mechanisms prior to initial HPN therapy.[1]

A detailed history is essential and beneficial in identifying psychological factors that hold impact or potential impact on the patient's HPEN teaching, plan of care, and long-term clinical outcomes. A patient's usual coping mechanisms may not be effective at this period of time due to the degree of illness, a prolonged illness or hospitalization, grief, sleep deprivation, pain, fear of death, perceived loss of independence, and lack of available family or care-partner support. The patient and care partner will psychologically benefit from an opportunity to meet with the nurse clinician or a member of the HNST to ask those immediate and priority questions that they hold as their primary concern about HPEN therapy.

Patients seldom initiate questions or discussion regarding their feelings regarding body image changes, feelings of self-worth, or their expression of sexuality toward their partners. The nurse clinician's open discussion of these possible concerns can facilitate further discussion by the patient and partner. Identifying HPEN support groups and local HPEN patients can be of benefit for the patient and partner as a source of information from others who are experiencing similar issues.[2]

Other psychosocial aspects that hold concern for patients are the changes in independence, mobility, comfort, and accommodating clothing (e.g., to cover central vascular catheters, ostomies, GI tubes) because of their HPEN therapy. These patients often have questions regarding the financial implications of HPEN therapy. Patients who are unable to eat are challenged, as many social gatherings revolve around food and beverages. These types of activities may be a challenge or a temptation for the patient who has been instructed to remain non per os (NPO) or has been instructed to avoid specific foods and beverages.

The nurse clinician and nutrition support team should coordinate community resources such as religious organizations, a local psychologist, a pain-management clinic, financial aide, and community counseling resources into the patient's plan of care. The role of the care partner in obtaining successful HPEN therapy outcomes cannot be overestimated; therefore, any factors that may affect the health and well being of that individual must be addressed.

TRANSITION FROM HOSPITAL TO HOME

Today's hospitalized patients are discharged to home more acutely ill. They are often experiencing a new medical diagnosis. There may be some degree of grieving once the patient realizes that they require HPEN therapy. They may struggle with body image issues and hold concerns regarding necessary lifestyle changes.[3] The patient has observed nursing care aspects of HPEN therapy throughout the hospitalization period and begins to question how this therapy will be administered within his or her home. Care coordination and continuity of HPEN therapy details provided by the nurse clinician assist the patient and care partner in the transition from hospital to home. The care partner is so vital to the patient's successful HPEN therapy and care outcomes that the role of the care partner cannot be overestimated.

The day of discharge from the hospital is an exhausting one for the patient and his or her entire family. For some, the travel distance to home can be significant by car or plane. Fatigue, generalized weakness due to hospitalization, and the excitement of actually going home combined with an element of apprehension about beginning HPEN therapy in his or home environment creates an overwhelming experience. The patient's emotions run the gamut from excitement to depression, and his or her coping skills may be stressed.

The nurse clinician may recommend or empower family members to minimize visitors and guests to the home for several days following the patient's discharge. This plan of action allows the patient and the care partner adequate periods of rest and relaxation and time to acclimate back to their home environment as well as to the new HPEN responsibilities. Oftentimes the initial home visit for start of care and assistance in the HPEN set-up and administration connection requires 2–3 hours of time. Patients and care partners express relief in knowing that clinical support, both pharmacy and nursing, are available for questions, concerns, and troubleshooting assistance by telephone 24 hours a day.

INITIAL PATIENT ASSESSMENT

Upon referral of a patient within the infusion therapy provider's system and prior to discharge home, the care coordination process begins. This process includes a patient assessment to determine if the patient is appropriate for HPEN therapy services and to ensure that the patient will receive these HPEN therapy services within a safe environment at home. With the primary goal being the patient and care partner's independence with HPEN therapy, it is important to ascertain that the patient and care partner are willing and physically and emotionally capable of learning the HPEN administration procedures and self-monitoring responsi-

---

TABLE 11–1   Factors Critical to the Successful Delivery of HPEN
Therapy

- Consent and agreement to receive therapy within home setting
- Safe home environment
  - secured area for supplies and sharps container
  - location of stairs or levels within home
- Electrical resource
- Refrigeration
- Running water to facilitate hand washing
- Telephone service
  - 911 or emergency medical service within region
- Participating care partner
- Local physician available for non-HPEN therapy needs

---

bilities of the therapy. There are a number of important factors that are critical to successful HPEN therapy delivery as seen in Table 11–1.[4]

The entire multidisciplinary HNST must address factors that may have a potential impact on the HPEN plan of care and the patient's clinical outcomes such as:

- history of substance abuse
- non-compliance
- negative physical and/or emotional behaviors
- frequent physician changes

Addressing those factors is of key importance for developing a customized treatment plan and for improving patient compliance. A team meeting or a care conference involving various members of the hospital health care staff and the HNST can provide resolutions to complex patient issues or environmental concerns. The HNST utilizes their clinical expertise, experiences, resources, and patient education to ensure individualized HPEN therapy that is safe and effective.

TEACHING ADMINISTRATION PROCEDURES

Patients and care partners usually receive written and verbal instructions regarding HPEN therapy followed by demonstration of various procedures such as catheter care, dressing changes, and HPEN set-up and administration. Providing detailed, written, step-by-step instructions for the patient and/or the care partner to read and actually follow aids in their ability to visually follow the various HPEN procedures as the nurse clinician provides verbal instruction and clinical demonstrations. This type of written material also enables the patient and care partner to read and review the various HPN procedures between teaching sessions with the nurse clinician. Encouraging the patient and care partner to immediately begin a "hands on" learning experience promotes a quicker and a higher level of self-confidence that will help to decrease their anxiety level.

This "hands on" teaching plan also allows the nurse clinician the opportunity to observe the patient and care partner functioning as a team. Patients and care partners often experience anxiety regarding their ability to correctly handle medical supplies and maintain asepsis. Patient observations of the medical team's handling equipment and/or supplies bring them an awareness of the potential for contamination; therefore, they experience stress because they have not had medical training and could potentially contaminate supplies without immediately knowing so.

The nurse clinician's attention to detail in identifying each of the HPN ancillary supply products by the correct medical product name, purpose, function, aseptic handling, and various components (e.g., bag spike, slide clamp, filter, distal tip) facilitates the patient's understanding, comfort level, and retention of procedure material presented.

SELF MONITORING

Patient monitoring of his or her own physical condition and symptoms while on HPEN therapy plays an important role in improving clinical outcomes. This includes monitoring of his or her HPEN equipment and ancillary supplies. Table 11–2 is an example of these monitoring processes.

INFUSION PUMP CONSIDERATIONS

Current infusion technology has provided the nutrition support team and HPN therapy patients with the opportunity for lightweight, compact infusion delivery pumps with variable therapy program modes.[5,6] These pumps, with their computerized capabilities, allow the patient a greater level of independence and mobility. The ambulatory infusion

---

TABLE 11–2   Patient Self-Monitoring

Daily:

1. Weight
   - same time, similar clothing, same scale
   - call clinician regarding any increase of 2 or more pounds in one day or increase of 5 pounds or more in one week

2. Temperature
   - same time of day
   - check any time feeling ill, chills, or warm
   - contact physician if greater than 100°F or 1.0 degree greater than usual temperature

3. Intake and Output
   - include any ostomy, fistula, wound and/or drainage tubes; contact clinician if there is a dramatic increase or decrease

Other:

4. Blood Glucose Monitoring
   - as instructed by health care or HNST
   - signs or symptoms of hypo- or hyperglycemia

---

pumps can be placed in an appropriately-sized backpack or "fanny pack," depending on the HPN volume to be administered. This allows the patient freedom of mobility and opportunity for increased flexibility in their activities of daily living, both at work and at home. Those patients infusing larger volumes of HPN with the ambulatory infusion pumps have several disadvantages. One disadvantage occurs when the larger HPN fluid volume tends to muffle pump alarms when the backpack is closed and zipped shut. A second disadvantage of larger HPN fluid volumes results in patients having a heavy HPN backpack. They may prefer hanging the backpack on a portable IV pole to ease the weight and stress on their backs. The nurse clinician can provide valuable recommendations and suggestions for the integration of HPN therapy into the patient's lifestyle. Community resources that are available to the nurse clinician, the patient, and family members regarding HPN therapy can be limited within many areas of the country; however, the Oley Foundation serves as a valuable informational resource through phone and internet access across the United States. (The Oley Foundation website is available at: www.oley.org.)

HPN THERAPY SUPPLY SELECTION AND PATIENT EDUCATION

With advancements in parenteral therapy technology there are many options available, such as ambulatory infusion pumps, pole-mounted infusion pumps, needleless, safety systems, and various administrative tubing connection products to meet the specific physical needs of the patient and/or care-partner. Consideration by the nurse clinician as to specific needs of the patient is required to identify the appropriate infusion therapy devices and products that will best meet those needs. The nurse clinician is responsible for ensuring that HPN infusion devices used to administer parenteral therapy are appropriate for the patient's needs, are safe and in proper working condition, and are used appropriately according to the agency's policies and procedures.

The selection process for HPN infusion therapy devices for a specific patient's use should include consideration as to the ease of equipment use for the patient or care partner, ease of patient or care-partner training, and equipment safety features (e.g., backup power system, occlusion recognition, air-in-line alarm, anti-free-flow potential, programming lockout capabilities, flow rate accuracy, and reliability).[5,6] It is essential that the patient and care partners are able to visually read the infusion device screen and that they can hear the device alarm. For blind patients the pump screen keys can be labeled with appropriate Braille symbols by Braille foundations located within many metro areas.

Patients and care partners require education and training that will enable them to safely and appropriately administer and manage the HPN therapy. During the initial visit, it is essential to assess the patient and care partner in their levels of willingness and in their abilities and capabilities to understand, comprehend, and perform the technical skills and procedures that are required to safely accomplish the administration procedures of HPN. It is paramount that the nurse clinician's assessment includes recognition of any cultural or religious practices or language barriers that necessitate a revised approach to patient education.[4] Communicating those factors to the multidisciplinary nutrition support team is of vital importance for creating an effective plan of care and for ensuring patient compliance. Printed patient instructions should be provided in a language or form that the patient and care partner can readily understand.

Patients and care partners must be informed of their infusion pump's purpose, function, and safe use, as well as troubleshooting measures. A nurse clinician's explanation and demonstration of the proper use of ancillary medical supplies and effective HPN product-ordering methods will enhance correct supply deliveries and eliminate unnecessary shortages. By contacting the patient on a routine basis and/or by reviewing the various therapy devices and product supplies during each nursing visits, the nurse clinician can ensure adequate therapy supplies are available without "overstocking" the patient's home environment. Patients and care partners frequently require direction and initial assistance in the organization and rotation of HPN therapy product and ancillary supplies to ensure that the oldest product or supply is used prior to any recent deliveries.

Basic information regarding home safety is important during the initial home visit. Physical environmental safety factors, as well as the home HPN therapy bags, supplies, sharps containers, and medical waste safety factors should be addressed and reviewed during each follow-up nursing visit. Printed safety information materials provided should be appropriate to the patient's language and reading comprehension, as well as to the specific HPN therapy.

Ongoing patient education and re-enforcement of administrative procedures are done throughout the HPN therapy during each follow-up nursing visit, based on assessment of the patient and care partner's compliance with the HPN therapy plan, response to therapy, and proficiency for performing and managing the technical requirements of the therapy.[4,7]

HPEN THERAPY EDUCATION

Explaining the HPEN therapy to the patient and care partner is important so they can understand the correlation between metabolic complications and physical signs and symptoms of improperly administered solution. It must be clearly explained that the patient owns as much of the responsibility in safely reaching the nutrition support goals as does the physician and nutrition support care team. It is the responsibility of the nurse to help the patient gain insight into the fact that the HPEN solution and its administration is an invasive medical therapy with associated risks and potential complications.

SAFETY & INFECTION CONTROL

Assessing and providing education for optimal safety and infection control measures in the home is necessary to ensure positive outcomes, as is education of the technical skills involved in administering the HPEN. The following are some of the safety issues to be addressed. The handling of HPN and additives is also included.

1. Fire Safety
   a. Working smoke detectors
   b. Exit routes established by each family member
   c. Knowledge of fire prevention
   d. Number to call in case of a fire
2. Electrical Safety
   a. Avoidance of overloading electrical outlets
   b. Grounded outlets or adapters
   c. Electrical cords free from frayed wires or loose connections
   d. Extension cords out of the way to prevent falls
   e. Operation of electrical appliances away from sources of water
3. Fall Prevention
   a. Nonskid surfaces in bathtub and shower
   b. Nonskid throw rugs
   c. Obstacle-free floors, steps, and stairs
   d. Steps with railings
   e. Infusion tubing secured in carrying case to prevent dragging on floor with potential for tripping, pulling on access device, or being chewed by a pet
4. Utilities Needed to Provide Appropriate Care and Emergency Help
   a. Telephone service with 911 access
   b. Electricity
      • Inform electric supply company regarding patient's infusion pump, if necessary
   c. Running water
      • Be aware whether it is private well water or city water. Well water can be a source of contamination (especially important in immune-compromised patients), which may cause diarrhea or coagulation of enteral formulas, which leads to clogged enteral

feeding tubes. (Calcium salts in well water can coagulate the proteins in enteral feedings.)

Infection Control Measures

1. Hand-washing procedure and supplies include soap, paper towel, and a clean working area.

2. A suggestion for preparing the work area when preparing HPEN is to use a cookie sheet or tray covered with paper towels. Place needed supplies on cookie sheet or tray for preparation of next infusion. Cover supplies with paper towel until ready to prepare infusion. This is important for organization and to ensure a clean area in a sometimes less-than-optimal home environment.

3. Avoid open windows, fans, air vents, and pets when preparing HPEN.

4. Appropriate disposal of waste—Materials grossly saturated with blood or body fluids are to be placed in red biohazard bag or sharps container. Other materials can be placed in a plastic bag in the patient's regular trash container.

5. Ensure that the patient and care partner understand the importance of following aseptic and sterile techniques—assess the patient's and care partner's techniques.

6. Supplies such as syringes, dressing kits, pump tubing, alcohol/betadine, gloves, sharps containers, and so on should be stored in a cool, dry area away from children and pets.

7. Enteral formulas are to be stored in a cool area out of the sun. The proteins in the formulas can coagulate if stored in very warm conditions.

8. HPN solutions need to be stored in the refrigerator. Additives should be stored as indicated on their labels.

    a. HPN solutions can be warmed at room temperature for at least 2 hours. If they need to be warmed quicker, wrap HPN bag in towel with a hot water bottle filled with warm, not hot water.

    b. Do not infuse HPN solutions or additives if they have not been stored properly. Make sure the patient understands when deliveries are made to place appropriate solutions/additives in the refrigerator.

    c. Do not infuse HPN 2-in-1 solutions that contain particles or appear cloudy at room temperature.

    d. Do not infuse HPN 3-in-1 solutions that contain an oily layer.

    e. Do not immerse HPN bags in water to warm. Tap water and sink or container are not sterile and will contaminate the HPN bag and injection ports.

    f. Do not place HPN bags or HEN formulas in a microwave, on heaters, or in direct sunlight.

    g. Do not leave HPN bags at room temperature for longer than 24 hours.

    h. Do not use an HPN bag if it has been spiked with the tubing for more than 24 hours.

Equipment and Supplies

The management of the patient's supplies and equipment is crucial to the success of the HPEN therapy and the sanity of everyone involved, not to mention the effect on the cost of the therapy. A quality, reputable, and experienced infusion provider will provide the following inventory control services:

1. Scheduled and on-time deliveries.
2. A call to the patient with the expected time of delivery. (This allows the patient to organize his or her day and shows respect for the patient's time. It also adds to the patient's quality of life.)
3. Inventory management providing sufficient supplies between scheduled deliveries preventing the patient from running out of supplies and preventing the added cost of extra deliveries.
4. Monitoring of the patient's usage of supplies, which helps in documenting the patient's adherence to the prescribed therapy or detect patient misunderstanding of the prescribed therapy. Misuse of supplies may indicate the need for further education regarding the prescribed therapy or the first indication that a patient is not tolerating a prescribed therapy. The clinical team is then alerted to the need for further assessment of the patient's response to the therapy and progress toward the nutrition therapy goals.
5. Routine maintenance of pumps/equipment to ensure the safe infusion and uninterrupted delivery of the nutrition therapy.
6. Patient notification in a timely manner of a back order or change in products by the manufacturer, with accompanying education when needed.

7. Seeks patient input as to ease of use and overall satisfaction with the equipment and supplies. Also troubleshoots patient complaints of equipment and supplies.

HPEN ACCESS AND MAINTENANCE

Patients receiving HPEN therapy may also have open abdominal wounds, incisions, enterocutaneous fistulas, stomas, or surgical drains that require frequent or daily site care, dressings, and appliance changes. These wounds can be potential sources of contamination and infection hazards for those patients with central vascular access devices.[8] It is of vital importance to maintain separation of GI catheters, tubes, ostomies, and drains from central vascular catheter devices to decrease the potential risk of cross contamination and infection. Patients and care partners are encouraged to separate central catheter site care and dressing care from wound, ostomy, or GI tube care by several hours and with thorough hand washing as a means to decrease potential bacterial contamination. It is recommended that the central venous catheter be anchored away from wounds, GI tubes, or stomas, by a securing device. This prevents the central venous catheter from lying in the vicinity of wounds, drains, or stomas, or allowing a potential pull on the central venous catheter itself.

Infection control should be individualized for each patient, his or her condition, ability to understand directions, and type of access (enteral or parenteral, peripheral versus central catheter). The following are some general guidelines for intravenous catheters:

- Keep the catheter anchored/clipped up to prevent pulling on the catheter.
- No swimming in lakes or unchlorinated pools, which are a source of many infectious agents.
- Use caution in hot tubs, whirlpools, and saunas, which could be potential sources of infectious agents.
- Catheter site care and dressing change procedures must be followed carefully. The physician and nurse will determine the best frequency for catheter site care and dressing changes based on the patient's unique condition, but is usually weekly for home care.
- Patients should be taught to monitor signs/symptoms of infection.

COMPLICATIONS OF HPEN THERAPY

The nurse clinician holds a vital role in the critical management and monitoring of the HPEN patient to ensure positive therapy outcomes. Potential complications can often be identified within early stages through frequent, focused assessments and detailed communication with the HNST and attending physician. By using investigative questioning and head-to-toe patient assessments, the nurse clinician can identify education needs, psychological needs, and physical condition changes. Prompt identification of condition changes can prevent the need for significant intervention and can reduce the severity of potential complications. The Oley Foundation has an excellent resource for clinicians and patients related to HEN and HPN complications on its website, www.oley.org. Chapter 6 and Chapter 9 provide more information on the complications of HEN.

It is important that the nurse clinician recognizes that potential complications may differ in those patients recently initiating HPEN therapy versus those long-term HPEN patients. Long-term HPEN patients can often identify the specific signs and symptoms of various imbalances or potential complications for the HNST staff. The incidence and severity of HPN therapy related complications are dependent on the underlying medical condition, the type of central vascular device, the patient's tolerance of HPN therapy, the skills and techniques of the patient and care partner, and compliance to the administration of the prescribed HPN therapy. Table 11–3 lists guidelines that patients can use for prevention of HPN complications.

TABLE 11–3   Potential Complications / Patient-Focused Monitoring
Guidelines and Actions

1) Systemic Infection
   a. Prevention—diligent practice of aseptic technique
      - thorough and frequent hand washing
      - recognition of touch contamination ("when in doubt, throw it out")
      - correct supply usage—one-time use
   b. Signs/Symptoms
      - fever
      - flu-like symptoms
      - headache
      - weakness
      - chills
      - shaking
      - diaphoresis
   c. Action
      - call physician
      - phone signs and symptoms to HNST clinician

2) Exit Site Infection
   a. Prevention
      - diligent aseptic technique
      - thorough and frequent hand washing
      - site care and dressing changes as instructed
      - use of sterile gloves for any nontunneled catheter
      - anchor catheter to prevent tension and pulling
   b. Signs/Symptoms
      - redness
      - tenderness
      - warmth
      - swelling
      - skin irritation
      - drainage at catheter exit site
   c. Action
      - call physician
      - call HNST clinician

3) Catheter Occlusion
   a. Prevention
      - Use physician-instructed prevention protocol
      - "push-pause" flush technique for venous access device
      - saline flush frequency as instructed by home NST clinician
      - heparinization of central catheter following completion of HPN
      - heparinization of dormant catheter/ports daily
      - heparinization following blood draws

b. Signs/Symptoms

- unable to infuse HPN solution
- increased resistance when attempting to flush or heparinize
- pump alarms "down occlusion"
- unable to aspirate from catheter

c. Action

- attempt to flush with saline
- attempt to aspire from catheter
- clamp catheter immediately if unsuccessful
- call HNST clinician
- call physician
- transport to nearest medical facility

4) Catheter Damage/Leaks

a. Prevention

- clamp over reinforced segment of catheter only
- never use scissors near catheter
- never use sharp, jagged, or tooth clamps near catheter
- do not use acetone on catheter
- do not pull on catheter
- do not use any needle longer than 1 inch through catheter hub
- do not allow catheter to hang free
- exhibit caution during contact activities or sports
- avoid excessive pressure when flushing
- use recommended size of syringe when flushing

b. Signs/Symptoms

- moist or wet dressing
- moisture or leaking outside of dressing along catheter or tubing
- pain or swelling at catheter exit site
- pain during HPN infusion or flushing

c. Action

- clamp catheter near exit site
- clamp catheter above catheter damage
- stop HPN infusion
- call physician
- call HNST clinician
- transport to nearest medical facility

5) Catheter Dislocation

a. Prevention

- keep catheter securely anchored to chest/skin
- avoid strenuous physical contact activities and sports
- do not allow catheter to hang free

b. Signs/Symptoms

- pain during HPN infusion or flushing
- swelling or pain in arm, neck, or face on same side of body as catheter

    c. Action
- discontinue the HPN infusion
- heparinize catheter
- clamp catheter
- call physician
- call HNST clinician

6) Blood Back-Up in Tubing

    a. Prevention
- catheter must be clamped immediately upon HPN infusion completion
- close the open catheter clamp
- possible loose injection cap—secure cap
- check catheter thoroughly for damage
- use back-check valves

    b. Signs/Symptoms
- blood visible within catheter or tubing

    c. Action
- clamp catheter immediately upon discontinuing HPN infusion
- attempt to flush or heparinize catheter
- turn on infusion pump
- clamp injection cap on reinforced portion of catheter
- tighten the injection cap
- evaluate catheter for cracks, tears, wear, or leaking
- call physician
- call HNST clinician

7) Air Embolism

    a. Prevention
- prime/purge all air from administration tubing
- use only luer-locking connections
- use proper clamping methods
- proper injection cap use on catheter
- avoid extension sets to administration tubing, if at all possible
- careful attention to all pump alarms
- use air elimination filters (preferably "in-line") on administration set

    b. Signs/Symptoms
- impending sense of doom
- chest pain and shortness of breath
- feeling of anxiety
- coughing
- loss of consciousness

    c. Action
- immediately clamp catheter
- immediately lie on left side, head down, chin on chest
- elevate legs slightly
- telephone 911—emergency medical system for transport
- call physician
- call HNST clinician

8) Dehydration
   a. Prevention
      - provide adequate fluids/electrolytes when dehydration is due to increased diarrhea, vomiting, fistula, wound, or ostomy output
      - do not skip HPN therapy days
      - sip oral rehydration fluids as ordered
   b. Signs/Symptoms
      - thirst
      - weakness
      - sudden weight loss
      - lightheadedness, dizziness
      - increased pulse rate
      - decreased urine output
      - muscle cramping, shakiness
      - numbness
   c. Action
      - sip oral rehydration solution as directed
      - telephone attending physician
      - infuse hydration fluids as instructed by physician
      - call physician
      - call HNST clinician
9) Hypoglycemia
   a. Prevention
      - complete HPN infusion as programmed through the taper down mode
      - avoid stopping HPN abruptly during the infusion
      - observe for pump malfunction causing over HPN infusion
      - avoid too much insulin within HPN solution
   b. Signs/Symptoms
      - sweating, clammy skin
      - heart pounding/palpitations
      - shaky sensation
      - nausea
      - headache
      - blurred vision
      - hunger
      - lightheadedness
   c. Action
      - check blood glucose level
      - drink orange juice with two teaspoons of sugar added if able to have fluids
      - allow 1–2 teaspoons of sugar to dissolve under tongue
      - stop activity and rest
      - call physician
      - call HNST clinician
10) Hyperglycemia
   a. Prevention
      - complete the HPN-programmed taper down mode
      - accurate insulin additive amount to HPN bag

- thoroughly mixing HPN bag additives
- never infuse HPN rate faster "to catch up"
- inform physician and home NST clinicians of any new medications, over-the-counter medications and herbal supplements taken

  b. Signs/Symptoms

- dehydration
- headache
- excessive urination
- nausea
- thirst
- confusion, irritability

  c. Action

- check blood glucose level
- call physician
- call HNST clinician

11) Phlebitis/Thrombophlebitis

  a. Prevention

- utilize aseptic technique
- avoid tension or pull on catheter

  b. Signs/Symptoms

- pain, tenderness, redness, warmth, hardness along the vein path
- bursitis symptoms

  c. Action

- apply warm, moist pack frequently throughout the day
- elevate extremity
- call physician
- call HNST clinician

12) Electrolyte Imbalance

  a. Prevention

- infusion HPN volume exactly as prescribed
- infusion rate of HPN as ordered
- infusing hydration fluids as prescribed
- self-monitoring of weight and fluid/stool outputs
- scheduled lab draws as prescribed

  b. Signs/Symptoms

- sudden weight loss
- edema
- unusual intake & output values

  c. Action

- call physician
- call HNST clinician
- closely self-monitor weight and fluid/stool outputs

COMPLICATIONS OF HPN THERAPY

Complications of HPN fall into three primary categories: 1) infection—both local site and systemic, 2) mechanical—relating to the central vascular access and the infusion pump devices, and 3) metabolic—relating to the infusion of the HPN admixture solution.[4]

Infectious Complications

Infections can occur at the catheter exit site, within the catheter tunnel, or in the circulatory system. The nurse clinician must be vigilant in watching for the typical and atypical presentation of signs and symptoms at each location. Recurring infections are an indication that aseptic techniques should be reviewed and evaluated with both the patient and the care partner. Patients and care partners often notice exit site and tunnel tract infections at the time of site care and dressing changes. Both the patient and the care partner need to understand the importance and purpose of exit site cultures or blood cultures that are done as prescribed by their physician.

Mechanical Complications

Vessel injury or irritation when the central catheter is inserted is usually related to the technical skill of the individual who places the catheter. Thrombus or fibrin sheath development can occur gradually or may cause a sudden occlusion of the central vascular catheter. The care and treatment of these types of occlusions require immediate attention and assessment by trained clinicians and physicians. The ability to resolve a central catheter occlusion lies in direct proportion to the amount of time that has passed from the initial report of the complication to the time treatment is initiated. The shorter this period of time is, the better the chance is for clearing the occlusion. Patients and care partners are encouraged to note and report immediately any resistance in flushing of the catheter, any changes noted in chest vein appearance, or any extremity edema or swelling on the side of the catheter placement. Any difficulty in swallowing, neck pain, shortness of breath, or a sudden change in chest vein distention indicates an emergency situation that requires immediate medical intervention.

Metabolic Complications

Metabolic complications are complex and also quite common for patients receiving HPN therapy. The nurse clinician must be astute as to the signs and symptoms of each potential metabolic complication. Specific disease states (e.g., renal disease, short-bowel syndrome, diabetes, congestive heart failure, and immune deficiency related to transplant) may also contribute to the occurrence of certain metabolic complications. Each of these states requires vigilant nursing assessment and a nursing response directing an appropriate patient plan of care. Metabolic complications can include, but are not limited to, electrolyte imbalance, fluid imbalance, hypo- and hyperglycemia, rebound hypoglycemia, refeeding syndrome, hypo- and hypermagnesemia, lipid intolerance, essential fatty acid deficiency, trace element abnormalities, liver enzyme elevation, and metabolic bone disease. Clinical management and monitoring by the HNST have been proven to decrease the incidence and severity of metabolic complications for the patient receiving HPN therapy.[9,10]

TROUBLESHOOTING PROBLEMS WITH PATIENTS ON HPEN

Troubleshooting common HPEN therapy associated problems as they occur can assist in the rapid resolution of the problem. Patient education is a key element of success. Another key element of success is that each member of the HNST uses a similar method of troubleshooting. Patients can readily learn from working through a troubleshooting measure with a member of the nutrition support team or nurse clinician. Having been led through a specific algorithm by the clinician to resolve an issue, the patient then learns how he or she may do the same troubleshooting assessment if and when the situation arises again.

Home parenteral and enteral nutrition therapy patient teaching materials provided at each home visit, especially the initial visit, are resources, and they hold essential information for the patient and the care partner. Emphasizing the importance of these resources to the patient and caregiver is of vital importance. A yellow highlighter is a valuable tool within the clinician's nursing bag. As the nurse clinician highlights important information and troubleshooting measures, it reinforces the location and importance of this information within the patient teaching materials.

PATIENT COMPLIANCE

During each follow-up nursing visit, the nurse clinician's attention to patient teaching materials reinforces their value as well as the need to keep these therapy tools readily at hand, within the home medical chart. Patients and care partners may be reluctant to ask a question that they know has been addressed previously. They may also require an explanation for information within the patient education material that they may not readily grasp. The nurse clinician will need to emphasize repeatedly that "there is no such thing as an unimportant question." It is important to recognize that every person values praise and recognition. This principle is especially true for patients and care partners. Extend praise for skills, techniques, and procedures that they have learned and perform well. Provide acknowledgement that they were correct in placing a telephone call to ask questions or to request assistance in troubleshooting. As the old nursing adage states, "They don't care how much you know until they know how much you care."

Emphasis must be placed on the self-monitoring components of HPEN therapy. The purpose and importance of monitoring daily weight, urine output, temperature, and other requirements (e.g., blood glucose monitoring, blood pressure) as directed by the attending physician must be conveyed to the patient and care partner. Providing the patient and care partner with a flow sheet or chart form to record the various necessary self-monitoring information will serve as visual reminders of what they are to monitor, the frequency of the monitoring, the importance of record keeping, and the need to keep this information contained together within their home medical chart. If the nutrition support team or the nurse clinician does not obtain this information from the patient and care partners on a routine basis, then the patient and the care partner soon may perceive that self-monitoring and record keeping are simply busy work that they feel they may not have the time or energy to do. Prevention of complications is the key to success.

CONCLUSION

Nursing care of the home nutrition support patient is multifaceted. The nutrition support nurse is involved in the coordination of the patient's discharge with the physician; the physician's nursing staff; hospital medical, pharmacy, and nursing staffs; the dietitian; social workers; discharge planners; the payor case manager; and the home infusion provider. The nurse also works closely with the above disciplines to assess the patient and care partner's readiness to learn and ability to understand and carry out the skills necessary to ensure safe and effective outcomes. The nurse is usually the primary clinician providing the patient and care partner teaching, continually evaluating the patient's and care partner's understanding of the procedures and the need for follow-up appointments, and working with the patient and the care partner in understanding and identifying the outcome goals.

The nurse has a primary role of being the patient's advocate. This includes clarifying information, promoting communication between the patient and his or her providers of care, and ensuring and helping the patient to share in decision-making in order to achieve the treatment goals.[11]

REFERENCES

1. Howard L. Home parenteral nutrition: clinical outcomes. In: Rombeau J, ed. *Parenteral Nutrition,* 3rd edition. Philadelphia: WB. Saunders, Co;2001: 503–510.
2. Smith CE, Curtas S, Werkowitch M, Kleinbeck SV, Howard L. Home parenteral nutrition: does affiliation with a national support and educational organization improve patient outcomes? *J Parenter Enteral Nutr.* 2002;26(3): 159–163.
3. Kindle R. Life with fred: 12 years of home parenteral nutrition. *Nutr Clin Pract.* 2003;18(3):235–237.
4. Ireton-Jones C, DeLegge M, Epperson L, Alexander J. Management of the home parenteral nutrition patient. *Nutr Clin Pract.* 2003;18:310–317.
5. http://www.baxter.com/products/medication_management/infusion_pumps/
6. http://www.curlinmedical.com/products.html
7. de Burgoa LJ, Seidner D, Hamilton C, Stafford J, Steiger E. Examination of factors that lead to complications for new home parenteral nutrition patients. *J Infus Nurs.* 2006;29(2):74–80.
8. Ryder M. Evidence-based practice in the management of vascular access devices for home parenteral nutrition therapy. *J Parenter Enteral Nutr.* 2006; 30(suppl 1):S82–S93.
9. Kovacevich DS, Frederick A, Kelly D, Nishikawa R, Young L, American Society for Parenteral and Enteral Nutrition Board of Directors, Standards for Specialized Nutrition Support Task Force. Standards for specialized nutrition support: home care patients. *Nutr Clin Pract.* 2005;20(5):579–590.

10. Monitoring home and other alternate site nutrition support. In: Gottsclich MM, ed. *The Science and Practice of Nutrition Support: A Case-based Core Curriculum*. Dubuque, IA: Kendall/Hunt Publishing Company;2001: 731–755.
11. Vermeire E, van Royen P, Coenen S, Wens J, Denekens J. The adherence of type 2 diabetes patients to their therapeutic regimens: a qualitative study from the patient's perspective, 2003. *Pract. Diab. Int.* 20(6):209–214.

READINGS

Infusion Nurses Society. Available at: http://www.ins1.org. Accessed 11/30/06.

Journal of Infusion Nursing. Available at: http://www.journalofin fusionnursing.com. Accessed 11/30/06.

The National Home Infusion Association. Available at: http://www. nhian et.org. Accessed 11/30/06.

CHAPTER 12

Specialized Nutrition Support at Home

Cynthia Hamilton, MS, RD, LD, CNSD
Melinda Parker, MS, RD, CNSD

INTRODUCTION

Patients requiring home specialized nutrition support (HSNS), for gastrointestinal disorders, frequently have co-morbid diseases that can affect their nutritional status and ability to tolerate nutrition support regimens. The type of nutrition support, enteral or parenteral, and the assimilation of macro- and micronutrients can be affected by the metabolic abnormalities of the disease, as well as by the various treatments and medications used in the medical management of these diseases. This chapter focuses on the use of HSNS in patients with hepatobiliary disease, renal disease, diabetes mellitus, pancreatitis, and cancer.

HEPATOBILIARY DISEASE

The liver is responsible for multiple functions in the body, including carbohydrate, protein, and fat metabolism; storage and activation of vitamins and minerals; formation and excretion of bile, hormone and steroid metabolism; and removal of toxins and bacteria.[1] Liver disease (LD) can be acute, defined as six months duration or less, or chronic, lasting more than six months. The diagnosis of hepatobiliary abnormalities can be made by laboratory evaluation of liver function tests (LFTs), specific diagnostic blood tests, radiographic tests, and by histologic liver biopsy.[1]

TABLE 12–1   Common Liver Function Tests[1]

Enzymes	Assessment
AST (aspartate aminotransferase)	hepatocellular injury
ALT (alanine aminotransferase)	hepatocellular injury
AP (alkaline phosphatase)	biliary obstruction, cholestasis, hepatocellular injury
GGT (γ-glutamyl transpeptidase)	hepatocellular injury
LDH (lactic dehydrogenase)	hepatocellular injury
Excretory	
Total bilirubin	biliary obstruction, cholestasis, hepatocellular injury
Indirect	bilirubin unconjugated, increased with excessive bilirubin production, inherited defects, drug effects
Direct bilirubin	conjugated, increased with depressed bilirubin excretion, hepatobiliary disease, cholestasis
Synthetic Products	
Albumin	decreased liver synthesis, chronic liver disease, malnutrition
Prothrombin Time	prolonged with decreased liver synthesis, severe liver damage, chronic liver disease, Vitamin K deficiency

LFTs, as outlined in Table 12–1, can indicate that there is an underlying pathological process that may require further investigation for the diagnosis of LD. Specific diagnostic laboratory tests, such as those for viral hepatitis, autoimmune liver disease, and inherited forms of liver disease including hemachromatosis, alpha 1-antitrypsin deficiency, and Wilson's disease may be necessary. A liver biopsy may be obtained to confirm the severity of liver damage and to provide histopathological information.

Radiographic tests that can detect biliary tree abnormalities, gallstones, and parenchymal disease include:[2]

• Computed tomography (CT)	• Magnetic resonance imaging (MRI)
• Ultrasound (U/S)	• Endoscopic retrograde cholangiopancreatography (ERCP)

The results of diagnostic tests may then help classify liver disorders as follows:[1]

- *Steatosis*—the accumulation of fat globules in hepatocytes, most commonly observed in patients with obesity, type 2 diabetes mellitus, and alcoholism.
- *Hepatitis*—inflammation of the liver with damage to hepatocytes. Causes include hepatitis A, B, C, D, E, Epstein-Barr virus, cytomegalovirus, and toxins such as drugs or alcohol. Chronic hepatitis can progress to fibrosis and cirrhosis.
- *Steatohepatitis*—the accumulation of fat globules in hepatocytes with inflammation.
- *Cholestasis*—biliary obstruction due to sludge or gallstones in the biliary tree (extrahepatic) or hepatocellular and cannicular (intrahepatic) dysfunction of bile acid secretion.
- *Cirrhosis*—formation of fibrotic tissue in the liver that can lead to end-stage liver disease with ascites, hepatic encephalopathy, and portal hypertension.
- *Fulminant Hepatic Failure*—sudden severe liver dysfunction characterized by hepatic encephalopathy that can progress to coma and death. It is most commonly caused by acute viral hepatitis.

Nutrition Assessment

Nutrition depletion is common among patients with LD, including protein-calorie malnutrition and vitamin and mineral deficiencies.[3] Malnutrition in LD is associated with metabolic abnormalities, malabsorption of fat, and poor oral intake. Nutrition assessment parameters such as visceral proteins and anthropometric data are frequently not useful in evaluating nutritional status in significant LD, due to the fluid fluctuations associated with ascites and decreased synthesis of proteins by the liver.[3] Nutrition support should include the provision of adequate calories, protein, vitamins, and minerals.

Hepatobiliary Disease in Parenteral Nutrition

Abnormal liver function in patients receiving parenteral nutrition (PN) may be associated with the patient's underlying disease, drug toxicity, sepsis, acute or chronic LD, or the PN itself. Abnormalities of liver function in patients receiving PN have been documented with steatosis as the predominant hepatobiliary disorder in patients receiving PN.[4–7] Biliary sludge accumulation is also very common in patients receiving PN and can develop within a few weeks of initiation of PN. In most instances, abnormal liver function is mild and resolves with cessation of the PN.[4–7] However, patients requiring PN for months or years are at risk for developing more serious liver abnormalities, and cessation of PN may not be an option without risking the development of severe malnutrition or dehydration.

Hepatobiliary Disease in Long-Term Parenteral Nutrition

The incidence of abnormal liver function has been reported to range from 39–87% in several studies in patients on long-term PN.[8–10] In a group of long-term PN patients, complicated liver disease, defined as portal hypertension, portal fibrosis, cirrhosis, serum bilirubin > 3.5 mg/dL, and hepatic encephalopathy was reported to occur in 26% of the patients after 2 years, 39% after 4 years, and 50% after 6 years.[9] Twenty-two percent of the deaths from this patient population were due to liver failure. Another report by Chan and associates[11] showed a 15% incidence of end-stage LD in their home PN patients.

Parenteral Nutrition-Associated Risk Factors

Several factors have shown to be related to PN-associated LD, including the macro- and micronutrients provided by the PN infusion, various medications, the length of remaining small bowel, and infections. These factors are summarized in Table 12–2.

Prevention and Treatment of Parenteral Nutrition-Induced Hepatobiliary Disease

Several measures should be considered, as listed in Table 12–2, to help prevent and treat LD in patients receiving PN. Patients with worsening LD who have failed treatment may need to be assessed for small bowel or combined small bowel-liver transplant.

TABLE 12–2   Parenteral Nutrition Associated Risk Factors in Hepatobiliary Disease[1,2,5,7–9,11–14]

Nutrient	Comment
Lipids	> 1 g/kg/day associated with LD [9,11] > 2.5 g/kg/day associated with steatosis and cholestasis [5,12]
Carbohydrate	> 50 kcal/kg associated with steatosis [7]
EFAD	linoleic and linolenic acid deficiency associated with steatosis [13]
Manganese	hypermanganesemia associated with cholestasis [13]
Copper	copper excess associated with cholestasis
Carnitine	deficiency associated with steatosis [13]
Choline	low blood levels associated with steatosis, increased ALT, AST. Currently not available as an additive to PN [13]
Other	
Medications	review patient medication profile for hepatotoxic drugs, commonly added medications to PN include histamine 2 receptors and octreotide, which are associated with cholestasis [2]
Short-Bowel Syndrome	shortest residual bowel at greatest risk for LD studies: < 50 cm, associated with LD mortality [9] < 100 cm, associated with abnormal LFTs [8] < 150 cm, associated with chronic cholestasis [14] partial colon resection or total colon resection associated with chronic cholestasis [14]
Infection	sepsis associated with increased bilirubin, AST, ALT, AP [1] catheter-related blood stream infection common complication in long-term PN

LD-liver disease, EFAD-essential fatty acid deficiency, ALT-alanine aminotransferase, AST-aspartate aminotransferase, AP-alkaline phosphatase, LFTs-liver function tests, PN-parenteral nutrition

- *Oral Intake*—If possible, even small amounts of oral intake or enteral feeding should be encouraged to stimulate gallbladder emptying and to help prevent biliary sludge and stones.[8,13]
- *Cyclic PN Administration*—Cycling of the PN solution over part of the day allows a "free" period from carbohydrate infusion, which al-

lows the mobilization of stored glycogen and lipid from the liver and promotes nitrogen retention. The use of cyclic PN in patients with mild to moderate impaired liver function was shown to prevent hepatocellular damage and progression of jaundice and maintained serum albumin better than those patients receiving a continuous infusion of PN.[15]

- *Over/Underfeeding*—Avoid overfeeding of macronutrients, including dextrose and fat. Excess dextrose calories are associated with steatosis and lipid overfeeding (> 1 gm/kg/day) is associated with steatosis and cholestasis.[5,7,12] Underfeeding and the development of severe protein calorie malnutrition is associated with insufficient production of very low density lipid synthesis and can lead to defective triglyceride transport from the liver, resulting in hepatic steatosis.[13]

- *Medications*—Ursodeoxycholic acid has been used in patients with cholestasis to improve bile flow and liver enzymes but has not been shown to prevent cholestasis.[13] Metronidazole has also been used to treat cholestasis in patients on PN with suspected bacterial overgrowth.[13]

- *Infection*—Sepsis is often associated with a rise in bilirubin, aspartate aminotransferase, alanine aminotransferase, and alkaline phosphatase.[1] Patients receiving PN who have recurrent catheter sepsis, intra-abdominal sepsis or inflammation may develop signs of abnormal liver function. Infection should be investigated as a possible cause of liver function abnormalities with appropriate treatment provided to clear the infection. Patients must be educated on proper care of their venous access device to prevent infections and sepsis.

- *Transplantation*—Patients with intestinal and liver failure may be candidates for a combined intestinal and liver transplant. Careful consideration and evaluation of this type of treatment modality may be necessary in those with impending liver failure or worsening liver function. These patients should be referred to an established small-bowel transplant center. Survival rates for this type of combined therapy are improving.[2]

TABLE 12–3   Guide for Managing Long-term PN Patients with Hepatobiliary Abnormalities

1. Monitor LFTs routinely (monthly), including AST, ALT, AP, bilirubin, albumin, prothrombin time. Refer patients with modest to severe abnormalities to a hepatologist for diagnostic testing.

2. Avoid overfeeding of dextrose calories (> 50 kcal/kg/day).

3. Avoid excessive lipid infusion (> 1 gm/kg/day).

4. Avoid essential fatty acid deficiency by providing 4% to 8% of calories from fat.

5. Monitor manganese and copper blood levels every 3–6 months, adjust PN formulas as needed.

6. Cycle PN.

7. Eliminate hepatoxic medications. Remove histamine 2 receptor antagonists and octreotide from the PN solution in patients with abnormal LFTs.

8. Control for infection risk. Promote proper venous catheter care.

9. Promote oral intake, if possible.

10. Refer for transplantation with impending liver failure or worsening liver tests despite formula changes.

AST-aspartate aminotransferase, ALT-alanine aminotransferase, AP-alkaline phosphatase,
PN-parenteral nutrition

Monitoring Hepatobiliary Function in the Home Parenteral Nutrition Patient

Patients on long-term PN should routinely be monitored for signs and symptoms of the development of hepatobiliary disease. Parenteral nutrition formulas should be modified as needed to reverse or reduce the risk of developing PN-associated LD. Guidelines for management are presented in Table 12–3.

Home Enteral Nutrition

Most patients with LD and adequate absorptive function can be given a standard enteral polymeric formula or a concentrated formula to meet protein, calorie, vitamin, mineral, and fluid needs.[3] Patients with advanced LD can be difficult to manage if fluid restriction or protein restriction is necessary. Special enteral formulas containing increased amounts of branched-chain amino acids and decreased amounts of aromatic amino acids have been designed to treat or prevent hepatic en-

TABLE 12–4   Features of Renal Replacement Therapies[16,17]

	Time	Frequency	Protein Losses	Glucose Load
Hemodialysis	3–4 hrs	3 times/week	10–13 gms/treatment	low
Peritoneal Dialysis	24 hrs	4–5 times/day	5–24 gms/day	high

cephalopathy; however, these can be costly for home use and must be managed carefully to obtain the highest efficacy.[3]

RENAL DISEASE

Nutrition support is an important component of treatment for patients with renal failure. The nutrition requirements of the home nutrition support (HSN) patient with renal disease will depend on the degree of renal failure present, including chronic renal failure (CRF) and end-stage renal disease requiring renal replacement therapy (RRT). Acute renal failure (ARF), the abrupt cessation or reduction of kidney function, requires hospitalization for immediate medical attention with kidney function usually returning to normal prior to discharge. Nutrition support in acute renal failure will not be covered in this chapter.

Diabetes, hypertension, vascular disease, urologic disorders, and primary glomerular or interstitial diseases of the kidney account for most causes of CRF.[16] The decline of renal function results in the loss of the body's ability to clear nitrogenous waste and metabolic by-products; regulate fluid, electrolytes, and acid-base balance; and produce hormones normally secreted by the kidney.[16] Due to the metabolic abnormalities of CRF, patients are prone to develop malnutrition and present many challenges to clinicians in formulating the HSNS regimen.

Renal Replacement Therapies

Renal replacement therapies for patients with end-stage renal disease (ESRD) include hemodialysis (HD) and peritoneal dialysis (PD). These therapies differ in time, frequency, removal of fluid, and effect on macronutrients[16,17] (see Table 12–4).

TABLE 12–5   Sample Calculation of Peritoneal Dialysis Glucose
Absorption

Peritoneal dialysis prescription: Two 1-L exchanges of 1.5%, one 2-L exchange of 2.5%, and 1-L exchange of 4.25%

Two 1-L exchanges 1.5% = 30 g of dextrose (15 g/L x 2)

One 2-L exchange of 2.5% = 50 g of dextrose (25 g/L x 2)

One 1-L exchange of 4.25% = 42.5 g of dextrose (42.5 g/L x 1)

Total grams of dextrose = 122.5 (30 + 50 + 42.5)

122.5 gm x 3.4 kcal/g = 416.5 kcal dextrose x .75 (absorption rate) = 312.4 kcal

Hemodialysis—The most common RRT used for patients with ESRD is intermittent HD. This method removes toxic waste from the blood through a venous catheter or arteriovenous fistula. Blood is pumped through a filter with a semi-permeable membrane and a dialysate solution pumped through the opposite side of the filter in the opposite direction. Diffusion and convection forces remove electrolytes, metabolic by-products, and fluid.[16,17]

Peritoneal Dialysis—PD is a therapy that the patient administers in the home. A dialysate fluid is instilled into the peritoneal cavity. The peritoneum acts as a semi-permeable membrane, and the high glucose concentration of the dialysate fluid forces convective losses by oncotic pressure. Because of the high dextrose concentration of PD solutions and prolonged dwell time, patients absorb nearly all of the glucose from the dialysate fluid. Approximately 75% of the calories from the administered dextrose are absorbed and should be considered when determining the NHS formula (see Table 12–5). Protein losses may be significant due to the permeability of the peritoneal membrane and range from 5 to 24 grams per day.[18] Adequate amounts of protein must be supplied in the NHS formula.

Nutrition Assessment

Patients with renal disease are frequently malnourished. Thirty percent of patients undergoing HD have mild to moderate protein-calorie malnutrition and 8% have severe protein-calorie malnutrition.[16] Eighteen to 51% of PD patients have signs of malnutrition.[19] Common symptoms in patients with CRF are uremia, anorexia, nausea, and vomiting, which can further contribute to malnutrition.

TABLE 12–6   Nutrient Requirements for Patients with Renal Failure* [20-23]

ENERGY	PROTEIN	FAT	FLUID
35 kcal/kg <60 yrs age	0.6–0.8 g/kg pre-dialysis	20–30% of kcal	intake match urine output *or* volume removal from RRT
30-35 kcal/kg >60 yrs age	1.2 g/kg HD		HD-1000 mL/d plus urine output
	1.2–1.3 g/kg PD		PD-1500 mL/d

HD-hemodialysis, PD-peritoneal dialysis

* Energy needs are stratified by age; protein and fluid recommendations are based on dialysis status

The National Kidney Foundation has published clinical practice guidelines for nutrition in CRF and recommends routine measures of body weight and serum albumin.[20] In patients receiving HD, a "dry" weight, or the usual post-dialysis weight in which there is no evidence of fluid overload, should be monitored monthly as well as pre-dialysis serum albumin. Serum albumin has been shown to be a predictor of mortality in patients with CRF with a relative risk of death five times greater when the albumin is between 3.0 and 3.4 g/dL compared to normal reference ranges.[21]

Nutrient requirements for energy, protein, fat, and fluid in patients with renal disease are listed in Table 12–6.[20-23]

Vitamin and Trace Element Requirements

Vitamin and trace element requirements for patients with CRF have not been well studied.[23] Reduced renal clearance of these nutrients may lead to toxicities; however, deficiencies of water soluble vitamins are common in patients receiving HD and PD due to dialysis losses.[22,23] Fat soluble vitamins are poorly cleared by dialysate membranes. Vitamins A and E can accumulate in CRF patients not receiving renal replacement therapy, and patients should not receive additional supplements of these vitamins.[22] Patients with CRF often require Vitamin D supplementation because the conversion to the active form (1, 25 dihydroxyvitamin D) normally produced in the kidney is impaired in kidney failure. The active form of Vitamin D helps facilitate calcium absorption from the intestines helps maintain normal serum calcium and, therefore, bone integrity.[22] Standard parenteral vitamin and trace element preparations are suggested for use in patients receiving PN.[22] Enteral formulas are designed for patients with renal failure and have adjusted amounts of vitamins and minerals. All patients receiving HSNS should be monitored for signs and symptoms of vitamin and mineral deficiencies.

Iron

Anemia is common in CRF due to blood loss with dialysis treatments, decreased red blood cell survival, and decreased production of the hormone erythropoetin normally produced by the kidney.[24] Erythropoetin is produced in response to decreased red blood cell production but requires sufficient amounts of iron in the bone marrow.[18] It is important to determine if the patient is iron- or erythropoetin-deficient and treat accordingly. Patients receiving recombinant erthyropoetin should have their iron status assessed by measuring serum ferritin and transferrin saturation. Serum ferritin should be maintained above 100 ng/mL and transferrin saturation above 20%.[24] Oral iron supplementation has generally been replaced with intravenous iron in patients receiving HD. Intravenous iron and erthyropoetin are given during the HD treatment when a deficiency has been determined.[23]

Electrolytes

Abnormal serum concentrations of electrolytes including sodium, potassium, phosphorus, calcium, and magnesium are observed in patients with CRF because of decreased urinary excretion. Metabolic acidosis may also occur due to loss of normal acid excretion.[25] Renal replacement therapies remove solutes such as urea, creatinine, potassium, magnesium, and phosphorus.[16] Patients undergoing HD will have increased accumulations of electrolytes between dialysis treatments. Alteration in calcium and phosphorus homeostasis occurs due to abnormal Vitamin D metabolism as previously reviewed. Patients taking oral or enteral nutrition (EN) will need phosphate binders to prevent intestinal absorption of dietary phosphorus. Acceptable laboratory ranges of electrolytes for patients with HD, drawn *prior* to treatment, have been established[26] (see Table 12–7). Serum electrolytes need to be closely monitored during HSNS with adjustments made to formulas based on laboratory values.

TABLE 12–7   Pre-Dialysis Laboratory Test Ranges[26]

Lab Test	Renal Range
BUN	60–120 mg/dL
Cr	4–20 mg/dL
Potassium	3.5–6.0 mEq/L
Phosphorus	4.5–6.5 mg/dL
Magnesium	1.6–2.4 mg/dL

BUN — blood urea nitrogen   Cr — creatinine

TABLE 12–8   Enteral Renal Disease Formulas

Product	kcal/mL	Protein (g)*	Potassium (mEq)*	Phosphorus (mg)*	Magnesium (mg)*
Magnacal Renal® (Mead Johnson)	2.0	37.5	16	400	100
Nepro® (Ross)	2.0	35	14	343	108
Novasource Renal™ (Novartis)	2.0	37	14	325	100
NutriRenal™ (Nestle)	2.0	35	16	350	100
Renalcal® (Nestle)	2.0	17**	ng	ng	ng
Suplena® (Ross)	2.0	15	14	365	108

* per 1000 kcal   ** protein source is 67% essential amino acids   ng-negligible

Home Enteral Nutrition

Home EN is provided to patients with CRF due to malnutrition or inability to consume adequate oral nutrition.[27] Specifically designed EN products for patients with CRF are available (Table 12–8). These products are generally concentrated to 2 kcal/mL and contain lower amounts of potassium, magnesium, and phosphorus due to altered metabolism and decreased excretion. The route of feeding will depend on the patient's available enteral access (nasogastric, gastrostomy, jejunostomy). The infusion method, continuous versus intermittent, can be determined based on patient tolerance and scheduled RRT treatments.

Home Parenteral Nutrition

Patients with CRF and gastrointestinal failure may require PN. Concentrated sources of dextrose, amino acids, and fat emulsions can be used to meet fluid restrictions of patients with CRF. (See Chapter 8 for parenteral macronutrient solutions.) Standard amino acid mixtures containing essential and nonessential amino acids are indicated for patients with CRF.[27]

Early studies using parenteral amino acid solutions containing only essential amino acids in patients with ARF did not improve survival, nitrogen balance, or uremia.[28] Patients on home parenteral nutrition (HPN) should have their serum electrolytes monitored weekly, with adjustments made to the HPN solution as needed to avoid electrolyte imbalances. Once serum electrolytes are stable, monitoring can be reduced to every 2–4 weeks.

Intradialytic Parenteral Nutrition

Intradialytic parenteral nutrition (IDPN) is the infusion of parenteral nutrients through the venous return line during HD treatment. Typical IDPN solutions will provide one liter consisting of 250 mL of concentrated amino acids, 250 mL of D70, and 500 mL of 20% intravenous fat emulsion.[18] The purpose of IDPN is to provide supplemental nutrition to malnourished patients who have not been able to meet their nutrient needs orally. Retrospective studies show IDPN improves serum albumin levels and decreases mortality in patients with low serum albumin concentrations.[29,30] Guidelines for patient selection for IDPN have been published and recommend its use for those with malnutrition, including serum albumin below normal reference range, and those with weight loss who have failed enteral supplementation.[20,31,32] Insurance reimbursement for this therapy can be difficult to obtain; therefore, IDPN is not frequently used.[31]

DIABETES MELLITUS

Diabetes Mellitus (DM) is a metabolic disorder characterized by an absolute or a relative lack of insulin manifested by hyperglycemia. It is estimated that over 13 million people in the United States are diagnosed with DM.[33] The American Diabetes Association classifies DM into type 1 and type 2 categories:[34]

- Type 1 DM is an absolute deficiency of insulin secretion due to pancreatic islet beta-cell destruction and most commonly occurs in children and young adults. Exogenous insulin is essential to achieve glycemic control and to prevent diabetic ketoacidosis.
- Type 2 DM is caused by a resistance of insulin action and/or an inadequate insulin secretory response. Type 2 DM is the most prevalent type of DM and is associated with increasing age, obesity, and lack of physical exercise.

Other types of DM are associated with pancreatic disease, drugs, endocrinopathies such as Cushing's syndrome or acromegaly, infections, and genetic disorders. Gestational DM is hyperglycemia during pregnancy with normalization of glucose metabolism usually following delivery.[34]

Diagnosis of DM is established when classic symptoms including polyuria, polydipsia, and weight loss, along with either a random plasma glucose of 200 mg/dL or more, a fasting glucose of 126 mg/dL or more, or a two hour plasma glucose > 200 mg/dL during an oral glucose tolerance test are observed.[34] Patients may also be asymptomatic, as commonly seen with type 2 DM, and are often found to be hyperglycemic during a routine health screening.[34]

Long-term complications are associated with all types of DM, and include retinopathy, neuropathy, nephropathy, macrovascular disease, coronary artery disease, and enteropathy such as diarrhea and gastroparesis.[35] Tight glucose control in patients who participated in the Diabetes Control and Complication Trial showed the onset of these complications can be delayed.[36]

Pharmacologic treatment for DM includes:[35]

- oral hypoglycemic agents, commonly used to treat type 2 DM, such as sulfonylureas, which stimulate insulin secretion, and biguanide (metformin), which reduces hepatic production and increases glucose uptake.
- insulin, classified by duration of action (see Table 12–9)

Dietary modification is also an important component of treatment, and evidence-based guidelines of the American Diabetes Association are available.[37] Controlling the total amount versus the source of carbohydrate, limiting saturated fat, and avoidance of excessive calories are emphasized.[37]

TABLE 12–9   Types of Insulin[35]

Type	Onset of Action	Peak	Duration of Action
Fast-Acting	< 0.5 hrs	0.5–2.5 hrs	3–4.5
Lispro			
Aspart			
Short-Acting	0.5–1 hr	1–4 hrs	4–8 hrs
Regular			
Intermediate-Acting	1–3 hrs	3–8 hrs	7–14 hrs
NPH			
Lente			
Long-Acting	2–4 hrs	6–12 hrs	24–28 hrs
Ultralente			
Glargine	1–2 hrs	**No peak**	**24 hrs**

Home Enteral and Parenteral Nutrition Support

The indications for HSNS in the diabetic patient do not differ from the nondiabetic patient. Home enteral nutrition (HEN) is used in patients with a functional gastrointestinal tract who cannot eat a sufficient amount of food, while HPN is reserved for patients in whom HEN is contraindicated or not tolerated. Diabetes alone is rarely a diagnosis associated with the absolute need for HEN or HPN. Most often, DM is a concomitant diagnosis with a disease process that affects the function of the GI tract. Diabetic gastroparesis, for example, is associated with DM and may require HEN distal to the stomach.

Management includes daily monitoring of blood glucose using a glucose meter to perform capillary blood glucose measurements, with the goal of avoiding hyper- and hypoglycemia. Critically ill patients receiving EN and/or PN with blood glucose levels maintained between 80–100 mg/dL had significantly less complications than patients with blood glucose maintained between 180–200 mg/dL.[38] However, blood glucose between 100–150 mg/dL in stable, noncritically ill patients is recommended to avoid symptoms of tight control and incidents of hypoglycemia.[39]

TABLE 12–10   Enteral Diabetic Formulas

Product*	%CHO kcal	%PRO kcal	%FAT kcal	Fiber g/1000 kcal	CHO source
Choice DM® (Mead Johnson)	40	17	43	14	maltodextrin
DiabetiSource® (Novartis)	36	20	44	4	maltodextrin, fructose, vegetables, fruit
Glucerna® (Ross)	34	17	49	14	maltodextrin, fructose
Glytrol® (Nestle)	40	18	42	15	maltodextrin, modified corn starch
Resource Diabetic® (Novartis)	36	24	40	13	hydrolyzed corn starch, fructose

* all products provide 1.0 kcal/mL

Home Enteral Formula Selection

Several diabetic enteral formulas are available (see Table 12–10). These formulas contain carbohydrate sources such as oligosaccharides, fructose, corn starch, fruits, vegetables, and fiber. The macronutrient distribution varies, but most provide fewer calories from carbohydrate and more from fat sources. The higher fat content of these formulas may impair gastric emptying, a concern for the diabetic patient with gastroparesis. Studies comparing diabetic formulas with standard polymeric formulas in ambulatory patients[40,41] and nursing home patients[42] showed a great deal of variability among individual patients and did not show consistently improved glycemic control. There is insufficient evidence to routinely use diabetic enteral formulas for all patients with DM, though they may be helpful for some patients.

Home Enteral Formula Delivery

Enteral formulas may be administered by continuous or intermittent method. Intermittent feedings are given over 20–30 minutes several times per day and are most commonly used in the stable home patient. The delivery method will depend on the location of the tube in the gastrointestinal tract and patient tolerance (see Chapter 6). Patients with gastric feeding tubes are usually given intermittent feedings while continuous feedings are administered to those with small-bowel feeding tubes. Patients with gastroparesis and delayed gastric emptying will need continuous feedings administered through a post-pyloric feeding tube.

Glycemic Management in Home Enteral Nutrition

The diabetic patient receiving HEN will need treatment with oral hypoglycemic agents or insulin. Oral hypoglycemic agents can be administered via the feeding tube. Frequently, type 2 diabetic patients who did not need insulin prior to illness and initiation of EN will need insulin added to their daily regimen. Insulin regimens (Table 12–9) will vary and may include the use of:[43]

- Intermediate-acting insulin as a single or split dose
- Short- or fast-acting insulin alone or in combination with intermediate-acting insulin
- Long-acting insulin alone or in combination with short- or fast-acting insulin

The home glucose management regimen (i.e., oral agent and/or insulin) is determined by the preadmission oral glucose management regimen, degree of physiologic stress, and additional medication such as corticosteroids known to affect glycemia. Patients receiving continuous feedings should check blood glucose every 4 to 6 hours, initially, then decrease to once or twice per day once stable. Patients receiving intermittent feedings should check blood glucose prior to each feeding and no sooner than 4 hours following the end of each feeding.[43]

Glycemic Management in Parenteral Nutrition

Glycemic control and the PN prescription should be established prior to hospital discharge in the diabetic patient. The majority of diabetic patients will require insulin coverage for the infused dextrose from the PN solution. A starting point for the diabetic patient is to provide no more than 200 grams of dextrose in the first day's bag of PN and to give 0.1 units of regular insulin per gram of dextrose (i.e., 20 units insulin for 200 grams dextrose) to meet basal insulin requirements.[43] Blood glucose should be monitored every 4 to 6 hours with subcutaneous regular insulin administered using an insulin algorithm such as one in Table 12–11. Blood glucose should be adjusted to 100–150 mg/dL. As blood glucose is controlled with subcutaneous insulin, the amount of regular insulin,

TABLE 12–11   Guidelines for SQ Regular Insulin Supplementation

Blood Glucose mg/dL	SQ Regular Insulin Dose (units)
200–250	2–3
251–300	4–6
301–350	6–9
>350	8–12

SQ-subcutaneous

or part of the amount, can then be added into the next day's PN solution. Patients with difficult blood glucose control while receiving 2-in-1 PN solutions (dextrose + protein) may experience better blood glucose control with 3-in-1 PN solutions (dextrose + protein + lipids).

Most patients to be discharged on HPN will be placed on a cyclic infusion schedule to allow part of the day free from intravenous fluids (see Chapter 8, Table 8–12). To avoid the incidence of hyperglycemia during the first 1–2 hours at initiation of HPN, and hypoglycemia after the last hour of infusion, a taper schedule is usually necessary. Blood glucose should be monitored throughout the HPN cycle (i.e., within the first hour of infusion, mid-cycle, and 1 hour after infusion) with adjustments made in the taper schedules and insulin requirements in order to achieve glycemic control prior to hospital discharge.

Glycemic Management in Home Parenteral Nutrition

Establishment of glycemic control during HPN infusion and when the HPN is not infusing (i.e., off cycle) is important. Regular insulin added to the HPN solution will help control blood glucose while PN is infusing, but the patient with DM will most likely need additional medication to establish glycemic control throughout the rest of the day. The medication may be any combination as previously outlined for the HEN patient, including the use of insulin and/or oral hypoglycemic agents. Adjustments will need to be made considering physiologic stress, previous hypoglycemic medications, and other prescribed medications such as corticosteroids and if an oral diet is consumed. Blood glucose should be monitored at least once or twice daily, including prior to starting HPN infusion and/or within an hour of stopping HPN.

Chromium, an essential trace element involved in carbohydrate metabolism, can impair glucose tolerance if depleted. Jeejeebhoy and associates[44] reported glucose intolerance, weight loss, and neuropathy associated with chromium depletion in a long-term HPN patient, which resolved with chromium supplementation. Chromium deficiency should be considered when glucose intolerance is unexpected or new in any patient on PN. Serum chromium levels may be measured along with other trace elements (copper, manganese, selenium, zinc) and supplemented in the HPN solution with evidence of low levels.

Diabetic patients receiving HSNS should be provided with specific guidelines for self-monitoring of DM and management of hyper- and hypoglycemia. Patients should be advised to contact their physician or HNS clinician if they experience inadequate glycemic control so adjustments can be made to their nutrition support prescription or glucose management medications.

PANCREATITIS

Pancreatitis is an inflamed condition of the pancreas associated with acinar cell injury and can be classified as either acute or chronic. Acute pancreatitis refers to an inflammatory process that usually resolves clinically and histologically to a normal condition. Chronic pancreatitis (CP) is also an inflammatory disorder; however, it is characterized by permanent damage to the pancreas, often resulting in malabsorption and maldigestion of nutrients.[45]

The pancreas is a gland, which has both exocrine and endocrine functions and is located in the upper retroperitoneum situated behind the stomach and close to the liver in a horizontal position. The head of the pancreas is attached to the duodenum, and its tail reaches towards the spleen. The common bile duct receives the main pancreatic duct as it passes through the pancreatic head. The pancreas measures approximately 12–20 cm in length, although it can vary widely among individuals. The endocrine function of the pancreas is to produce insulin, glucagon, and somatostatin, hormones necessary for the metabolism of glucose, fats, and amino acids. The exocrine function, made up of acinar cells, produces the digestive enzymes, amylase, trypsin, and lipase. The pancreas has small ducts that eventually drain 1.5 to 4 liters per day of alkaline digestive fluid into the main pancreatic ducts, which connect to the duodenum at the ampulla where the enzymes are activated.[46] The function of the pancreatic enzymes is to neutralize the gastric juices entering

TABLE 12–12   Physiology and Functions of the Pancreas [46-47]

Endocrine	Exocrine
Islets of Langerhans: clusters of alpha, beta, and delta cells between the ancinar tissue	Acinar cells connected to the pancreatic duct
• Secretes hormones, insulin, glucagons, somatastatin • Secretes hormones necessary for the metabolism of fats, glucose, and amino acids	• Secretes bicarbonate-rich juices • Secretes juices or digestive enzymes, protease, lipase, amylase that aid in digestion. • Secretes enzymes into the ductular system and flow into the duodenum

the duodenum and to help with the continued breakdown of food parti-
cles in the small intestine.[47–50] The endocrine and exocrine functions of
the pancreas are listed in Table 12–12.[46,50] Because of the important role
the pancreas plays in digestion, pancreatitis can result in high nutritional
risk.

Pancreatitis

The pathogenesis of acute and chronic pancreatitis is poorly understood,
but it is thought that intrapancreatic, premature activation of enzymes
into the interstitium may lead to autodigestion of the pancreas. The primary and secondary causes of pancreatitis are listed on Table 12–13.[51,52]

Acute Pancreatitis

Over 80% of hospital admissions for acute pancreatitis are mild cases of
pancreatitis. The hospital course is limited, and there is a rather quick
return to normal pancreatic function. Patients typically present with a
history of abdominal pain and tenderness and elevations in serum pancreatic enzymes, amylase, and lipase. Twenty percent of acute pancreatitis cases, however, are classified as severe and are characterized by organ
failure, pancreatic necrosis, abscess, pseudocyst, and/or acute fluid collections. Patients with mild acute pancreatitis generally recover with supportive care of IV fluids, repletion of electrolytes, bowel rest, and antibiotics as indicated and analgesia.[49] These patients generally transition to
an oral diet within 5–7 days, although patients with more severe pancreatitis may require HSNS as a therapeutic management tool that may
favorably alter the patient's hospital course. The prevalence of acute pancreatitis is approximately 80,000 cases per year.[47,51]

TABLE 12–13   Primary and Secondary Causes of Pancreatitis[51,52]

Primary	Secondary
Gallstones: common cause of acute pancreatitis and associated with chronic pancreatitis 20–25% of the time	Hyperlipidemia (usually Type I and Type V)
Alcohol abuse: associated with chronic pancreatitis about 60% of the time	Blunt abdominal trauma from accidents involving motor vehicles, bicycles, horses
Idiopathic: 20% of the cases	Hereditary pancreatitis: autosomal dominant disorder
	Cystic Fibrosis
	Uremia
	Medications: <1.4% of cases and usually acute form
	Pancreatic cancer
	Obesity
	Viral trigger (mumps, CMV)
	Congenital causes: abnormality of fusion, pancreas divisum

Chronic Pancreatitis

Chronic pancreatitis (CP) refers to a condition that is characterized by relapsing inflammation, which results in permanent damage to the pancreas and destruction of the exocrine and eventually endocrine tissue and function of the pancreas. Patients with prolonged CP or with complications as a result of pancreatitis may require long-term HSNS long-term and are often managed in the home care setting.[52,53]

The diagnosis of CP is based on the patient's history and signs and symptoms of pancreatitis (listed on Table 12–14) that is then confirmed by imaging studies that can assess morphology for abnormalities. Examples of imaging studies include: abdominal x-ray, ultrasonography, endoscopic ultrasonography, computed axial tomography, magnetic resonance cholangiopanreatography, and endoscopic retrograde cholangiopancreatography, the most accurate visualization of the pancreatic ductal system. Additionally, specific laboratory tests may be ordered to diagnose CP and assess pancreatic function; however, elevations in serum amylase and lipase found during acute attacks and early in the course of the disease are not reliable diagnostic indicators for CP.[54,55]

TABLE 12–14   Signs and Symptoms of Chronic Pancreatitis[54,55]

- Upper abdominal pain radiating to the back
- Fever
- Bloating, gas, distention, tenderness
- Loose stools/diarrhea
- Dehydration
- Steatorrhea with <10% exocrine function
- Hyperglycemia
- Abnormal lipid metabolism
- Abnormalities in gastric emptying
- Decreased appetite
- Weight loss
- Loss of lean body mass, temporal wasting
- Jaundice with common bile duct obstruction
- Maldigestion
- Malabsorption noted in 25% to 45% of patients
- Malnutrition

Malnutrition and nutritional alterations are known complications associated with pancreatitis. The causes are multifactorial and are listed in Table 12–15.[47,48] When the destruction of islet cells and the insulin-secreting beta cells occur, diabetes can develop. The occurrence of diabetes in CP has been reported in 70–90% of patients.[56] Insulin may be required to maintain good glycemic control. Diabetes management in CP can be challenging for patients on HSNS. (Please refer to the section on Diabetes Mellitus in this chapter for more complete management protocols.)

Nutrition Support in Chronic Pancreatitis

Pancreatic enzyme replacement, titrated to minimize steatorrhea, and a moderate fat oral diet, customized to alleviate symptoms, are recommended for those patients who can eat. For patients who are unable to eat, have secondary to pain, worsening symptoms or digestive disturbances due to pancreatic insufficiency, HSNS may be indicated.[57,58]

Nutritional Assessment of Chronic Pancreatitis Patients

Patients with pancreatitis are at high nutritional risk. When oral intake is anticipated to be inadequate for longer than 5–7 days, patients should receive a comprehensive nutrition assessment to set nutrition goals, to establish the patient's plan of care, and to determine the most appropriate nutrition support intervention, using either the enteral or parenteral

TABLE 12–15   Potential Causes of Malnutrition in Chronic
Pancreatitis[48, 50]

Hypermetabolism:	Related to chronic inflammation, but hypermetabolism is primarily associated with acute pancreatitis
Reduced oral intake:	Secondary to pain, nausea, vomiting, gastric atony, paralytic ileus, partial duodenal obstruction, bowel rest, fear of eating
Maldigestion and malabsorption:	Secondary to pancreatic insufficiency, small bowel changes. Specifically malabsorption of fat-soluble vitamins (A,D,E,K), calcium, zinc, selenium
Errors in carbohydrate metabolism:	Secondary to the loss of endocrine function seen in 40%–90% of patients

route.[58] The nutrition support professional should consider the cause as well as the symptoms of pancreatitis to determine the best plan of care. For instance, those with a history of alcohol use may benefit from therapeutic supplementation of thiamine and folate, and patients with protracted vomiting may require supplementation of micronutrients, such as zinc, magnesium, and potassium. Table 12–16 outlines the nutrition assessment considerations for the patient with CP.[47,58] The goals for HSNS intervention are to avoid catabolism, to provide adequate macronutrients and micronutrients to meet an individual's needs, and to minimize pancreatic stimulation and pain.

When patients are clinically stable, they can be considered candidates for receiving their infusion therapies in the home or outpatient setting. Pancreatitis patients often receive multiple therapies, and discharge planning and/or home care delivery is challenging. Monitoring patients on PN or EN in the home care setting should be therapy specific, ongoing, collaborative, and multidisciplinary. It is imperative that patients and care partners receive education regarding CP and supportive therapies. HSNS can be cost-effective and safely delivered in the home with proper patient selection and close monitoring by a nutrition support team working with therapy and disease-specific standards of care.

TABLE 12–16   Nutrition Assessment Considerations in Chronic Pancreatitis [47,58]

Alcoholic pancreatitis:	Consider thiamine, folate supplementation; consider deficiencies in water-soluble vitamins as well as magnesium, zinc
Vomiting, diarrhea:	Evaluate micronutrient needs for supplementation
Steatorrhea:	Consider risk for fat-soluble vitamin malabsorption, need for pancreatitic enzyme supplementation containing 30,000 units of lipase activity, and addition of MCT for calories
Hyperglycemia:	Consider balanced carbohydrate intake and need for insulin to maintain good glycemic control
Multiple therapies:	Consider the need for pain therapy, antibiotics, or enteral therapy transition; consider need for multiple lumen catheter

Home Enteral Nutrition

Postpyloric placement of access for EN has shown to be efficacious in pancreatitis, as it is presumed that negligible stimulation occurs in the distal jejunum due to the elimination of the cephalic and gastric phases of digestion. According to Giger and associates,[59] feeding beyond the Ligament of Treitz through a percutaneous endoscopic gastrojejunostomy (PEG/J) or a direct percutaneous endoscopic jejunostomy (DEPJ) tube minimizes pancreatic stimulation and appears to be well tolerated. Stanga and colleagues[60] reported that jejunal feeding in symptomatic patients with CP, improved weight decreased the degree of malnutrition, pain, nausea, and vomiting. Several other studies have shown jejunal feeding in CP to be effective and less expensive than HPN.[57] Although it has been reported that some patients tolerate standard polymeric formulas well,[59] other reports suggest less pancreatic stimulation and therefore pain occurs with formulas containing medium chain triglycerides and hydrolyzed peptides.[61] Formula selection should be based on pancreatic function and the established goals for nutrition support and patient care. Patients with less than 10% exocrine function, however, may benefit from a predigested formula containing a lower fat content and pancreatic enzyme replacement in conjunction with the enteral feeding.[62] Monitoring of HEN for patients with acute pancreatitis or CP should be done by experienced nutrition support clinicians (see Chapter 6). It is impor-

TABLE 12–17   Parenteral Nutrition Prescription for Pancreatitis[50,61]

Calories	Generally normometabolic, 33% hypermetabolic with needs 1.5 times Harris-Benedict equation or 120% of REE
Protein	Consider, per renal, liver tolerance, increased protein needs: 1.4–2.0 g/kg body weight
Lipids	1 gm/kg/BW Can be used safely as a source of calories and essential fatty acids for patients if serum TG levels are monitored and remain below 400 mg/dL
Fluids	35 ml/kg 20–55 yr 30 ml/kg 55–75 yr 25 ml/kg >75 yr
Vitamins/minerals	Meet the AMA-NAG recommended amounts of the Nutrition Advisory Group (NAG) of the Department of Foods and Nutrition of the American Medical Association (AMA)

tant to ensure that pain and symptoms are managed so that HEN is successful. Care should be taken to ensure that the feeding tube is not malpositioned and is in the optimal location. If pain and symptoms persist, a change to HPN may be warranted to prevent malnutrition.

Home Parenteral Nutrition

Patients who have poor tolerance to HEN or who experience an exacerbation of symptoms may benefit from HPN to promote bowel rest and maintain or restore nutritional status and positive nitrogen balance. Controversy has persisted about the use of fat emulsions; however, unless the pancreatitis is caused by a lipid disorder, IV lipids can be safely administered at 1 gm/kg body weight. Dextrose infusion should be titrated to provide adequate, balanced calories while maintaining glycemic control between 80–150 mg/dl. It has been recommended that infusion of dextrose not exceed 5–7 mg/kg/minute for patients in the acute care setting;[56] however, stable patients in the home care setting may be able to tolerate a higher infusion rate. Ultimately, glycemic control should be the guide for dextrose infusion in the stable, home care patient. Table 12–17 lists PN prescription recommendations.[47,61]

Monitoring pancreatitis patients on HPN is similar to that of any patient on HPN (see Chapter 6). As with the HEN patient, pain and symptom assessment should be a standard component of care. Concomitant pain medications may affect GI motility and therefore this should be considered in the HPN or HEN monitoring protocol.

In addition to these guidelines, the oral diet progression should be monitored, as well as any pain exacerbation associated with eating. The HPN patient with pancreatitis should begin to be challenged with an oral diet. Because there is no problem with the mechanism of getting food into the GI tract, there is no need to progress from HPN to an enteral tube feeding to an oral diet. It has been suggested that patients begin with clear liquids and advance to a diet low in fat, high in protein, low-residue, low fiber, and moderate to high carbohydrate with alcohol abstinence. A registered dietitian can assist the patients in increasing their oral intake while decreasing the enteral or parenteral intake. An oral vitamin and mineral supplement should be provided as HSNS is weaned. Pancreatic enzyme replacement (30,000 units of lipase activity per meal suggested) is recommended when steatorrhea is present, and if persistent, then fat should be lowered to 30% of caloric intake or less.[59] It has been reported that over 95% of patients with CP experience abdominal pain; therefore, the pain will interfere with the ability to optimize nutrition.[63] Monitoring of pain, using assessment tools such as a pain diary and a pain rating scale, should be completed weekly for all pancreatitis patients on HSNS.

CANCER

Cancer is a general term for more than 250 diseases and is the second leading cause of death in the United States.[64] It is characterized by disorganized, uncontrolled abnormal cell growth that spreads locally through the bloodstream and lymphatic system to other parts of the body. Malnutrition frequently occurs in cancer patients; therefore, nutrition can play an important role throughout the clinical course of the disease.

Malnutrition

Forty to 80% of cancer patients have some degree of malnutrition.[67,68] Malnourished cancer patients are at risk for increased morbidity and mortality when undergoing major surgical procedures, and malnutrition

TABLE 12–18   Risk Factors Associated with Malnutrition in Cancer Patients[64-66]

Type of tumor
Stage of disease
Side effects of radiation or chemotherapy (i.e., mucositis, dysgeusia, xerostomia, stomatitis, nausea, vomiting, anorexia)
Effects of surgery (i.e., gastrectomy, intestinal resections, esophagectomy)
Bowel obstruction
Increased nutritional needs
Diminished nutrient intake
Depression/anxiety
Abnormal nutrient metabolism
Pain
Cytokine activity
Cytoreduction

is a poor prognostic indicator for patients undergoing various cancer treatments.[64] Additionally, malnutrition results in delayed wound healing, weight loss, muscle weakness, compromised organ function, impaired immune function, increased hospital stay, decreased quality of life, and an increased use of health care dollars.[65] Several factors increase the risk of malnutrition in the cancer patient and are outlined in Table 12–18.[64,66]

Cancer cachexia is a maladaptive response to starvation, resulting in extreme weight loss of both lean and fat tissue. It results in anorexia and early satiety and cannot be reversed by nutrition alone. The inability of feeding to reverse the weight loss in cancer cachexia is a fundamental difference between simple starvation and cancer cachexia.[69] Cytokines promote increased demands for energy and have been implicated in the pathophysiology of cancer cachexia and may cause the metabolic aberrations seen not only in cancer patients, but also in patients who are stressed or critically ill. Cytokines play a part in the activation of the immune response as well as the inflammatory response and are produced by the tumor or by the host's response to the tumor. Approximately 50% of cancer patients suffer from cancer cachexia, and it has been reported that 20% of all cancer patients die of cachexia.[70] Nutrition support alone in the cachectic patient has not been shown to be an effective treatment for poor nutrition.[71]

Not all cancers are associated with weight loss and malnutrition. A lower frequency of weight loss is associated with breast and hematologic cancers. However, a high frequency of weight loss is associated with solid tumors of the pancreas and stomach. With pancreatic cancer, greater than 50% suffer weight loss and 30% exhibit weight loss greater than 10% within the previous 6 months.[72] Esophageal and head and neck cancers are also associated with significant nutritional deficits primarily due to the inability to eat secondary to obstruction.[72]

Nutrition Assessment in the Cancer Patient

A comprehensive nutritional assessment that includes an evaluation of anthropometrics, laboratory values, diet history, medication profile, functionality, cancer treatment, and other supportive care modalities must be completed to identify the degree of malnutrition or the risk for malnutrition and to determine a patient's macronutrient and micronutrient needs.[73] A patient-specific care plan should be developed to monitor and evaluate the patient's progress. The PG-SGA has been tested and utilized in the cancer population and can be useful when assessing baseline nutritional deficits and determining nutrition needs around the time of diagnosis.[74] The PG-SGA was adopted from the Subjective Global Assessment clinical tool, but with the PG-SGA the patient has input and answers questions regarding weight changes, food intake, gastrointestinal symptoms, and functional status.[74] Monitoring weight changes alone, however, can provide a meaningful and quick way to assess nutritional status, especially in the home care patient (see Table 12–19[75]). Roy and associates[76] suggest that simply monitoring patients for weight loss of 6% or greater can be used as a quick and effective way to predict postoperative complications in cancer patients.

Home Nutrition Support Recommendations for the Cancer Patient

It is important to provide adequate calories to spare reserves of body fat and muscle and enough protein to meet protein needs and reduce catabolism. When determining micronutrient needs, it is imperative that a thorough review of antineoplastic medications be conducted to evaluate for potential metabolic derangements caused by the medications. For example, cytotoxic agents such as cisplatin may cause wasting of magne-

TABLE 12–19   Evaluating Adult Weight Loss [75]

Percentage of Ideal Body Weight

- 80–90% mild malnutrition
- 70–79% moderate malnutrition
- < 69% severe malnutrition

Percentage of Usual Body Weight

- 85–95% mild malnutrition
- 75–84% moderate malnutrition
- < 74% severe malnutrition

Weight Loss Over Time

• 1 week	1–2% significant loss	>2% severe loss
• 1 month	5% significant loss	>5% severe loss
• 3 months	7.5% significant loss	>7.5% severe loss
• 6 months	10% significant loss	>10% severe loss

sium, and methotrexate is associated with folate deficiency. Provisions in the plan of care must be made for short- and long-term effects of all cancer treatments, including medications that may trigger a need to re-evaluate the nutrition prescription to ensure that the patient's needs are met. Nutrient recommendations and considerations for cancer patients are outlined in Table 12–20.[66]

Goals of Nutrition Therapy

The use of HSNS in the cancer patient is adjuvant and is meant to be a part of the patient's overall treatment plan. Routine use of HSNS in the cancer patient has not been shown to change clinical outcome; however, HSNS is used when oral intake is inadequate or impossible to support the "host" (the patient with cancer) in maintaining or regaining optimal nutritional status.[66] Although nutrition support alone will not change the outcome of the cancer, it will allow the patient to retain lean body mass, which is associated with improved functional status and quality of life. It has become a standard of practice to use PN support in the bone marrow transplant (BMT) patient where its use during and immediately following BMT has been shown to increase survival.[66,72] It is imperative to give careful consideration to the benefits and the risks of HSNS in the cancer population.[77]

TABLE 12–20   Nutrient Recommendations and Considerations for Cancer Patients[68]

Energy:	Use actual body weight	
	Refeeding	20 kcal/kg
	Obese	21–25 kcal/kg
	Maintenance	25–30 kcal/kg
	Weight loss	30–35 kcal/kg
	Depleted	35 kcal/kg and adjusted upwards
Protein:	0.5–0.8 g/kg with hepatic or renal compromise	
	1.0–1.5 g/kg most non-stressed cancer patients	
	1.5 g/kg bone marrow transplant	
	1.5–2.0 g/kg depleted/increased demands	
Lipids:	30% of calories or 1 gm/kg BW	
Fluids:	35 ml/kg/day	20–55 yr
	30 ml/kg/day	55–75 yr
	25 ml/kg/day	>75 yr
Micronutrients:	Enteral: 1–2 times RDA/DRI	
	Parenteral: AMA-NAG daily	
	Appropriate dose per deficiency/toxicity	
	Avoid megadosing[7-9]	
Drug Treatments:	Immunotherapy	
	TNF	Hypotension, Nausea Vomiting, Diarrhea
	Interferons	Anorexia, Nausea Vomiting, Diarrhea
	Corticosteroids	Sodium retention; Potassium, calcium Magnesium, zinc Retention, Hyperglycemia, Nitrogen losses
	Megestrol Acetate	Fluid retention
	Cytotoxic Agents	Drug dependent, but includes: Hypoglycemia, mucositis, Fluid retention, folate and calcium deficiency

The nutrition goals for cancer patients are not dissimilar to the goals that are made for other disease states, but the goals should consider the effects of various treatments and any nutritional implications of those treatments. The overall goal in cancer patients is to minimize or stop weight loss, preserve or improve lean body mass, prevent micronutrient deficiencies, reduce complications associated with malnutrition, and improve functional capacity as well as quality of life.[78,79]

Home Specialized Nutrition Support

Oral Nutrition/Appetite Stimulation

Many cancer patients may benefit from oral nutritional supplements, which provide a source of calories, protein, vitamins, and minerals. They can be used as a meal replacement or as a supplement. There is an array of standard oral supplements, as well as immune-enhancing supplements specifically modulated for the cancer patient available on the market.

The use of appetite-stimulating agents has been evaluated as a means to treat the anorexia associated with cancer. Few have shown to be effective at sustaining weight gain or improving nutritional status over time, with the exception of megesterol acetate (Megace®).[66,80] Megace® is both immunosuppressive and anti-inflammatory and was first used to treat hormone-sensitive tumors. Studies have reported that patients on Megace® experienced weight gain and appetite stimulation.[80] Anabolic agents, such as oxandrolone and growth hormone may also prove to be beneficial in maintaining and promoting lean body mass; however, more studies are needed to provide clinicians with better direction in the use of these agents.[66]

Home Enteral Nutrition

Home enteral nutrition should be considered when a patient is unable to meet nutrient needs by the oral route alone but has a functional GI tract.

Indications for HEN include:

- Dysphagia
- Anatomical defect that would normally allow food to reach the small intestine (esophageal resection or obstruction, gastric outlet obstruction, glossectomy)
- Anorexia
- Dysmotility
- Fistula
- Nausea and vomiting

If short-duration EN is anticipated (< 4 weeks), then HEN can be easily delivered by a nasogastric or nasoenteric tube. Longer-term op-

TABLE 12–21   Monthly Monitoring Checklist for the Cancer Patient on Enteral Tube Feeding[77,80]

Monitoring Parameter	Checklist
Anthropometrics	Determine if there have been any weight changes and cause
Vital signs	Determine if history of a fever
Gastrointestinal complaints	Determine if there are complaints of nausea, vomiting, constipation, and diarrhea. Determine frequency and discern cause.
Medication list	Any medication deletions or additions. Review side effects.
Hydration status	Determine fluid intake and compare to need and the amount in tube feeding formula. Ask about urine frequency and color, skin turgor.
Compliance to prescription	Review and calculate the average daily intake and compare to prescription
Tube patency and stoma site	Assess tube for patency and inspect stoma site for drainage, redness
Insurance changes	Inquire if there has been a change in insurance coverage
Quality of life	Measure functional and performance status once per month using a quality of life assessment tool such as Karnofsky Performance Status Scale

tions, generally more appropriate for home care, include gastrostomy or jejunostomy feeding tubes inserted endoscopically or surgically. Formula selection should be made based on a patient's clinical status (see Chapter 6). The patient's initial assessment dictates the plan of care and the initial monitoring guidelines. Once the patient is stable, monthly monitoring that relies on patient participation is generally adequate. Monitoring guidelines for EN in cancer patients are provided in Table 12–21.[77,80]

Parenteral Nutrition

When HEN is contraindicated, HPN may be considered.
    Indications for HPN include:[76,81]

- Bowel obstruction
- High output fistula (> 500 ml)
- Severe malabsorption
- Intractable vomiting
- GI bleeding
- Inability to meet nutrient needs with enteral nutrition[13,18]

Common reasons for HPN therapy in the cancer patient include obstruction secondary to ovarian cancer, radiation enteritis, cancers of the small intestine, pancreatic cancer, BMT, and chronic graft versus host disease (GVHD).[82] Nutrition therapy plays an important role in all phases of solid organ and BMTs. Transplant patients who are malnourished have been shown to have poorer outcomes and reduced survival.[83] In particular, GVHD is a leading cause of morbidity and mortality in allogeneic stem cell transplant patients. Intestinal GVHD manifests as high output diarrhea, nausea, pain, vomiting, and malabsorption, which causes further compromise of a patient's nutritional status.[84] Patients with GVHD have increased nutritional needs secondary to hypermetabolism and tissue regeneration. Both acute and chronic GVHD may be treated with PN support, and often patients with chronic GVHD are on longer-term PN support in the home care setting.[85] For a more complete description of GVHD and its management, please refer to Chapter 15.

Home PN may be initiated in an acute care setting with discharge occurring after the patient is tolerating the recommended amount. Cycling, if appropriate, can be done before discharge or by the infusion provider. With careful patient selection, PN may be initiated in the home care setting. A checklist to assist with determining clinical appropriateness for home PN is provided in Table 12–22. There are a variety of venous access devices available to the oncologist for providing chemotherapy as well as nutrition therapy.[81,82] For a full description of vascular access devices, see Chapter 7.

Monitoring guidelines for HPN are outlined in Chapter 8 and are applicable to the cancer patient. For both HPN and HEN patients, it may be important to measure functional and performance status once per month using a quality of life assessment tool such as the Karnofsky Performance Status Scale.[86] A baseline measurement taken at the start of care allows for monthly comparison to determine functionality and performance status for patients receiving home nutrition support therapies. These scores may be used as an indicator to report quality of life out-

TABLE 12–22   Checklist for Determining Appropriateness for Initiation of Parenteral Nutrition in the Cancer Patient

1. Prescribing physician of record has seen the patient in the last week, and the risks and benefits of parenteral nutrition therapy as adjuvant to cancer treatment have been discussed with the patient.

2. The patient is clinically stable with no renal failure, congestive heart failure, liver failure, or insulin-dependent diabetes.

3. The patient does not have output losses of greater than 1 liter per day.

4. No history of substance abuse.

5. No history of egg allergy.

6. The patient or care partner is willing and able to become independent with all aspects of parenteral nutrition administration.

7. The patient has a venous access device.

8. The patient has a home environment suitable for the administration of parenteral nutrition.

9. Current laboratory values are available and include the following:

    - CBC with differential
    - Electrolyte panel
    - BUN/Creatinine
    - LFTs
    - Total protein
    - Albumin
    - Calcium, phosphorus, magnesium, glucose
    - PT

10. Medication and cancer treatment regimens have been reviewed for wasting and concentration of micronutrients and other potential metabolic aberrations such as hyperglycemia, fluid retention.

11. The risk of *refeeding syndrome* has been evaluated, and the nutrition support team or clinician has completed a comprehensive nutrition assessment to determine appropriate initiation protocol.

12. The ability to improve or maintain quality of life has been evaluated, and goals for maintaining or improving quality of life, using measurement tools such as Karnofsky, have been established.

13. Goals of therapy have been established.

14. Patient consents to treatment.

comes in cancer patients receiving parenteral and/or enteral nutrition in the home and perhaps be useful in determining the efficacy of HSNS as an adjuvant therapy. Monitoring patients for response to HSNS, as well as attempting to quantify the impact on quality of life, may allow for better clinical guidance when determining the appropriateness of nutrition support interventions in the cancer population at risk for malnutrition as well as determining the efficacy of HSNS.[79,87]

CONCLUSION

Patients suffering from intestinal failure and requiring nutrition support in the home often have co-morbid conditions that have a significant impact on the selection and management of enteral and parenteral nutrition therapies. While the overall goal of home nutrition support for all patients is the provision of adequate nutrients and fluid in a safe manner, this can be especially challenging in patients with liver and renal disease, diabetes mellitus, pancreatitis, and cancer. Home care clinicians must be familiar with the effects of altered metabolism, and the various treatments and medications of these diseases when developing, managing, and monitoring HSNS.

REFERENCES

1. Hayes PC, Simpson KJ, Gorden OJ. Liver and biliary tract disease. In: Haslet C, Chilvers ER, Boon NA, Colledge NR, Hunter JAA, eds. *Davidson's Principles and Practice of Medicine*, 19th edition. New York: Churchill Livingston; 2002:831–888.
2. Steiger E, Hamilton C. Hepatobiliary associated complications of home parenteral nutrition. *Support Line*. 2003;25(5):3–5.
3. Raup SM, Kaproth P. Hepatic failure. In: Matarese LM, Gottsclich MM, eds. *Contemporary Nutrition Support Practice, A Clinical Guide*. Philadelphia: W.B. Saunders Company;1998:441–446.
4. Lindor KD, Fleming CR, Abrams A, Hirschkorn MA. Liver function values in adults receiving total parenteral nutrition. *JAMA*. 1979;241(22): 2398–2400.
5. Salvian AJ, Allardyce DB. Impaired bilirubin secretion during total parenteral nutrition. *J Surg Res*. 1980;28:547–555.
6. Grant JP, Cox CE, Kleinman LM, et al. Serum hepatic enzyme and bilirubin elevations during parenteral nutrition. *Surg Gynecol Obstet*. 1977;145: 573–580.

7. Lowry SF, Brennan MF. Abnormal liver function during parenteral nutrition. Relation to infusion excess. *J Surg Res.* 1979; 26:300–307.

8. Luman W, Shaffer JL. Prevalence, outcome and associated factors of deranged liver function tests in patients on home parenteral nutrition. *Clin Nutr.* 2002;21:337–343.

9. Cavicchi M, Beau P, Crenn P, et al. Prevalence of liver disease and contributing factors in patients receiving home parenteral nutrition for permanent intestinal failure. *Ann Intern Med.* 2000;132:525–532.

10. Seidner DL, Salvino RM, Ghanta RK, Steiger E, Mascha E. Liver failure is uncommon in adults on home TPN. *JPEN.* 2003;27(1): S3 abstract.

11. Chan S, McGowen KC, Bistrian BR, et al. Incidence, prognosis, and etiology of end-stage liver disease in patients receiving home total parenteral nutrition. *Surgery.* 1999;126:28–34.

12. Allardyce DB. Cholestasis caused by lipid emulsions. *Surg Gynecol Obstet.* 1982;154:641–647.

13. Buchman A. Total parenteral nutrition-associated liver disease. *J Parenter Enteral Nutr.* 2002;26(suppl 5):S43–S48.

14. Chambrier C, Lemann M, Vahedi M, et al. Chronic cholestasis in patients supported by prolonged parenteral nutrition. (abstr) *J Parenter Enteral Nutr.* 1998;22(1):S16.

15. Hwang T, Lue M, Chen L. Early use of cyclic TPN prevents further deterioration of liver functions for TPN patients with impaired liver function. *Hepatogastroenterology.* 2000;47:1347–1350.

16. Wolk R. Nutrition in renal failure. In: Gottsclich MM, ed. *The Science and Practice of Nutrition Support, A Case-Based Core Curriculum.* Dubuque: Kendall/Hunt Publishing Company;2001:575–599.

17. Charney DI. Medical treatment in renal disease: basic concept in dialysis. *Support Line.* 1998;20(1):3–7.

18. Charney P, Charney D. Nutrition support in renal failure. *Nutr Clin Pract.* 2002;17(4):226–236.

19. Birnbaum B. Protein status in chronic dialysis patients. *Support Line.* 1999; 21(1):16–22.

20. National Kidney Foundation. Clinical practice guidelines for nutrition in chronic renal failure. *Am J Kidney Dis.* 2000;35(suppl 6):S1–S140.

21. Lowrie EG, Lew NL. Death risk in hemodialysis patients: the predictive value of commonly measured variables and an evaluation of death rate differences between facilities. *Am J Kidney Dis.* 1990;15:458–482.

22. Barco K. Total parenteral nutrition for adults with renal failure in acute care. *Support Line.* 200224(4):22–28.

23. Beto JA, Bansal VK. Medical nutrition therapy in chronic kidney failure: integrating clinical practice guidelines. *J Am Diet Assoc.* 2004;104(3):404–409.

24. Kalista-Richards M, Cook HC. Iron as an essential micronutrient. *Support Line.* 2002;24(6):17–22.

25. Duerksen DR, Papineau N. Electrolyte abnormalities in patients with chronic renal failure receiving parenteral nutrition. *J Parenter Enteral Nutr.* 1998; 22(2):102–104.

26. McCann L, Nelson P, Fedje F, Wang M, eds. *Pocket Guide to Nutrition Assessment of the Renal Patient.* 2nd ed. New York: National Kidney Foundation; 1998.

27. Kopple JD. Therapeutic approaches to malnutrition in chronic dialysis patients: the different modalities of nutritional support. *Am J Kidney Dis.* 1999; 33(1):180–185.

28. Mirtallo JM, Schneider PJ, Mavko K, et al. A comparison of essential and general amino acid infusions in the nutrition support of patients with compromised renal function. *J Parenter Enteral Nutr.* 1982;6:109–113.

29. Capelli JP, Kushner H, Camiscioli TC, et al. Effect of intradialytic parenteral nutrition on mortality rates in end-stage renal disease care. *Am J Kidney Dis.* 1994;23:808–816.

30. Chertow GM, Ling J, Lew NL, et al. The association of intradialytic parenteral nutrition administration with survival in hemodialysis patients. *Am J Kidney Dis.* 1994;24:912–920.

31. Lazarus JM. Recommended criteria for initiating and discontinuing intradialytic parenteral nutrition. *Am J Kidney Dis.* 1999;33:211–216.

32. Foulks CJ. An evidence-based evaluation of intradialytic parenteral nutrition. *Am J Kidney Dis.* 1999;33(1):186–192.

33. National diabetes statistics. [National Diabetes Information Clearinghouse Website]. Available at: http://www.diabetes.niddk.nih.gov. Accessed February 28, 2005.

34. The Expert Committee on the Diagnosis and Classification of Diabetes Mellitus. Report of the expert committee on the diagnosis and classification of diabetes mellitus. *Diabetes Care.* 1997;20:1183–1197.

35. Frier BM, Fisher BM. Diabetes mellitus. In: Haslett C, Chilvers ER, Boon NA, Colledge NR, Hunter JAA, eds. *Davidson's Principles and Practice of Medicine*, 19th edition. New York: Churchill Livingston;2002:641–682.

36. Diabetes Control and Complications Trial Research Group. The effect of intensive treatment of diabetes on the development and progression of long-term complications in insulin-dependent diabetes mellitus. *N Engl J Med.* 1993;329:977–986.

37. Franz MJ, Bantle JP, Beebe CA, et al. Evidence-based nutrition principles and recommendations for the treatment and prevention of diabetes and related complications. *Diabetes Care.* 2002;25:148–198.

38. Van Den Berghe G, Wouters P, Weekers F, et al. Intensive insulin therapy in critically ill patients. *N Engl J Med.* 2001;345:1359–1367.

39. McMahon MM. Management of parenteral nutrition in acutely ill patients with hyperglycemia. *Nutr Clin Pract.* 2004;19:120–128.

40. Peters AL, Davidson MB, Isaac RM. Lack of glucose elevation after simulated tube feeding with low carbohydrate, high-fat enteral formula in patients with type I diabetes. *Am J Med.* 1989;87:178–182.

41. Peters AL, Davidson MB. Effects of various enteral feeding products on post-prandial blood glucose response in patients with type I diabetes. *J Parenter Enteral Nutr.* 1992;16:69–74.

42. Craig LD, Nicholson S, Silverstone FA, Kennedy RD. Use of a reduced-carbohydrate, modified-fat enteral formula for improving metabolic control and clinical outcomes in long-term care residents with type 2 diabetes: results of a pilot trial. *Nutrition.* 1998;14:529–534.

43. Hurley DL, Neven AK, McMahon MM. Diabetes mellitus. In: Gottsclich MM, ed. *The Science and Practice of Nutrition Support, A Core-Based Curriculum.* Dubuque: Kendall/Hunt Publishing Company;2001:663–675.

44. Jeejeebhoy KN, Chu RC, Marliss EB, et al. Chromium deficiency, glucose intolerance, and neuropathy reversed by chromium supplementation, in a patient receiving long-term total parenteral nutrition. *Am J Clin Nutr.* 1977;30: 531–538.

45. Khokar AS, Seidner DL. The pathophysiology of pancreatitis. *Nutr Clin Pract.* 2004;19(1):5–15.

46. Crawford JM, Cotran RS. The pancreas. In: Komar V, Cotran R, Collins T, eds. *Robbins Pathologic Basis of Disease.* 6th ed. Philadelphia, PA: WB Saunders;1999:902–913.

47. Wall-Alonso E, Sullivan MM, Byrne TA. Gastrointestinal and pancreatic disease. In: Matarese LE, Gottsclich MM, eds. *Contemporary Nutrition Support Practice A Clinical Guide.* Saunders Publishing; 2003:412–444.

48. Holthouse B. Pancreatitis: a comprehensive review. *Support Line.* 2000;22(1): 3–10.

49. Banks, PA. Practice guidelines in acute pancreatitis. *Am J Gastroenterol.* 1997; 92:377–386.

50. Weber CK, Adler G. From acinar cell damage to systemic inflammatory response: current concepts in pancreatitis. *Pancreatology.* 2001;1(4):356–362.

51. Cano NJM. Nutrition in acute pancreatitis. *Crit Care & Shock.* 2004;7: 69–76.

52. Yakseh P. eMedicine Journal. Pancreatitis, chronic. March 4, 2002, Volume 3, Number 3.

53. The Merck Manual of Diagnosis and Therapy. Chronic pancreatitis. Section 3 Gastrointestinal Disorders; Chapter 26 Pancreatitis. 2005.

54. Niederau C, Grendell JH. Diagnosis of chronic pancreatitis. *Gastroenterology.* 1985;88:1973–1995.

55. Niederau C, Schonberg M. New developments in the pathophysiology of inflammatory pancreatic disease. *Hepatogastroenterology.* 1999;46:2722.

56. McMahon MM. Management of parenteral nutrition in acutely ill patients with hyperglycemia. *Nutr Clin Pract.* 2004;19:120–128.

57. McClave SA. Defining the new gold standard for nutrition support in acute pancreatitis. *Nutr Clin Pract.* 2004;19(1):1–4.
58. A.S.P.E.N. Board of Directors and The Clinical Guidelines Task Force Guidelines for the use of parenteral and enteral nutrition in adult and pediatric patients: pancreatitis. *J Parenter Enteral Nutr.* 2002;26(1):S69–S70.
59. Giger U, Stanga Z, DeLegge MH. Management of chronic pancreatitis. *Nutr Clin Pract.* 2004;19(1):37–49.
60. Stanga Z, Giger U, Marx A, DeLegge MH. Effect of jejunal long-term feeding in chronic pancreatitis. *J Parenter Enteral Nutr.* 2005;29(1):12–20.
61. Kaushik N, O'Keefe SJ. Severe acute pancreatitis: nutritional management in the ICU. *Nutr Clin Pract.* 2004;19(1):25–30.
62. Fang JC, DiSario JA. Strategies in managing chronic pancreatitis-placement of direct percutaneous endoscopic jejunostomy feeding tubes. *Nutr Clin Pract.* 2004;19(1):50–55.
63. Rothley B. Unraveling the mystery of pain in chronic pancreatitis. *Nutr Clin Pract.* 2004;19(1):56–59.
64. Yeatman TJ. Nutritional support for the surgical oncology patient. *Cancer Control.* 2000;7(6):563–565.
65. Ollenschlager G, Viell B, Thomas W, et al. Tumor anorexia: causes, assessment, treatment. *Recent Results Cancer Res.* 1991;121:249–259.
66. Bloch, AS. Cancer. In: Matarese LE, Gottsclich MM, eds. *Contemporary Nutrition Support Practice, A Clinical Guide.* Philadelphia: W.B. Saunders Publishing;2003:484–508.
67. Kern KA, Norton JA. Cancer cachexia. *J Parenter Enteral Nutr.* 1988;12:286–298.
68. van Bokhorst-de van der Schuer, van Leewen PA, Kuik DJ, et al. The impact of nutritional status on the prognoses of patients with advanced head and neck cancer. *Cancer.* 1999;86:519–527.
69. Nebeling L. Changes in carbohydrate, protein and fat metabolism in cancer. In: McCallum PD, Polisena CG, eds. *The Clinical Guide to Oncology Nutrition.* Chicago: American Dietetic Association; 2000.
70. Barber, MD. The pathophysiology and treatment of cancer cachexia. *Nutr Clin Pract.* 2002;17(4):203–209.
71. Brennan MF. Uncomplicated starvation versus cancer cachexia. *Cancer Res.* 1977;37:2359–2364.
72. Barrera R. Nutritional support in cancer patients. *J Parenter Enteral Nutr.* 2002;26(suppl 5):S63–S71.
73. A.S.P.E.N. Board of Directors: Standards for home nutrition support. *Nutr Clin Pract.* 1999;14:151–162.
74. Ottery FD. Cancer cachexia prevention, early diagnosis, and management. *Cancer Pract.* 1994;2(2):123–131.
75. Shopbell JM, Hopkins B, Shronts EP. Nutrition screening and assessment. In: *The Science and Practice of Nutrition Support, A Case Based Core Curriculum.* Dubuque: Kendall/Hunt Publishing Company;2001:107–140.

76. Roy LB, Edwards PA, Barr LH. The value of nutritional assessment in the surgical patient. *J Parenter Enteral Nutr.* 1985;9:170–172.

77. Martin C. Calorie, protein, fluid and micronutrient requirements. In McCallum PD, Polisena CG, eds. *The clinical guide to oncology nutrition.* Chicago: American Dietetic Association; 2000.

78. August DA, Thorn D, Fisher RL, Welchek CM. Home parenteral nutrition for patients with inoperable malignant bowel obstruction. *J Parenter Enteral Nutr.* 1991;15(3):323–327.

79. Ireton-Jones C, Cox-Davis S, DeLegge M. Quality of life outcomes in cancer patients receiving home parenteral nutrition support. *Nutr Clin Pract.* 2002; 17(1):59 (abstr.)

80. McGuire M. Nutritional care of surgical oncology patients. *Semin Oncol Nurs.* 2000;16(2):128–134.

81. Allison G, Dixon D, et al. Nutrition implications of surgical oncology. In: McCallum PD, Polisena CG, eds. *The clinical guide to oncology nutrition.* Chicago: The American Dietetic Association; 2000.

82. Braunschweig CL, Levy P, Sheean PM, et al. Enteral compared with parenteral nutrition: a meta-analysis. *Am J Clin Nutr.* 2001;74:534–542.

83. Pikul, J, Sharpe MD, Lowndes R, Ghent CN. Degree of preoperative malnutrition is predictive of postoperative morbidity and mortality in liver transplant recipients. *Transplantation.* 1994;57:469–472.

84. Allard JP. The role of nutrition before and after transplantation. *Curr Opin Clin Nutr Metab Care.* 1999;2(4):313–314.

85. Weisdorf S, Lysne J, Wind D, et al. Positive effect of prophylactic total parenteral nutrition on long-term outcome of bone marrow transplantation. *Transplantation.* 1987;43:833–838.

86. Karnofsky DA. Meaningful clinical classification of therapeutic responses to anticancer drugs. Editorial. *Clin Pharmacol Ther.* 1961;2:709–712.

87. Capra S, Bauer J, Davidson W, Ash S. Nutritional therapy for cancer-induced weight loss. *Nutr Clin Pract.* 2002;17(4):210–213.

CHAPTER 13

Home Nutrition Support of Hyperemesis Gravidarum

Karen Hamilton, MS, RD, LD, CNSD

HYPEREMESIS GRAVIDARUM

Medical conditions in pregnant women requiring nutrition support generally include the same conditions that would require nutrition support in non-pregnant adults. However, one condition that is unique to pregnancy is hyperemesis gravidarum (HG).

Hyperemesis gravidarum is a persistent, severe form of nausea and vomiting that affects approximately 1% of pregnant women. Nausea and vomiting commonly occurs in early pregnancy, affecting 50–90% of women.[1] Generalized nausea and vomiting symptoms usually begin between the 4th and 7th weeks of pregnancy, with a majority of women experiencing symptoms peaking by the 12th week. Nausea and vomiting as a result of hyperemesis gravidarum symptoms, however, may extend into the second and third trimesters.

Etiology

The etiology of HG during pregnancy remains unclear, although numerous theories exist. Proposed mechanisms include gastric pacesetter dysfunction, hepatic dysfunction, elevated levels of gestational hormones, thyroid dysfunction, gastrointestinal abnormalities, fetal anomalies, and psychological and social factors.[2] The risk factors for the development of HG are listed in Table 13–1.[3,4,5]

TABLE 13-1   Risk Factors for Developing Hyperemesis Gravidarum

- Nulliparity
- HG in a prior pregnancy
- Obesity
- Multiple gestations
- Smoking
- Gestational trophoblastic disease
- Maternal age > 35 years

Clinical Presentation

The clinical presentation of HG includes:

- Persistent vomiting that occurs before the 20th week of gestation
- > 5% weight loss or inability to gain weight
- Fluid and electrolyte abnormalities
- Acid-base disturbances
- Ketonuria

In the past, this condition has often required hospitalization. Current advances in home care practice have allowed for safe and effective nutrition initiation and fluid and electrolyte management in the home setting.[6,7]

Diagnosis of Hyperemesis Gravidarum

Hyperemesis gravidarum is a diagnosis of exclusion. There are no specific confirmatory laboratory or radiographic findings. The patient assessment must exclude the likelihood of other disorders, including pancreatitis, peptic ulcer disease, hepatobiliary disease, gastroenteritis, appendicitis, molar pregnancy, intestinal obstruction, hyperthyroidism, and *Heliobacter pylori* infection.[1,8,9]

Morbidity and Mortality Related to Hyperemesis Gravidarum

Hyperemesis gravidarum was once a leading cause of maternal mortality, leading to the practice of pregnancy termination in most severe cases.[10]

Today, maternal death from HG can occur as a result of fluid, electrolyte, and metabolic disturbances associated with malnutrition.

Fluid, Electrolyte, and Metabolic Derangements in Hyperemesis Gravidarum

Clinical symptoms of dehydration include increases in blood urea nitrogen, hematocrit levels, and urine specific gravity. Maternal hypovolemia can become severe before it is clinically manifested. During pregnancy, plasma blood volume expands considerably; thus, blood pressure and pulse rate are not always reliable indicators of hemodynamic stability. Additionally, catecholamines secreted in response to hypovolemia result in vasoconstriction and reduction of uterine perfusion by up to 20% without a change in maternal blood pressure.[11]

Ketonuria in HG is a result of the metabolism of fatty acids as an adaptive phase in response to nutrient deprivation. Ketosis can further lead to acidemia, electrolyte abnormalities, and pH disturbances.[12]

Other serum alterations that are noted during HG include minor elevations of aspartate aminotransferase and alanine transferase. These increases usually reverse rapidly with adequate hydration, improved nutrition, and cessation of vomiting.[13]

Biochemical Alterations in Pregnancy and Hyperemesis Gravidarum

In addition to specific serum alterations noted in the pregnant patient who is experiencing HG, standard biochemical indices used for nonpregnant women are frequently not applicable in pregnancy. Two biochemical indices commonly used in nutritional assessment are serum albumin and total iron-binding capacity. In normal pregnancy, serum albumin concentrations fall rapidly in the first trimester and then decline gradually during the third trimester.[14] Serum total iron-binding capacity levels gradually increase throughout gestation and peak during the last trimester. The increase is noted to be less pronounced in women receiving iron supplements. An elevated total iron-binding capacity should not be mistaken for iron deficiency.[15] In pregnancy, a serum iron level of < 60 or 70 micrograms/100ml or a transferrin saturation of 16% is considered indicative of iron deficiency.[15]

Hemoglobin and hematocrit levels decline the first and second trimesters and then rise again in the third trimester. As a result, it is recommended by the Centers for Disease Control Pregnancy Nutrition Surveillance System that anemia is categorized by the stage of pregnancy.[16]

Other biochemical changes occurring during pregnancy include fasting hypoglycemia and post-prandial hyperglycemia. Fasting blood glucose levels decrease in the first trimester and continue to gradually decrease throughout the remaining gestation. Alternatively, impaired glucose tolerance is noted in some pregnant women during the second and third trimesters.[17]

Hypertriglyceridemia is also characteristic of pregnancy, with serum triglyceride levels increasing to 250–400% greater than normal. Cholesterol and phospholipid levels each increase by approximately 25% each, but can increase to as much as 180% of usual levels. Complications associated with hyperlipidemia in pregnancy are rare, and long-term effects on health are thought to be nonexistent.[15,18,19]

Vitamin and mineral deficiencies can occur with severe nausea and vomiting. Iron deficiency anemia is the most common mineral deficiency of HG, but is also common in pregnancy without HG. Vitamin B[6] and B[12] deficiency is also commonly noted in HG, and may result in the development of peripheral neuropathy.[9] The most serious of all vitamin and mineral deficiencies noted in HG is a deficiency of thiamin. It has been estimated that suboptimal thiamin levels may occur in as many as 60% of patients with HG.[16] Suboptimal thiamine intake coupled with prolonged administration of dextrose-containing fluids without simultaneous thiamin supplementation can result in Wernickes encephalopathy. This syndrome is characterized by disorientation, ataxia, vision disturbance, and ultimately may lead to coma and death.[20] Other maternal complications related to HG and malnutrition are listed in Table 13–2.[20,21,23–25] Reduced plasma inorganic iodide and thyroid clearance rates that are diagnostic of iodine deficiency in a non-pregnant female are normal during pregnancy. Low levels of T3 and T4 may aid in the diagnosis of iodine deficiency in pregnancy because they are normally elevated in pregnancy.[18]

Economic Impact of Hyperemesis Gravidarum

Significant negative economic impact is also a byproduct of HG. It is estimated that as a result of HG's debilitating nature, in excess of eight million hours of paid employment and five million hours of housework are lost per year.[26]

TABLE 13–2 Other Maternal Complications Associated with Hyperemesis Gravidarum and Malnutrition

- Malaise
- Fatigue
- Dizziness
- Hypoalbuminemia
- Ptyalism (increased salivation)
- Inappropriate weight gain or weight loss
- Mucosal bleeding
- Spontaneous pneumomediastinum (rarely)
- Esophageal perforation (rarely)

Fetal Complications

There is much debate regarding the impact of HG on fetal outcome. Evidence indicates that poor nutrition before and during pregnancy may lead to adverse pregnancy outcomes; however, HG itself has not been definitively linked to such outcomes. The variables that consistently appear to determine risk in the fetus may be the degree of weight loss combined with prepregnancy nutritional status and weight. It has also been noted that ketones readily cross the placenta. Prolonged maternal ketosis is thought to impair fetal development and may lead to impairment in neuropsychological development.[22]

Nutritional Requirements in Hyperemesis Gravidarum

Despite the metabolic, physiologic, and immunologic changes that occur with a HG patient, nutrient absorption and utilization do not differ from those who experience a normal HG-free pregnancy. Interestingly, pregnancy itself may be a condition whereby enhanced nutrient absorption occurs. It has also been documented in anecdotal case studies that improved nutrient absorption during pregnancy occurs among women with normally pre-existent impaired nutrient absorption.[26] It has been noted that absorption is enhanced for the mineral iron during pregnancy. Because iron requirements are elevated, a greater percentage of dietary iron intake is absorbed.[27] Nutritional requirements for the pregnant individual are generally altered by two factors: nutrient utilization and nutrient loss. Pregnancy is an anabolic state with approximately 925 grams of protein and 3,825 grams of fat accumulated in the mother and fetus during gestation.[26] Energy requirements are elevated as a result of both increased oxygen consumption and tissue growth. Oxygen consumption increases steadily throughout pregnancy, with 80% of the increase secondary to tissue metabolism and body function (cardiac output, uterus muscles, breast, kidneys, respiration).[28] The remaining 20% of the increased oxygen consumption is as a result of the developing fetus.

The altered utilization of energy results in an average increase in energy requirements by approximately 300 kcal/d. This energy requirement is not steady from the first to third trimester, but rather, increases proportionally with increasing oxygen consumption.[26] Additional calories are required in cases of stress, trauma, and sepsis, or during a teen pregnancy. Women with HG may also have additional energy needs in excess of 300 kcal/d to achieve the desired weight gain.[28] The estimation of energy needs during pregnancy of a normal-weight individual is 36 kcal per kilogram of current body weight (CBW) per day. Protein intake should be increased by 10g/d above the recommended dietary allowances or should be sufficient to achieve positive nitrogen balance. The estimation of protein needs during pregnancy of a normal-weight individual is 1.3 grams of protein per kilogram CBW per day. When protein deficiency is a concern, 1.4 to 1.7 grams of protein per kilogram CBW per day for repletion is suggested.[28] As with energy, the increased utilization of protein is greater in late pregnancy.

Nutrient losses during a normal healthy pregnancy are not greater than in a non-pregnant state. However, in HG patients, frequent emesis may result in electrolyte and fluid imbalance. In severe cases, protein and iron loss may also occur due to blood loss with esophageal damage from persistent emesis.

Maternal Weight Status

As nutrient utilization increases in pregnancy, so must energy intake increase to compensate for increased needs while promoting essential weight gain. Weight gain throughout pregnancy is the most important indicator of the adequacy of the nutritional status of the mother and fetus. Maternal weight gain is not linear over the course of the pregnancy and is not solely caused by the gain of new tissue. Weight gain also represents an increase in extracellular fluid, a rise in blood volume, and an accumulation of amniotic fluid. The child's birth weight is directly asso-

TABLE 13–3 Weight Goals Based on Prepregnancy BMI (kg/m^2)

BMI	Normal BMI= 19.8–26 (90–120% IBW)	Underweight BMI=<19.8 (<90% IBW)	Overweight BMI=26–29 (120–130% IBW)	Obese BMI=>29 (>135% IBW)	Twin Pregnancy	Triplet Pregnancy
Goal	25–25 lbs	28–40 lbs	15–25 lbs	15 lbs	34–45 lbs	50 lbs

1. MacBurney M, Matarese L. Pregnancy. In: Matarese L, Gottlisch M, eds. *Contemporary Nutrition Support Practice*. New York: Saunders;2002:337–343.
2. Kaiser L, Allen L. Position of the American Dietetic Association: Nutrition and lifestyle for a healthy pregnancy outcome. *J Am Diet Assoc*. 2002;102:1479–1490.

ciated with total gestational maternal weight gain. Maternal weight gain is also directly correlated with a decreased risk of intrauterine growth retardation.[28]

Except in the very obese, a total pregnancy weight gain of less than 5 kilograms or weight gains of less than 0.5 pounds per week during weeks 20–40 of gestation may be detrimental to fetal outcome.[28,29] The frequency of perinatal deaths and prematurity diminishes as maternal weight gain increases, up to approximately 15 kilograms. Weight gain beyond this point does not exert any further beneficial effect, and may in fact correlate with increased incidence of gestational hypertension, diabetes, and pre-eclampsia.[29,30]

In addition to total weight gain during pregnancy, prepregnancy weight for height is thought to influence infant outcome. Both factors emphasize the importance of maternal body mass for fetal growth. The committee on Nutritional Status and Weight Gain During Pregnancy suggests that maternal prepregnancy weight for height or body mass is the simplest and most useful index for assessment of maternal prepregnancy nutritional status.[31] Body mass index is calculated in weight (kg) divided by height squared (m^2). Energy intake should be adjusted up or down to achieve weight-gain goals based on prepregnancy body mass. Total maternal body mass, not weight gain alone, may influence fetal growth. Therefore, the fetus of an underweight mother is at greater risk than a fetus of a normal or overweight mother if a feeding problem such as HG arises (see Table 13–3).

Management of the Hyperemesis Gravidarum Patient at Home

Several reports suggest that home therapy for this population is safe and effective.[6,7,9,32–34] Successful management of HG in the home care setting

TABLE 13–4   Home Admission Criteria

Patients are admitted to home care services based on a reasonable expectation that care can be provided in a safe and timely manner appropriate to the patient's needs and level of care required by the patient's condition.

- Patient is under direct and continuing medical supervision by a licensed physician
- Care/services ordered by the physician are necessary and reasonable for the patient's condition
- Patient consents to treatment in the home setting
- Patient's residence has adequate facilities for safely meeting the patient's health care needs:
  - Adequate clean storage space for mediations and supplies
  - Telephone access if no home phone available
  - Adequate facilities to allow for hand washing prior to self-administration of medication
  - Care partner who is available and willing to participate in patient's care

is dependent upon careful patient selection and assessment of her home environment and support (see Table 13–4). Benefits of home care management for HG patients include less family disruption, a comfortable environment, improved quality of life, and reduced health care costs.

Home Nutrition Assessment

Targeted nutrition assessment will aid in accurate identification of maternal under-nutrition and the application of appropriate nutrition support. This information will provide a baseline to compare the adequacy and effectiveness of the nutrition support regimen.

Initial nutrition assessments for pregnant women should include:

- *Weight History*: height; prepregnancy weight; current weight; and weight history with previous pregnancies, as applicable
- *Past Medical and Gestational History*: ascertain if there is history of previous HG; if so, duration of symptoms and treatment; birth history; and significant past medical history that may impact nutrition status
- *Diet/Intake*: allergies; intolerances; foods and liquids avoided; symptoms affecting intake; 24–72 hour recall (including questions regarding alcohol consumption); food cravings; quantify nausea level; quantify number of emesis episodes/day and timing; food preparer

and financial resources to obtain nutritious food; dietary supplements / prenatal vitamins / herbal use.

- *Physical Examination*: oral cavity examination for moisture content; color and turgor of skin; vital signs; sclera of eyes to determine if they are icteric; evaluation for other clinical signs and symptoms of dehydration.
- *Laboratory*: urinalysis for specific gravity and ketones; complete metabolic profile taking into consideration weeks of gestation and pregnancy normal values; complete blood count.

Clinical Management & Nutrition Support

Oral Nutrition

The first step in ensuring adequate oral nutrition intake with HG is to control nausea and vomiting. There are a variety of oral and suppository forms of antiemetics. However, because of the concern related to the potential teratogenicity of these medications and the lack of controlled safety trials, especially in the HG population, their use is often limited. Ideally, the selection of antiemetic medications from a variety of drug classes that have a different mechanism of action will result in the greatest nausea control and allow resumption of adequate oral intake.[35,36]

The time-aged approach to managing HG with oral diet has been to withhold solids for 1–2 days, with gradual initiation of a B.R.A.T. (bananas, rice, apple sauce, tea or toast) diet or a low-fat, high-carbohydrate diet. Small, frequent meals are encouraged as tolerated.[1,35] Room-temperature, clear liquids are also encouraged between meals and in small, frequent quantities. An alternative approach encourages women with HG to follow their cravings and eat to quell nausea. Tart, sour, and salty foods have also been noted to be tolerated by some afflicted with HG.[37]

Ginger root has also been suggested to provide relief for nausea and vomiting associated with HG, as reported in a double-blind, randomized cross-over trial.[38] The etiology of the relief may be due to a direct effect on the gastrointestinal tract and reduced stimulation of the emetic center.

Intravenous Hydration

If severe dehydration occurs as a result of uncontrolled emesis, additional treatment with correction of fluid, electrolyte, and metabolic distur-

TABLE 13-5   IV Antiemetic Guide for Hyperemesis Gravidarum

Medication Type	Generic Name	Pregnancy Risk Category	Suggested Rx Range	Comments
Motility	Metoclopramide hydrochloride 5 mg/ml 2 ml *SDV	B	30 mg max	Start and max dose is the same
Phenothiazine	Promethazine hydrochloride 25 mg/ml 1ml SDV	C	25–100 mg/L max	Sedating in higher doses, unstable in 3-in-1
Antacid	Raniditine 25 mg/ml 6 ml *MDV	B	40–150 mg max	Not an antiemetic, but may reduce heartburn related nausea
5-HT₃ receptor antagonist	Ondansetron 2 mg/ml 20 ml MDV	B	8–24 mg max	Not usually used before 9 wks gestation
Phenothiazine	Prochlorperazine 5mg/ml 10ml MDV	C		Not stable in PPN/TPN. No advantage over Phenergan.
Antacid	Famotidine 10 mg/ml 20 ml MDV	B	20–40 mg/d	

*Key: SDV=single does vial (preservative free)
      MDV=multi-dose vial (has preservatives)

1. Sullivan CA, Johnson CA, et al. A pilot study of intravenous ondansetron for hyperemesis gravidarum. *Am J Obstet Gynecol*. 1996;174:1565–1568.

2. Tincello DG, Johnstone MJ. Treatment of hyperemesis gravidarum with 5HT3 antagonist ondansetron (Zofran). *Postgrad Med*. 1996;72(853):688–689.

3. Mazzotta P, Magee LA. A risk benefit assessment of pharmacological and nonpharmacological treatments for nausea and vomiting in pregnancy. *Drugs*. 2000;59(4):781–800.

bances is indicated. Initial treatment with intravenous (IV) hydration and antiemetic (see Table 13–5) therapy may be indicated if any of the following conditions exist:

- Weight loss > 2 kg in 1 week or > 5% prepregnancy weight loss
- Electrolyte abnormalities
- Ketosis > 24 hrs
- Clinical manifestations of dehydration
- Urine specific gravity > 1030

Consideration should be made for vitamin repletion via IV hydration if a greater than 5 day period of poor oral intake is noted or if a patient is at nutritional risk prior to pregnancy. Repletion of thiamine is indicat-

TABLE 13-6   Indications for IV Fluid and Antiemetic Use

- Weight loss > 2 kg in 1 week or > 5% prepregnancy weight loss
- Electrolyte abnormalities
- Ketosis > 24 hr
- Clinical manifestations of dehydration
- Urine specific gravity > 1030

ed to decrease the risk of encephalopathy with initiation of nutrition support. The provision of adequate folic acid during organogenesis to help prevent the occurrence of neural tube defects may also be indicated.

When clinical management with IV hydration, antiemetics, and oral diet fails to prevent ketosis, and continued weight loss is evident, considerations must be made to provide enteral or parenteral therapy. Correction of fluid, electrolytes, glucose, and vitamin abnormalities before initiating specialized nutrition support is beneficial for the prevention of refeeding syndrome.[39]

In the home care setting, initiation of IV fluids and antiemetic therapy via peripheral venous access (PVA) can safely deliver hydration and promote positive clinical outcomes (see Table 13–6). Optimal home management will be monitored and accomplished through the efforts of the patients' primary physician or obstetrician and the home nutrition support team clinicians. These clinicians will closely monitor the patient's clinical status and tolerance to therapy and the patient's ability to reestablish an optimal oral diet. If attainment of an adequate oral diet is not possible in a reasonable timeframe, then transition to other, more invasive nutrition modalities can also be accomplished without hospitalization.

Enteral Nutrition

Women who experience HG are known to have a functional gastrointestinal tract and ideally would benefit from the application of enteral tube feeding when the oral route is not possible. In practice, however, obtaining and maintaining a nasogastric (NG) feeding access is fraught with difficulties, including patient resistance to placement, due to their exaggerated gag reflex, and the discomfort of maintaining even a small-bore feeding tube for an indefinite period of time. Frequent tube dislodgement can occur with the retching associated with HG. This results in the need for multiple home care visits or patient trips to their physician, emergency room, or clinic for NG tube replacement. In published case reports and in small, clinical studies, the use of enteral nutrition through an NG tube in HG patients resulted in a prompt cessation of their nausea. It is believed this is as a result of the patients not being required to smell, taste, or swallow foods.

In most published cases of enteral nutrition in HG, the patients received standard, isotonic, polymeric formulas (with or without fiber). The NG feedings were delivered continuously with an initiation at 20–50ml/hr, and a gradual increase as tolerated to 90–130 ml/hr.[33,34,39,40] Cyclic feedings were gradually accomplished and tolerated in a few cases.[34] Reported cases of the use of nasojejunal feedings are even fewer, with frequent tube dislodgement noted, and varying success of emesis suppression.[41]

When NG tubes are placed in the home setting, an 8 Fr, unweighted feeding tube is measured for gastric placement by adding the distance length from the tip of the nose to the earlobe to the xyphoid process. Radiographic confirmation of proper tube position prior to use should be obtained with an abdominal radiograph. This radiograph should be obtained with shielding of the lower abdomen (see Table 13–7). Generally, patients are asked to remain nil per os (Latin for "nothing by mouth") after NG tubes are placed to allow for tube feeding initiation. Intermittent warm water flushes are encouraged to prevent cramping and intolerance. Feedings are generally provided continuously via an ambulatory pump. Cycling of the enteral feedings can be accomplished. Many women prefer to infuse feedings during the day when their nausea is at its peak, and discontinue feedings at night while sleeping.[42]

Enteral nutrition can be safely managed in the home setting. With proper patient selection and thorough education and monitoring, women with HG can experience significant cessation of nausea and vomiting. The patients' physician and home care nutrition team must be available, not only to replace displaced tubes, but also to monitor patient clinical outcomes and to provide patient contact at least 1–2 times per week for emotional support and reinforcement of education. This includes a review of the signs and symptoms of potential complications (see Table 13–8).

TABLE 13-7   Inserting Nasogastric Tubes

1. Explain procedure and purpose.
2. Place patient in sitting position with neck flexed slightly and head of bed elevated 45°.
3. Estimate distance for placement into stomach by measuring the length from tip of patient's nose to earlobe and then from earlobe to xyphoid process.
4. Observe markings on shaft of tube for guidance.
5. Inspect nares and determine optimal patency by having patient breathe through one nostril while the other is occluded temporarily. Lubricate chosen nostril with water-soluble lubricant or local anesthetic jelly.
6. Lubricate end of tube or activate self-lubricant with water and pass it posteriorly. Ask the patient to facilitate tube passage by swallowing water.
7. After tube is beyond the nasopharynx, allow patient to rest.
8. Have patient flex neck and swallow while tube is being advanced.
9. If patient begins to cough, withdraw tube into nasopharynx and reattempt passage.
10. Confirm passage into stomach using organizational guidelines. If x-ray confirmation is chosen, then pregnant patients' abdomens should be shielded.
11. Secure tube to bridge of nose with nonallergenic tape or tube attachment device.
12. After tube placement is confirmed, remove stylet. Do not try to reinsert stylet after removal.

Gunther P, Jones S, Seed M, Ericson M. Delivery systems and administration of enteral nutrition. In: Rombeau J, ed. *Enteral Nutrition and Tube Feeding*, 3rd ed. Philadelphia: WB Saunders Co; 1997:240–252.

Parenteral Nutrition

If the gastrointestinal route of access is not feasible or refused, and the patient is at risk for malnutrition, parenteral nutrition (PN) is an appropriate therapy to support patient needs until resumption of an adequate oral diet occurs. Examples of risk factors associated with maternal malnutrition that would warrant consideration of PN initiation can be found in Table 13–6.

Contraindication for PN use during pregnancy may include:

- Uncontrolled preeclampsia or eclampsia
- Uncontrolled gestational diabetes or diabetes mellitus
- Uncontrolled cardiac disease
- Diminished renal function
- A home, physical, or psychosocial environment that is not suitable for the delivery of home PN.
- Absence of a willing care partner
- Good tolerance to enteral feedings
- Inability to obtain venous access

TABLE 13–8   Complications of Home Enteral Therapy for the Patient with HG

Complication	Causes	Interventions
Nasal bleeding	Direct trauma to the vasculature of the nasal passages	• Place a water-soluble lubricant on the first few inches of the tube tip prior to inserting • Use a soft, small-bore tube, if possible • Advance the tube slowly and gently, stopping if resistance is met
Laryngeal edema	Irritation to the mucosal surfaces that line the nasopharyngeal structures initiate the inflammatory response, resulting in edema	• During insertion, when the tube is just above the larynx and epiglottis, have the patient flex head forward. This will promote passage into the esophagus, as opposed to the trachea. • Use a soft, small-bore tube • Advance slowly and gently, stopping if resistance is met
Nasal ulceration, necrosis	Tube is pressing against the nasal cartilage	• Identify patients at greatest risk, including malnourished or dehydrated patients, as well as those with a history of inhaled drug abuse. • Use of water soluble lubricant can help prevent mucosal drying. • Avoid angulation of tube as it exits the nose. • Use a soft small-bore tube, if possible • If reinsertion is necessary, use opposite nare
Rhinitis/sinusitis	Inflammation and infection of the paranasal sinuses can occur when sinus drainage is obstructed.	• Use a soft, small-bore tube • Monitor patient for signs/symptoms of sinus drainage, pain
Otitis media	Middle ear irritation or infection	• Monitor patient for signs/symptoms. Notify the physician for appropriate medication • Consider another route for tube placement and/or TPN
Occlusion	Feeding tube kinks, control clamp in off position, pump malfunction or formula clogged tube	• Unkink tubing • Check flow control clamps • Flush with warm water before and after feeding and medications • Replace tube

Eisenberg PG. Nasoenteral tubes. *RN*. 1994;10:62–69.

Vento BA, Durrant JD, Palmer CV, Smith EK. Middle ear effects secondary to nasogastric intubation. *Am J Otol*. 1995;16:820–822.

Rouby J, Laurent P, Gosnach M, et al. Risk factors and clinical relevance of nosocomial maxillary sinusitis in the critically ill. *Am J Respir Crit Care Med*. 1994;150:776–783.

Goals of Parenteral Nutrition

Goals of PN in the pregnant patient should include:

- Provision of sufficient fluid, electrolytes, vitamins, minerals, calories, and amino acids to restore hydration status and prevent negative energy and nitrogen balances
- Prevent complications related to PN therapy, with an emphasis on stringent blood glucose management and fluid status to avoid fetal complications
- Provide optimal nourishment for mother and baby as a replacement for, or supplement to, oral intake

Vascular Access

Appropriate vascular access is an essential component to successful PN therapy. Before selecting a venous access device, several criteria must be evaluated, including:

- Expected duration of therapy
- Requirement for multiple infusions
- Thrombogenicity of catheter material
- Preexisting blood clotting disorders of the patient
- Patient/caregiver ability to manage access care
- Nutrient needs (complete or supplemental)

Pregnancy is a hypercoagulable state that may enhance the risk for thrombosis for patients with venous access devices. The patient with HG who requires PN is at particular risk, not only because of their thrombogenic state, but also due to dehydration contributing to blood stasis and vessel wall injury due to access device placement and/or hypertonic solutions. If a thrombus were to form, partial or total catheter occlusion may result in the need for catheter removal and replacement.

In the home care setting, peripherally inserted catheter (PIC) lines can be placed by PIC certified home health agency nurses, thus preventing hospitalization. These access devices generally have smaller lumens than PIC lines placed in the hospital to allow for ease of insertion (3 Fr vs. 4 Fr or larger). Due to the smaller lumen size and the patients' hypercoagulable state, the need for prophylactic anticoagulation therapy may be indicated. Heparin (1,000 U) may be added safely to the peripheral parenteral nutrition or central parenteral nutrition solution at 1 U/ml, and may aid in PIC line retention and decreased fibrin sheath development.

De-clotting of central venous catheters utilizing Streptokinase[R]/Anistreplase[R] generally occurs in a controlled setting such as a hospital with close supervision because of its highly antigenic nature in humans.[43] Recombinant tissue plasminogen activator (t-PA) has been a safer alternative to restore lumen patency due to thrombotic catheter dysfunction. However, to date, no controlled trials have been completed on pregnant patients.

In many instances, women who suffer from HG may not require full calorie PN to support their needs. Peripheral parenteral nutrition can optimally meet their needs during the early stages of pregnancy. The use of peripheral parenteral nutrition avoids the need for central venous access. However, standard PVA devices will require frequent catheter changes. The most common associated complications associated with the delivery of peripheral parenteral nutrition through a peripheral IV include infection and phlebitis. This limits the use of PVA catheters to very short-term hydration or peripheral parenteral nutrition therapy (1–3 days per PVA device). Peripheral parenteral nutrition may be more optimally delivered via a mid-line or long-line PIC. These PVA devices do not require frequent catheter changes. They also may reduce the potential for infectious complications.

When infusing PN peripherally, proper attention to the PN formula osmolarity must be made to reduce the potential for vessel wall injury. When infusing PN through a centrally placed, peripherally inserted catheter (PICC) and/or other central venous access devices, osmolarity limitations are not present, and goal energy and protein needs of pregnant patients can be more easily obtained with the PN solution.

Parenteral Formulations

Home parenteral nutrition (HPN) administration during pregnancy does not differ significantly from HPN in other adult populations. Caution must be used in administering dextrose, as a persistent state of hyperglycemia from PN can mimic gestational diabetes and increases the risk of fetal complications. Consideration of the following areas should be made when devising an optimal PN formulation:

- *Caloric Appropriation*: 40–60% in dextrose calories, 10–20% in amino acid calories, and 10–30% in lipid calories.

- *Dextrose*: No greater than 5 mg/kg/min should be infused to prevent hyperglycemia. Serum blood glucose levels must be strictly maintained between 70–120 mg/dl. Closely monitor finger stick blood glucoses 1–2 hours into the start of the PN infusion and ½ hour after PN infusion. Discontinuation is indicated to ensure tight glycemic control.[3,21]
- *Lipids*: The minimum amount required to meet essential fatty acid requirements is 4.5% of total PN calories. However, it is suggested that not > 40% of total calories are provided as lipid, or approximately 1g/kg of prepregnancy ideal body weight.
- *Fluid*: Adequate fluid administration is important for a host of metabolic activities. The maintenance requirement for free water is 30–35 ml/kg/day, plus any losses associated with gastrointestinal symptoms such as excessive vomiting or diarrhea.[29]
- *Amino Acids*: The ideal composition of amino acids during pregnancy is not known. The amino acid profile of commercially available solutions varies, but generally provides a balance of essential and nonessential amino acids. Special consideration may be made for women known to be at risk for delivering an infant with metabolic abnormalities, as select amino acids such as phenylalanine and methionine may be neurotoxic.[44]
- *Electrolytes*: Calcium, phosphate, and magnesium requirements are increased in pregnancy. Both phosphate and calcium are crucial for fetal bone development. Seven to ten mMol of phosphate must be administered per 1,000 calories of glucose to aid in glucose metabolism.[45]
- *Vitamins*: The current IV multivitamin formulation with vitamin K meets or exceeds the requirements for pregnancy. Additional thiamine may be considered if the patient has experienced poor oral intake for > 2 weeks to prevent Wernicke's encephalopathy.
- *Trace elements*: The current multitrace element preparation (MTE-5) meets the requirements for pregnancy. If no oral or tube feeding intake is ingested or tolerated, then consideration for the addition of 50 ug of iodine is indicated.
- *Minerals*: When severe iron deficiency anemia is present, and no oral iron can be taken or tolerated, consideration for IV iron may be indicated. Iron dextran is a pregnancy risk category C. It may

cause anaphylaxis. Precaution must be taken to deliver IV iron in a safe, supervised setting for the initial dose.

Monitoring

Aspects of monitoring pregnant patient tolerance to the prescribed PN regimen do not significantly differ from that of the non-pregnant patient (see Table 13–9). Particular attention, however, must be paid to finger stick blood glucose monitoring to ensure tight glucose management while receiving PN. Laboratory monitoring and frequency of lab assessment does not differ. Careful attention must be made to pregnancy "normal" laboratory values, versus normal laboratory values in the non-pregnant state. Fetal growth and development should be monitored. Fundal height, presence of fetal heart sounds, and periodic ultrasound

TABLE 13–9   Home Monitoring of the PN Patient

Parameter	Monitoring Guideline
Temperature	Measured each afternoon. Report to physician if > 100° F.
Glucose Monitoring	Finger stick blood glucose 1–2 hours into infusion, ½ hour after discontinuation. Maintain between 70–120 mg/dl.
Body Weight	Measured daily until goal nutrition prescription is attained, twice weekly thereafter.
Catheter/Exit Site	Observed daily or with every dressing change for redness, swelling, drainage, migration.
Laboratory Monitoring	Baseline: Chemistry panel, Mg, Phos, PT/INR, Transferrin, Prealbumin, TG, and CBC with differential
	Weekly until stable: Chemistry panel, Mg, Phos, and CBC with differential
	As stable, reduce labs to every 2–4 weeks
	If symptomatic, consider iron panel to determine presence of iron deficiency (CBC, iron, ferritin, reticulocyte count).
Compliance Monitoring	Supply usage, compliance to visit schedule and physician appointments.
PN Solution Inventory	At home visit, evaluate the number of bags remaining, adequacy of storage facilities, evidence of stock rotation, and expiration dates.
Signs and Symptoms of Complications from PN	To include hypo/hyperglycemia, and instructions to contact physician and/or home care immediately with problems and concerns.

testing are important information that may speak to the adequacy of the nutrition therapy.

As tolerance to oral intake improves, gradual tapering of PN or PPN therapy should occur. Calorie counts of all oral intake and concurrent supportive diet counseling are indicated. When oral intake meets 75% of estimated fluid and energy needs, discontinuation of PN therapy is indicated.

CONCLUSION

The clinical needs of women who experience HG are numerous and complex. Successful home management of the HG patient is dependent upon the availability of qualified personnel resources that have experience in home nutrition and obstetrical management. An experienced home nutrition support team can effectively evaluate the patients' stability, appropriateness for home care, unique nutritional needs, and optimal nutrition therapy modality that can ensure the most positive outcome.

REFERENCES

1. Broussard CN, Richter JE. Nausea and vomiting of pregnancy. *Gastroenterol Clin North Am.* 1998;27:123–151.
2. Gardner DK. Parenteral nutrition in pregnancy. Editorial NCP 2000;15(2): 63–64.
3. Klebanoff MA, Koslowe PA, Kaslow R, et al. Epidemiology of vomiting in early pregnancy. *Obstet Gynecol.* 1985;66:612–616.
4. Kallen B. Hyperemesis during pregnancy and delivery outcome: a registry study. *Eur J Obstet Gynecol Reprod Biol.* 1987;26:291–302.
5. Tierson FD, Olsen CL, Hook EB. Nausea and vomiting of pregnancy. *Am J Obstet Gynecol.* 1986;155:1017–22.
6. Cowan MJ. Hyperemesis gravidarum: implications for home care and infusion therapies. *J Intraven Nurs.* 1996;19:46–58.
7. Chevreau N, Anthony PS, Kessinger K. Managing hyperemesis gravidarum with home parenteral nutrition: treatment parameters and clinical outcomes. *Infusion.* 1999;5:22–28.
8. Scott LD. Gastrointestinal disease in pregnancy. In: Creasy RK, Resnik R eds., *Maternal-Fetal Medicine.* 4th ed. Philadelphia: WB Saunders; 1999: 1038–1051.
9. Goodwin TM. Hyperemesis gravidarum. *Clin Obstet Gynecol.* 1998;41: 597–605.

10. Fairweather DV: Nausea and vomiting in pregnancy. *Am J Obstet Gynecol.* 1968;102:135–175.
11. Hamoavi E, Hamaovi M. Nutritional assessment and support during pregnancy. *Gastroenterol Clin North Am.* 1998;27:89–121.
12. van Stuijevenberg ME, Schabort I, Labadarios D, Nel JT. The nutritional status and treatment of patients with hyperemesis gravidarum. *Am J Obstet Gynecol.* 1995;172:1585–1591.
13. Fagan EA. Diseases of the liver, biliary system and pancreas. In: Creasy RK, Resnick R, eds. *Maternal-Fetal Medicine*, 4th ed. Philadelphia, PA: WB Saunders;1999:1056–1591.
14. Robertson EG, Cheyne GA. Plasma biochemistry in relation to edema of pregnancy. *J Obstet Gynaecol Br Commonw.* 1972;79:769–776.
15. National Research Council: Laboratory Indices of Nutritional Status in Pregnancy. Washington DC, National Academy of Sciences, 1989.
16. CDC. Criteria for anemia in children and childbearing-aged women. *MMWR Morb Mortal Wkly Rep.* 1989;38:400–404.
17. O'Sullivan JB, Mahan CM. Criteria for the oral glucose tolerance test in pregnancy. *Diabetes.* 1964;13:278–285.
18. MacBurney M, Wilmore DW. Parenteral nutrition in pregnancy. In: Rombeau J, Caldwell M, eds. Philadelphia: WB Saunders;1986:615–633.
19. Biezenski JJ. Maternal lipid metabolism. *Obstet Gynecol Annu.* 1974;3:203–233.
20. Lavin PJ, Smith D, Kori SH, Ellenberger C Jr. Wernicke's encephalopathy: a predictable complication of hyperemesis gravidarum. *Obstet Gynecol.* 1983;62(suppl 3):13S-15S.
21. Moore TR. Diabetes in pregnancy. In: Creasy RK, Resnik R, eds. *Maternal-Fetal Medicine.* 4th ed. Philadelphia: W.B. Saunders;1999:964–965.
22. Hod M, Orvieto R, Kaplan B, et al. Hyperemesis gravidarum: a review. *J Reprod Med.* 1994;39(8):605–612.
23. Gorbach JS, Counselman FL, Mendelson MH. Spontaneous pneumomediastinum secondary to hyperemesis gravidarum. *J Emerg Med.* 1997;15:639–643.
24. Woolford TJ, Birzgalis AR, Lundell C, Farrington WT. Vomiting in pregnancy resulting in esophageal perforation in a 15-year-old. *J Laryngol Otol.* 1993;107:1059–1060.
25. Montgomery TL, Pincus IJ. A nutritional problem in pregnancy resulting from extensive resection of the small bowel; case report. *Am J Obstet Gynecol.* 1995;69:865–868.
26. Gadsby R, Barnie-Adshead AM, Jagger C. A prospective study of nausea and vomiting during pregnancy. *Br J Gen Pract.*1993;43:245–248.
27. Svanberg B. Absorption of iron in pregnancy. *Acta Obstet Gynecol Scand Suppl.* 1975;48:1–108.
28. Hytten FE. Nutrition. In: Hytten FE, Chamberlain G, eds. *Clinical Physiology and Obstetrics.* Oxford: Blackwell Scientific Publications;1980:147–162.

29. Food and Nutrition Board: Recommended Dietary Allowances (10th ed.). National Academy of Science. Washington DC, 1989.

30. Klotz R. Parenteral nutrition therapy plan in the pregnant patient. *OB Pharmacy.* 1989;2(4):1–5.

31. Institute of Medicine Subcommittee on Nutritional Status and Weight Gain during Pregnancy: Nutrition During Pregnancy. National Academy Press, Washington, DC, 1990.

32. Barclay BA. Experience with enteral nutrition in the treatment of hyperemesis gravidarum. *Nutr Clin Pract.* 1990;5(4):153–155.

33. Sanders SL, Greenspoon JS. New protocol to manage hyperemesis gravidarum. *J Am Diet Assoc.* 1994;94:1367–1368.

34. Hsu JJ, Clark-Glena R, Nelson DK, Kim CH. Nasogastric enteral feeding in the management of hyperemesis gravidarum. *Obstet Gynecol.* 1996;88: 343–346.

35. Newman V, Fullerton JT, Anderson PO. Clinical advances in the management of severe nausea during pregnancy. *J Obstet Gynecol Neonatal Nurs.* 1993;22:483–490.

36. American Hospital Formulary Service: Drug Information. American Society of Health System Pharmacists. Bethesda, MD, 2002.

37. Erick M. *No More Morning Sickness: A Survival Guide for Pregnant Women.* New York: Plume;1993.

38. Fischer-Rasmussen W, Kjaer SK, Dahl C, Asping U. Ginger treatment of hyperemesis gravidarum. *Eur J Obstet Gynecol Reprod Biol.* 1991;38:19–24.

39. Solomon SM, Kirby DF. The refeeding syndrome: a review. *J Parenter Enteral Nutr.* 1990;14(1):90–97.

40. Gulley RM, Vander Pleog N, Gulley JM. Treatment of hyperemesis gravidarum with nasogastric feeding. *Nutr Clin Pract.* 1993;8:33–35.

41. Boyce RA: Enteral nutrition in hyperemesis gravidarum: a new development. *J Am Diet Assoc.* 1992;92:733–736.

42. Barclay BA. Experience with enteral nutrition in the treatment of hyperemesis gravidarum. *Nutr Clin Pract.* 1990;5(4):153–155.

43. Food and Drug Administration. Important Drug Warning. Center for Biologics Evaluation and Research. Streptokinase. December 10, 1999.

44. Grant JP. *Handbook of TPN.* Philadelphia: WB Saunders;1992:99–100.

45. National Academies Press. "Dietary Reference Intakes for Calcium, Phosphorus, Magnesium, Vitamin D and Fluoride." 1997.

READINGS

Kramer MS. Intrauterine growth and gestational duration determinants. *Pediatrics.* 1987;80:502–511.

Simpson JW, Lawless RW, Mitchell AC. Responsibility of the obstetrician to the fetus. II. Influence of prepregnancy weight and pregnancy weight gain on birthweight. *Obstet Gynecol.* 1975;45:481–487.

van der Berg BJ. Maternal variables affecting fetal growth. *Am J Clin Nutr.* 1981;34(suppl 4):722–726.

Shepard MJ, Hellenbrand KG, Bracken MB. Proportional weight gain and complications of pregnancy, labor, and delivery in healthy women of normal prepregnant stature. *Am J Obstet Gynecol.* 1986;155:947–954.

CHAPTER 14

Transitioning the Home Nutrition Support Patient to an Oral Diet

Carol S. Ireton-Jones, PhD, RD, LD, CNSD, FACN

Home nutrition support is an important component of the continuum of care for many patients. A 2002 report indicated that 344,000 people receive home enteral nutrition (HEN) and another 39,000 receive home parenteral nutrition (HPN).[1] Certainly, all of these individuals will not be lifetime patients on home parenteral or enteral nutrition (HPEN). The goal of nutrition support is to transition patients to the oral nutrition route if at all possible, not only to meet nutritional goals, but also to improve quality of life.

Diet or nutrition intervention via diet instruction, meal planning assistance, and follow up has traditionally been the role of the hospital dietitian and outpatient clinical dietitian. Often, the dietitian working with the hospital nutrition support team transfers care to another dietitian when the patient no longer requires parenteral or enteral nutrition and transitions to an oral diet. Although often previously relegated to a less important facet of a HPN or HEN patient's care, diet therapy has now moved to a more important intervention. Oral intake can greatly affect gastrointestinal (GI) adaptation, secretion, and output and can, therefore, greatly influence the patient's ability to transition off of HPEN.[2] The dietitian's role in transitioning the patient from HPEN to an oral diet, either partially or completely, involves an understanding of GI physiology and anatomy, GI diseases, and food and nutrient actions within the GI system.

HEN patients may receive therapy because of head and neck cancer or a stroke, or because of debilitating diseases that affect the ability to swallow. Transition from HEN to an oral diet will be most successful with instruction and monitoring provided by a dietitian and other clinicians, such as a speech therapist, as well as family or care partner involvement and encouragement.[3] A study of HEN patient outcomes after one year of therapy indicated that 19–30% are able to transition to an oral diet while 45–60% die from their primary disease process during this time.[4]

Transitioning the patient from HPN or HEN to oral nutrition is a challenge because the underlying disease process causing the patient to rely on HPN must be considered as well as variations in GI function and the amount of bowel remaining. The clinical expertise of the team working to assist the patient in transitioning off HPN to enteral nutrition or an oral diet will also be a factor. Short-bowel syndrome (SBS), defined as a collection of signs and symptoms occurring after surgical intestinal resection, is characterized by weight loss and malabsorption of fluids and micro- and macronutrients.[4] Short-bowel syndrome is one of the most common reasons for long-term HPN.[5] Other intestinal diagnoses that may result in HPN dependence include Crohn's disease, ischemic bowel, congenital disorders, and motility disorders.[6] Functional SBS has been defined as a condition where patients have a diseased small bowel interfering with adequate nutrient and water absorption, thus resulting in an inability to maintain normal nutritional status. Whereas previously patients with SBS were thought to be dependent on HPN for a lifetime, it has been shown that the small bowel has the ability to compensate after massive small-bowel resection with elongation and dilation of the remnant bowel and hypertrophy of the intestinal villi, which can therefore enhance the area of absorption and prolong transit time.[7-9] This may occur in other disease states where adaptation occurs even after prolonged periods on HPN.

Transitioning a patient from complete reliance on HPN to a partial or complete oral diet requires individualized medical and dietary management provided by skilled clinicians, particularly dietitians. Furthermore, it requires a motivated individual willing to try many manipula-

TABLE 14–1 Evaluation of Ability to Transition from HPN

- Determine the anatomical status of the patient's remaining GI tract
- Evaluate length of small bowel as well as amount of remaining colon
- Review of past medical history and hospital discharge notes
- Obtain patient's physician's office records and relevant hospital admissions
- Review patient's food and fluid tolerances.

tions of the diet, an individual who will maintain compliance with his or her diet, an individual who will maintain detailed fluid/stool output and symptom records, and an individual who has a readiness to participate in his or her own care and recovery. Though patients who have had an intestinal resection or have been on HPN for many years may not be able to absorb 100% of their required nutrients everyday, some do absorb enough nutrients to decrease HPN administration from daily to 4–6 days per week. Others may be able to decrease the amount of fluid administered daily, which can be an important goal of transition. A day "off" from HPN can improve a patient's quality of life and provide an overall savings in health care costs.

The first step in evaluating the potential for a patient's transition from HPN is to determine the anatomical status of the patient's remaining GI tract. Review of the past medical history and hospital discharge notes can be helpful in determining bowel status. Information should be obtained from the patient's physician's office records and relevant hospital admissions (see Table 14–1). Data has shown that the length of small bowel as well as the amount of remaining colon can provide the basis for determining the optimal nutritional intervention. Patients with less than 150–200 cm of remaining small intestine without a colon may have significant fluid and nutrient losses and may need HPN to survive, whereas patients with a partial or complete colon in continuity with the small intestine may not have significant fluid and energy loss unless the length of small intestine is less than 50–70 cm.[5,10] For patients with SBS or functional SBS, transition to an oral diet may be a much longer-term endeavor. According to Scolapio and associates, specific dietary interventions should be based on the presence or absence of a colon.[8]

NUTRITION INTERVENTIONS

A vital component of the transition plan is a complete nutrition assessment by a registered dietitian (see Chapter 4). The nutrition assessment must include a thorough diet history and recall with an evaluation not only of intake but also of output related to foods consumed.[11] A review of current medications that could affect GI status or output is also important. Combining the status of the GI tract (length and function) with the diet and medication history will provide the experienced clinician with a starting point for diet manipulation and intervention.

Diet intervention for transitioning from HPN will vary, depending on the reason for HPN therapy. For short-term HPN patients, such as those recovering, GI function after chemotherapy or radiation therapy, diet intervention will be a matter of trialing specific foods that are more bland and soft and then progressing to a "normal" diet if absorption is adequate. Additionally, several small meals plus adequate provision of nutrient and electrolyte containing fluids may be necessary. In most cases, transition can occur over a period of 30–60 days.

If the small bowel has been damaged significantly, then nutrient intake may need to be much higher than usual to account for the decreased ability to efficiently absorb nutrients. One other important facet of organizing the appropriate diet for a patient with SBS is if there is a colon present in continuity with the small intestine. In general, all short-bowel patients should be maintained on a low-fat diet. If a patient has a colon or partial colon remaining, then a relatively high carbohydrate diet should be developed. Carbohydrates are metabolized to short-chain fatty acids in the colon. These short-chain fatty acids are trophic for the colonic mucosa, leading to an improvement in fluid and electrolyte absorption. Patients who have a full or partial colon should receive a high-carbohydrate, low-fat diet (60%:20%) with restricted oxalate.[8] Medium chain triglycerides can be used to supplement energy intake. Nightingale has reported that short-bowel patients maintained on an oral diet need to consume as much as 50% more calories than their normal counterparts because of the presence of malabsorption.[12] Failure to recognize this higher energy need may result in decreased muscle mass and low body fat, which may cause decreased functional status.

Lactose intolerance may be evident in some patients returning to an oral diet. The degree of lactose deficiency may allow for some intake in small amounts. Lactose-free milk products can be used. Vitamin B-12 should be given intramuscularly for patients if > 60 cm of terminal ileum is diseased or has been resected.[8] Anti-diarrheal medications may slow motility, allowing for increased absorptive capacity and decreased fluid output.[8]

A 1993 study evaluated the quality of life of SBS patients over the first year of HPN. The average body weight at the start of HPN for the SBS patients was 82% of usual body weight for the males and 86% of usual body weight for the females, indicating a state of undernutrition prior to initiating HPN.[13] Quality of life and functional status are diminished in a state of undernutrition, which further demonstrates the importance of close clinical monitoring for the patient who is transitioning from HPN. While it is a goal to completely eliminate HPN, it is important to note that even decreasing one day per week should be considered a success.

Oral rehydration solutions should be evaluated and implemented for patients with continued fluid losses.[8,14] Oral rehydration solutions (ORS) are used when patients have extensive fluid losses such as those with a jejunostomy or extreme SBS to prevent or correct dehydration. These are used in place of water because they contain sodium, water, and some level of glucose. Sodium concentrations in ORS are suggested to contain between 90 and 120 mMol, and the concentration of glucose is recommended at levels of 20–40 grams/liter.[15] These are best when mixed and sipped throughout the day.

Along with dietary management intervention, optimizing medical management is important in employing not only anti-diarrheals but also pharmacological treatments such as proton pump inhibitors and somatostatin analogues.[8,14,16] Other interventions that may be implemented include anticholinergics, pancreatic enzyme replacements, antimicrobials, and probiotics.[17,18] Furthermore, surgical procedures may be employed to lengthen the GI tract or to modify GI physiology to enhance absorption.[19]

Putting all of these components together will provide the clinician with a transition checklist to ensure that all components have been considered and the appropriate therapy implemented (see Table 14–2).

TABLE 14–2   Transition Checklist

---

1. Underlying cause for HPN:
    ☐ SBS   ☐ Resection   ☐ Congenital malformation   ☐ Other: _____

2. Length of remaining SB:
    ☐ >200 cm   ☐ 200–150 cm   ☐ <150 cm   ☐ Unknown

3. Intact colon?
    ☐ Yes   ☐ No

4. No colon?
    ☐ Yes   ☐ No

5. Ileocecal valve:
    ☐ Yes   ☐ No

6. Quantifiable fluid losses:
    ☐ Yes   ☐ No

7. Fluid requirements >2500 ml/day:
    ☐ Yes   ☐ No

8. Urine output >1 liter/day:
    ☐ Yes   ☐ No

9. Complete nutrition assessment completed:
    ☐ Yes   ☐ No

10. Patient is motivated to follow modified diet:
    ☐ Yes   ☐ No

11. Dietitian available to provide continued follow up:
    ☐ Yes   ☐ No

12. Pharmacological treatments optimized?
    Anti-diarrheals?   ☐ Yes   ☐ No
    Anti-cholinergics?   ☐ Yes   ☐ No
    Pancreatic enzyme replacements: ☐ Yes   ☐ No
    Antimicrobials: ☐ Yes   ☐ No
    Probiotics: ☐ Yes   ☐ No
    Growth hormone: ☐ Yes   ☐ No
    Other factors: _____

QUALITY OF LIFE AND FINANCIAL IMPLICATIONS

Quality of life issues are an extremely important determinant of the success of any therapy. Howard and associates have determined that having an experienced supervising clinician and patient and family interaction with an effective education and peer support organization is vital to improving quality of life for HPN patients.[6]

Transitioning off HPN is a lofty goal for an HPN-dependent person; however, it can be accomplished.[5,7,8,14] It is important to recognize that transitioning an individual from daily HPN to 6, 5, or 4 days per week can have a positive effect in quality of life and can probably be accomplished in many HPN patients. In a survey of long-term HPN patients, 63% infused daily, 8% infused 6 days per week, 5%, infused 5 days per week, 13% infused 4 days per week, 8% infused 3 days per week, and 5% infused 2 days per week.[20] Additionally, because these individuals were able to absorb some oral nutrients, 19% did not infuse lipids at all. Quality of life changes are easy to quantify when a person is able to go from daily infusions to 4–6 days per week infusions. Even with one day (or night) off HPN per week, there is no rush to return home to "hook-up" for the days' nutrients. If the person infuses during the night, then the night off of HPN can be more restful. Even when fewer kilocalories of protein, and therefore fluid, are infused, there is less output and again potentially a more restful sleep. Financial outcomes are also affected. Receiving HPN for 6 days per week rather than 7 decreases this annual expenditure, which is beneficial to the reimbursement resource for the patient whether it is a commercial payer or a governmental agency.

Clinical and objective data related to transition of patients from parenteral or enteral nutrition to an oral diet has been presented previously. However, often the most profound advice on "what to eat" comes from the consumers.[21] The information in Tables 14–3 through 14–5 come from consumers and clinicians as to suggestions for foods to eat. This is not all objective, but rather includes some subjective data. However, lessons from consumers can be very helpful. *These are only suggestions taken from comments from people with digestive disorders and are not a substitute for a physician or dietitian's advice.*

TABLE 14–3   Food and Eating Suggestions

- Fruits
  - Remove the skin; most canned is fine
  - Fruits that aren't always tolerated:
    Pineapple (including pineapple juice)
    Orange Juice (try low acid without pulp)
- Veggies
  - Cook until soft — remove skin
    Try: steamed squash — yellow zucchini
    Tomatoes (no skin), mushrooms, green beans (cooked well), etc.
  - Veggies that aren't always tolerated:
    Carrots (even cooked)
    Corn, black olives, spinach (raw or cooked)
- Breads and cereals
  - Learn how much fiber you can tolerate (take it slow & easy)
  - Try ground whole wheat rather than whole grain, use flour tortillas instead of whole wheat or corn
  - Pick the highest nutrition you can find
- Fat — low to moderate fat intake
- Dairy — low to moderate intakes for lactose intolerance
  - Cheeses:
    The harder the cheese, the less lactose it contains
  - Milk — Try skim or 1%
  - Yogurt — before trying yogurt with active cultures, contact your physician

In general, consume small amounts of:
  - Concentrated sweets
  - Juices, regular sodas, other sugar-sweetened beverages, beverages containing caffeine
- To decrease output — try increasing fiber intake to slow motility and increase absorption — commercial fibers are available as is liquid pectin. This works best if the patient has colon left in continuity with the small intestine.
- When you are having increased output/diarrhea, a good choice of foods is:
    B-bananas — for the pectin content
    R-rice — easy to digest and is a binding starch
    A-apple sauce — to provide energy and soluble (water-holding) fiber
    T-toast — easy to tolerate and is a binding starch
- When these foods are being well tolerated, then you can start adding other foods. Choose bland low-fiber foods, such as:
    White-chicken meat without the skin, scrambled eggs
    Crackers, white bread, and pasta noodles without sauce
    Canned or cooked fruits without skins

TABLE 14–4   Lessons from Patients: What to Eat?

- Sometimes the foods suggested "work" (are tolerated) well, but what works for one may not work for another.
- In addition, what didn't work last month may work this month.
- Physical issues can affect the outcome of whether or not a particular food works.
- Mental health is also something to consider; how much effort is the patient willing to invest in this diet?
- Several small meals eaten over the day are usually better tolerated.
- For sweetened beverages (including juice), drink slowly over as much time as possible.
- Use low-sugar foods or dilute high-sugar foods (such as juices). Watch out for sorbitol-containing sweeteners.

TABLE 14–5   Top Ten Things to Know About Eating if You Are on HPN

1. First and foremost, enjoy your food!

2. Don't overdo anything—you may overwhelm you digestive system.

3. Beverages should be low in sugar because fluids empty from the stomach faster than solid food. Try sugar-free sweetened, powdered drink flavorings to enhance beverages such as ORS. Avoid diet beverages sweetened with sorbitol or xylitol because these sweeteners are not absorbed and may stimulate stool output. Fruit juices should be diluted and are best when they don't have sugar added to them (such as most fruit punches, fruit drinks, and fruit juice cocktails). To include juices in your diet, try mixing grapefruit juice and Fresca™, or orange juice and diet Sprite™. By doing this you decrease the amount of concentrated sugar in these beverages.

4. Beverages should be sipped continuously, with the largest amounts taken between meals and smaller amounts taken with meals.

5. Include sources of soluble fiber like bananas, rice, applesauce, toast, tapioca, and oatmeal. Foods containing large amounts of insoluble fiber may or may not be tolerated, depending upon your risk of intestinal obstruction. Foods with higher insoluble fiber are green leafy vegetables and whole grains such as high-fiber cereals and breads—all greater than 3 grams per serving.

6. Eat small frequent meals rather than large meals.

7. Fatty foods (i.e., eggs, sausage, whole milk dairy products, and fried foods) may be better tolerated in the morning rather than later in the day.

8. Unless you have been told otherwise by your physician, it s okay to salt your foods and to eat salty foods, because loss of gastrointestinal flu d is also loss of salt.

9. You can eat the foods that you like unless they make you sick. Try small amounts first!

10. Caffeine can be a potent gastric stimulator and increase output by causing diarrhea. This should be considered not only in coffee intake but also in soft drink intake as well.

Individuals dependent on HPN may be able to be transitioned partially or totally off therapy. This requires a multidisciplinary approach with significant diet manipulation and nutrition intervention, monitoring by a skilled home nutrition support team, and a motivated HPN patient. The home nutrition support team has demonstrated effectiveness in transitioning patients from HPN to an oral or enteral diet in both pediatric and adult patients.[22]

REFERENCES

1. Ireton-Jones C, DeLegge M, Epperson L, Alexander J. Management of the home parenteral nutrition patient. *Nutr Clin Pract.* 2003:18:310–317.
2. Matarese LE, O'Keefe SJ, Kandil HM, et al. Short bowel syndrome: guidelines for management. *Nutr Clin Pract.* 2005,20(5):493–502.
3. Guenter P, Silkroski M. *Tube Feeding: Practical Guidelines and Nursing Protocols.* Gaithersburg, MD: Aspen Publishers; 2001.
4. DeLegge MH, Kirby DF: Enteral feeding, formula, delivery, and complications. *Pract Gastroenterol.* 1992;16:32–44.
5. Scolapio JS. Short bowel syndrome. *J Parenter Enteral Nutr.* 2002;26(suppl 5):S11–S16.
6. Howard LJ. Length of life and quality of life on home parenteral nutrition. *J Parenter Enteral Nutr.* 2002;26(suppl 5):S55–S59.
7. Wilmore DW, Dudrick SJ, Daley JM, et al. The role of nutrition in the adaptation of the small intestine after massive resection. *Surg Gynecol Obstet.* 1971;132(4):673–680.
8. Byrne TA, Persinger RL, Young LS, et al. A new treatment for patients with short-bowel syndrome. Growth hormone, glutamine, and a modified diet. *Ann Surg.* 1995;222(3):243–254.
9. Dowling RH. Small bowel adaptation and its regulation. *Scand J Gastroenterol.* 1982;74:53–74.
10. Nordgaard I, Hansen BS, Mortensen PB. Importance of colonic support for energy absorption as small-bowel failure proceeds. *Am J Clin Nutr.* 1996; 64(2):222–231.
11. Ireton-Jones CS, Hasse JM. Comprehensive nutritional assessment: the dietitian's contribution to the team effort. *Nutrition.* 1992;8(2):75–81.
12. Nightingale JMD. The short bowel. In: Nightingale J, ed. *Intestinal Failure.* Cornwall, UK: MPG Books Ltd, Bodmin; 2001:186.
13. Ireton-Jones C, Cox-Davis S, DeLegge M. Nutritional Status of Adult Patients with Short Bowel Syndrome at Initiation of HPN. Abstract submitted to Nutrition Week, 2003.
14. Johnson MD. Management of Short Bowel Syndrome – A Review. Support Line 22(6): 11–25, 2000.

15. Ukleja A, Scolapio J. Abnormalities in fluid and electrolytes absorption in intestinal failure. In: Matarese L, Steiger E, Seidner D, eds. *Intestinal Failure and Rehabilitation: A Clinical Guide.* Boca Raton, FL: CRC Press;2005: 58–59.

16. Kandil HM, O'Keefe SJD. Medications: antidiarrheals, H2 blockers, proton pump inhibitors and antisecretory therapy. In: Matarese L, Steiger E, Seidner D, eds. *Intestinal Failure and Rehabilitation: A Clinical Guide.* Boca Raton, FL: CRC Press;2005:149–160.

17. Stevens, T, Conwell DL. Pancreatitic enzyme replacement and bile acid therapy. In: Matarese L, Steiger E, Seidner D, eds. *Intestinal Failure and Rehabilitation: A Clinical Guide.* Boca Raton, FL: CRC Press;2005:161–176.

18. Vanderhoof J, Young R. Antimicrobials and probiotics. In: Matarese L, Steiger E, Seidner D, eds. *Intestinal Failure and Rehabilitation: A Clinical Guide.* Boca Raton, FL: CRC Press;2005:177–186.

19. Iyer KR, Richard M. Surgery for intestinal failure. In: Matarese L, Steiger E, Seidner D, eds. *Intestinal Failure and Rehabilitation: A Clinical Guide.* Boca Raton, FL: CRC Press; 2005:279–294.

20. Ireton-Jones C, Anthony P, Parker M, et al. Factors associated with the quality of life and long-term nutrition support consumer satisfaction. Presented at the 2000 A.S.P.E.N. Clinical Congress, Nashville, TN, January 2000.

21. Suneson J, Ireton-Jones C. Gutsy Issues in Nutrition. Oley Foundation Lifeline Letter, May/June 1997.

22. Hamilton K, Newton A, Ireton-Jones C. Home nutrition support team advanced nutrition management outcomes for home parenteral nutrition patients. *Nutr Clin Pract.* 2003:18(2):186.

CHAPTER 15

Home Nutrition Management in the Transplant Patient

Lecia Snell, RN, MSN
Susan Randolph, RN, MSN
Tess Artig-Brown, RN, MN

INTRODUCTION

Solid organ and blood and marrow transplantation has evolved from a few experimental procedures in the 1960s to an accepted treatment modality for many individuals suffering from end-stage organ failure, congenital disorders, and select malignancies. The development of advanced surgical techniques and an improved understanding of the immune system have significantly fueled this growth, making transplantation a promising option for many patients. However, rejection in solid organ transplantation, graft-versus-host disease (GVHD) in allogeneic blood and marrow transplantation, and infection in all types of transplantation remain significant obstacles to successful patient and graft survival.

During the past decade, research has focused on the development of new pharmaceuticals, advanced laboratory testing, and immune modulating techniques to help overcome these challenges. Though both patient and graft survival rates have improved significantly, there is also a growing body of literature documenting the need to evaluate other factors that may impact outcomes.

The role of nutrition and nutrition support in transplantation is one such factor and is increasingly recognized as an essential supportive care therapy to help maintain maximum wellness throughout the transplant continuum. Understanding the potential for nutritional disability in transplant patients allows the clinician to be proactive in applying nutrition support. The purpose of this chapter is to review the physiology and clinical features of transplantation and the potential impact on home nutrition management. An overview of both solid organ and blood cell/bone marrow transplantation will be followed by a review of immunosuppression, infectious complications, rejection, GVHD, metabolic disorders, and long-term complications.

TRANSPLANTATION OVERVIEW

Solid Organ Transplantation

Solid organ transplant has become an accepted treatment modality for end-stage organ failure associated with a variety of diseases. The number of transplants being done continues to grow, limited only by the shortage of organ donors. Graft and patient survival rates continue to improve, positively impacted by improved surgical techniques, better donor matching, enhanced immunosuppressive medications and management, and improved prevention and treatment of infectious complications (see Table 15–1).

Indications

The indications for solid organ transplant vary by organ (see Table 15–2). The underlying disease process for transplantation is a major consideration in the nutritional management of the patient and will follow disease specific guidelines. For example, the management of the pre-renal transplant patient will be guided by principles for any end-stage renal patient.

The Transplant Process

The transplant process, outlined in Table 15–3, includes the evaluation, waiting period, surgical procedure, and posttransplantation. Each phase is critical in the process, and careful assessment, monitoring, and communication are essential for success.

TABLE 15-1   Number of Organ Transplants and Survival

Transplants by Type*		Survival			
		Patient		Graft	
		1 yr	5 yr	1 yr	5 yr
Heart	2,056	85	69	85	69
Lung	1,085	78	43	77	43
Heart/Lung	25	*	*	*	*
Kidney	15,134	90	70	90	70
Liver	5,670	80	64	80	64
Pancreas	502	*	*	*	*
Intestine	116	69	40	69	40

* Indicates not available

2003 Annual Report of the U.S. Scientific Registry of Transplant Recipients and the Organ Procurement and Transplantation Network: Transplant Date 1988–2004. (2005, February 4). Rockville, MD and Richmond, VA: HHA/HRSA/DOT and UNOS

Pretransplant Evaluation. The pretransplant evaluation is a critical component of the transplant process. The goal of this phase is to assess any actual or potential problems that may negatively impact outcomes and either 1) determine that the patient is not a candidate, 2) design interventions to minimize or correct the problems prior to transplant, or 3) adjust posttransplant protocols to compensate for results. Patients undergo a battery of laboratory and radiologic tests to determine baseline clinical status and identify any areas of risk or required intervention. Necessary consults are obtained, including a psychosocial evaluation. A financial evaluation is important in order to ensure sufficient coverage for both the transplant and posttransplant care needs. Detailed education is essential so that patients and families are informed of the processes, the potential complications, and their responsibilities throughout. Nutrition assessment is also critical prior to transplant. Depending on the disease process and the individual patient, many patients likely have not had adequate nutrition management during their pretransplant illness.

Contraindications to Transplant. Ultimately, patient candidacy is determined after interpreting all evaluation results, designing pretransplant interventions as appropriate, and determining the risk/benefit ratio. Certain evaluation outcomes will likely make a patient ineligible for

TABLE 15-2   Indications for Solid Organ Transplant

Heart	Lung	Kidney	Liver	Intestine	Pancreas
• Ischemic cardiomyopathy	• COPD	• Diabetes mellitus	• Hepatitis B & C	• Vovulus	• Juvenile onset diabetes mellitus
• Non-ischemic cardiomyopathy	• Bronchiectasis	• Hypertension	• Alcoholic liver disease	• Gastroschisis	
• Congenital anomalies	• Cystic fibrosis	• Chronic glomerulo-nephritis	• Primary biliary cirrhosis	• Hirschsprungs disease	
• Refractory ventricular dysrhythmnias	• Primary hypertension	• Systemic lupus erythematosus	• Primary sclerosing cholangitis	• Chronic intestinal pseudo-obstruction	
• Valvular disease	• Pulmonary fibrosis	• Vasculitis	• Autoimmune hepatitis	• Crohns diease	
• Retransplantation	• Eosinophilic granuloma	• Plycystic kidney disease	• Biliary atresia	• Vascular insufficiency	
	• Idiopathic pulmonary fibrosis	• Chronic pyelonephritis	• Metabolic disorders	• Radiation enteritis	
	• Hemosiderosis				
	• Goodpasture's Syndrome				

Adapted from Cupples, S. & Ohler, L. (eds.) (2003). Transplantation Nursing Secrets. Hanley & Belfus, Inc: Philadelphia, PA transplant. The "absolute" contraindications, listed in Table 15–4, are generally viewed as creating a risk/benefit ratio that is weighted too heavily toward risk. For example, a patient who does not complete the pre-transplant work-up should not be placed on the list; a patient with acute or chronic serious infection or malignancy will only become more ill when immunosuppressed; severe heart disease may cause a patient not to survive the surgical procedure; or other major issues. However, with a few exceptions, each "absolute" contraindication taken by itself may or may not rule out a candidate. The patient must be evaluated as a whole. Candidacy generally depends on a combination of factors, both medical and psychosocial. Other conditions exist that may have a negative impact on patient survival but not to the extent that transplant should not be considered. These relative contraindications to organ transplantation are listed in Table 15–5.

Donor Sources. There are three potential donor sources for organ transplantation: deceased donor, living related, or living non-related donors. The most common source of organs is from deceased donors. A deceased donor is a person who has undergone a traumatic death, has neither brain stem function nor any potential to regain brain stem function, and has been declared brain dead. Common causes of brain death include motor vehicle accidents, cerebrovascular accidents, and gunshot wounds to the head. Living donation occurs when a related or unrelated person donates an organ to someone needing a transplant. Living donation has decreased the need for deceased donations, thus expanding the donor pool. Based on the Organ Procurement and Transplant Network,[1] the number of living donors continues to increase annually; 49 percent of the kidney transplants performed in 2005 were from living donors. Many people, however, in need of an organ transplant either do not have an acceptable living donor or a living donor cannot donate the organ needed. Patients, then, must wait until a deceased donor organ becomes available. The advantages of a living related donor transplant generally include fewer complications, especially if the donor is "matched" to the recipient. Matching of a donor refers to the number of human leukocyte antigens (HLA) from the donors that match the potential recipient. HLA matching has been found to be critical in bone marrow transplantation, important in kidney and pancreas transplantation, and valuable but not essential in liver and heart transplantation. When HLAs are matched between donor and recipient in these organs, there is gener-

TABLE 15–3   The Transplant Process

Pre-Op Evaluation	Waiting Period	Surgical Procedure	Post-Op
History & Physical	Donor sources	General anesthesia	ICU
Laboratory studies	Impact on:	Process and length	Transplant unit infection precautions
Consultants:	• clinical		
• anesthesia	• psychosocial		Potential complications:
• dental	• financial		• infection
• surgery			• bleeding
• social work			• rejection
• psychiatry			• altered nutritional status
• cardiology			• fluid and electrolyte imbalance
• gynecology			
• other organ specific			• other organ specific
• other patient specific			
Patient/family teaching:			Discharge teaching:
• informed consent			• short and long term f/u
• compliance			• medications
• post-tx responsibilities			• compliance
			• s/s infection
			• s/s rejection
			• activities/rehab

ally less reaction to donor tissue and therefore less of a rejection response.

The Waiting List.   Upon completion of the evaluation, the patient is placed on the waiting list until an appropriate donor is available. For many patients, the wait can be weeks, months, or even years, depending on the organ needed and other medical factors of the patient. It is a challenging time medically. There is risk for deterioration of their clinical status, including progressive nutritional decline. Optimizing nutritional status during this waiting period is essential to ensure that the patient is in as good a condition at the time of transplant as possible.

Once an appropriate organ is found, the patient is brought to the center for transplantation. Hospital length of stays vary between organ and transplant center. Rejection and infection are significant potential post-

TABLE 15–4 Absolute Contraindications to Organ Transplantation

Psychosocial	Physical
Active drug, tobacco, or alcohol abuse	Active infection
	Chronic infection
Evidence of psychotherapy	AIDS
Inability to comply with regimen	
Inability to understand risks	Hemophilia
Non-adherence to the evaluation requirements	Active peptic ulcer disease
	GI bleeding
	Recent malignancy
Severe, irreversible organ system damage other than organ(s) to be transplanted	

Adapted from Donaldson, T. (2003). The role of the transplant coordinator. In Cupples and Ohler (eds.). Transplantation Nursing Secrets. Hanley & Belfus: Philadelphia: PA.

TABLE 15–5 Relative Contraindications to Organ Transplantation

Age*

HIV

Lack of financial support to cover any aspect of the transplant process

Morbid obesity (>140% IBW)

Severe osteoporosis

Cachexia

* An age criterion varies by organ and transplant center.
Generally, age is based on biological vs. chronological age.

Adapted from Donaldson, T. (2003). The role of the transplant coordinator. In Cupples and Ohler (eds.). Transplantation Nursing Secrets. Hanley & Belfus: Philadelphia: PA.

TABLE 15–6 Discharge Criteria for Solid Organ Transplant Patients

Organ function within acceptable limits	Adequate caloric intake
Stable immunosuppression levels without rejection	(may require EN/PN)
	Safe home environment
Afebrile (may be on anti-microbials)	Adequate understanding of posttransplant care

transplant problems and will be discussed later in this chapter. Discharge criteria are dependent upon transplant center protocol, availability of support services, and the organ transplanted (see Table 15–6).

Pretransplant Nutritional Management Considerations

Poor nutritional management is prevalent in the pretransplantation phase, often due to end-stage organ failure, metabolic alterations, and poor dietary intake.[2,3] Malnutrition compromises posttransplant survival, and prolonged waiting times worsen outcomes when patients are already malnourished.[2] Timely nutrition assessment and intervention may improve posttransplant outcomes.

There are many factors that contribute to malnutrition in the organ transplant candidate, including anorexia, nausea, vomiting, difficulty chewing or swallowing, limited access to food, depression, fatigue, restricted diets, and hypermetabolic states due to disease and/or surgery.[3] End-stage organ disease specific to each body system will also influence nutrition status. For example, a lung transplant candidate will experience increased work of breathing, hyperinflation resulting in early satiety, and increased energy expenditures due to chronic infections.

Intestinal transplant candidates are unique among solid organ recipients. All pre-intestinal transplant candidates have been on parenteral nutrition for a period of time due to gut dysfunction/malabsorption. Currently, these patients are considered for transplant only when they have developed significant complications from PN (parenteral nutrition), such as liver failure, lack of vascular access, and frequent sepsis. The goal of intestinal transplantation, then, is to get the patient off PN and reverse and treat the complications.

Approximately 70% of intestinal transplant candidates are waiting at home at the time of transplant.[4] The home nutrition support team, therefore, plays an integral role in optimizing the patient's nutritional status and decreasing complications prior to transplant.

Management of the pretransplant patient in the home requires prompt nutritional screening and consistent, detailed follow-up to ensure that the patient is in a top nutritional state prior to transplant to ensure the best outcomes. Nutritional screening should include an evaluation of subjective and objective parameters such as current weight, weigh loss, appetite, and any symptoms affecting the ability to eat or absorb nutrients. Follow-up by the home care dietitian, especially if the patient is receiving home nutrition support, should be done with close communication with the transplant team.

Hematopoietic Stem Cell Transplantation

Hematopoietic stem cell transplantation (HSCT) is an increasingly used treatment for a variety of disorders (see Table 15–7). Hematopoietic stem cell transplantation is a procedure consisting of the administration of high-dose chemotherapy and/or radiation therapy followed by intravenous infusion of hematopoietic stem cells to reestablish marrow function. The high-dose therapy will not only ablate the tumor or diseased cells, but has the consequence of ablating the patient's bone marrow, that is, their red cells, white blood cells, and platelets. Patients cannot sustain life after this destruction and must have a chance to renew their cell lines.

The two types of HSCT are bone marrow transplantation and peripheral blood stem cell transplantation, indicating from where the cells are collected. Hematopoietic stem cell transplantation can be further defined by the source of the stem cells (see Table 15–9). Allogeneic HSCT involves the transfer of marrow from a related or unrelated donor to a recipient, whereas autologous HSCT uses the patient's own stem cells for re-infusion.

Allogeneic donors can be HLA matched or mismatched. Just as in solid organ transplant, allogeneic transplantation of cells from a sibling donor who is an HLA match generally results in better outcomes.[5]

After the donor is identified, the patient undergoes high-dose radiation and/or chemotherapy to destroy any residual cancer cells and to provide space for the new marrow to grow. The major disadvantages of allogeneic HSCT include the difficulty in finding an appropriate HLA-matched donor and the occurrence of a higher rate of complications, including toxicities from the conditioning regimen, infectious complications, and graft-versus-host disease (GVHD).

Autologous HSCT uses the patient's own marrow to reestablish hematopoietic cell function after the administration of myeloablative therapy. The major advantages of autologous transplantation include the ready availability of a stem cell product and the absence of GVHD, which translates into lower morbidity, mortality, and cost. However, the incidence of disease relapse is higher in autologous HSCT.[6]

HSCT may be performed inpatient and/or outpatient, depending on center protocols. If performed inpatient, hospital length of stay and discharge criteria will vary by center, depending on available, trained ancillary services, which may include home infusion. Discharge criteria for

TABLE 15–7   Common Diseases Treated with Hematopoetic Stem Cell Transplant

Autologous	Allogeneic
Acute myelogenous leukemia	Acute and chronic myeloid leukemia
Non-Hodgkin's lymphoma	Myelodysplastic syndromes
Hodgkin's disease	Immune deficiencies
Multiple myeloma	Severe aplastic anemia
Solid tumors	Red cell aplasias: Sickle Cell Disease
Auto-immune diseases: Multiple Sclerosis, Sclera Derma, SLE	Inborne errors of metabolism: Hurlers, ALD

Adapted from Mattox, T. (1999). Specialized nutrition management of patients receiving hematopoietic stem cell transplantation, Nutrition in Clinical Practice, 14, 5–15.

TABLE 15–8   Types of Hematopoietic Stem Cell Transplants

Type of Transplantation	Source of Cells
Autologous transplant	• Patient (self)
Allogeneic transplant	
• Related	• Human leukocyte antigen-matched (HLA-matched) family member, usually a sibling
• Syngeneic	• Patient's identical twin (HLA identical)
• Unrelated	• HLA-matched nonfamily member
• Mismatched	• Partially HLA-matched family or nonfamily member
• Cord blood	• Related and unrelated donors

Adapted from Poliquin, C. (1997). Overview of Bone Marrow and Peripheral Blood Stem Cell Transplantation. Clinical Journal of Oncology Nursing, (1)1, 11–17.

the HSCT mirror that of the solid organ transplant patient (see Table 15–6).

POSTTRANSPLANT CONSIDERATIONS

Rejection in solid organ and GVHD in HSCT, as well as infection in both types of transplant, are leading causes of morbidity and mortality posttransplant. GVHD is prevented and/or treated by pharmacologic

TABLE 15–9   Common Immunosuppressive Medications Used in Transplantation

Medication	Therapeutic Drug Monitoring	Potential Adverse Effects
Prednisone (Deltasone®) Methlyprenisolone (Solu-Medrol®)	• White blood cell • Blood sugar • Blood pressure	• Incrased susceptibility to infection • Hypertension • Cardiomyopathy • Sodium retention • Fluid retention • Hypokalemia • Mood swings, depression • Diabetes • Hyperlipidemia • Growth retardation • Truncal obesity • Osteoporosis • Lymphocytosis • Glaucoma, cataracts • Gastritis, GI bleeding • Increased appetite • Acne, striae
Cyclosporine USP (Sandimmune®, Neoral®, Gengraf®) Generics available — are not always equivalent	• 12-hour trough blood level • Renal function	• Increased susceptibility to infection • Nephrotoxicity • Hepatotoxicity • Hypertension • Tremors, parathesias, seizures • Hyperglycemia/diabetes • Hyperlipidemia • Hirsutism • Increased susceptibility to malignancy • Gingival hyperplasia
Tacrolimus, FK506 (Prograf®)	• 12-hour trough blood level • Renal function	• Increased susceptibility to infection • Nephrotoxicity • Hepatotoxicity • Hypertension • Tremors, parathesias, seizures • Hyperglycemia/diabetes • Hyperlipidemia • Alopecia • Increased susceptibility to malignancy

TABLE 15–9   Common Immunosuppressive Medications Used in
Transplantation (Continued)

Medication	Therapeutic Drug Monitoring	Potential Adverse Effects
Azathioprine (Imuran®)	• WBC • Platelets	• Increased susceptibility to infection • Leukopenia
Mycophenolate mofetil (CellCept®)	• 12- hour trough blood level • White blood cell counts • Platelet count	• Increased susceptibility to infection • Diarrhea • Leukopenia, neutropenia • Vomiting • Abdominal pain
Cyclophosphamide (Cytoxan®)	• CBC • Renal function	• Nephrotoxicity • Cardiotoxicity
Antithymocyte globulin (Atgam®, Thymoglobulin®)		• Increased susceptibility to infection • Bone marrow suppression • Thrombocytopenia • Local inflammation, rxns • Fever, chills • Serum sickness • Anaphylaxis
Muromonab-CD-3 (Orthoclone OKT®3)	• CBC • Renal function • Weight • Fluid status	• Increased susceptibility to infection • Pyrexia, rigors, malaise (first 3 doses) • Diarrhea (first 3 doses) • Hyper/hypotension • Resp. distress if fluid overloaded (dose 1)
Daclizumab (Zenapax ®)		• Increased susceptibility to infection • Constipation, nausea, diarrhea, vomiting • Hyper/hypotension • Peripheral edema • Headache, tremor
Basiliximab (Simulect ®)		• Increased susceptibility to infection • Data are still very limited • Does not increase the incidence of side effects that are usually observed with standard immuno-suppressive regimen

Adapted from Dumas-Hicks, D. (2003). Immunosupppression. In Cupples and Ohler (eds). *Transplantation Nursing Secrets*. Hanley and Belfus: Philadelphia, PA suppression of the immune system. Simultaneously, however, immuno-suppression can increase the risk for infectious complications. In addition, potential complications related to the type of chemotherapy administered in the conditioning regimen of the HSCT process can have lasting effects. Therefore, it is important to know what conditioning regimen the patient received and the potential adverse effects of that regimen.

Immunosuppression

Suppression of the immune system is required to prevent rejection in the solid organ transplant recipient and GVHD in the allogeneic HSCT patient. Significant advances in immunosuppressive therapy have certainly resulted in improved transplant-related outcomes; however, immuno-suppression and the resulting side effects add considerable complexity to the posttransplant management of the patient.

The term immunosuppression refers to the pharmacologic alteration of immune system functions to prevent rejection of the allograft while maintaining sufficient immunity to prevent infection.[7] Balanced control of the immune system is the cornerstone of transplantation.[8] If the patient is underdosed, then rejection or GVHD will ensue. On the other hand, if the patient is overdosed, then infectious complications and drug toxicities will occur.

Management of immunosuppression varies among transplant centers, depending on clinical experience, patient population, and the type of transplant performed. In addition, gender, race, age, center protocol, and HLA incompatibility are considered.[7] Table 15–9 provides a listing of common immunosuppressants and their potential adverse effects.

Dosing of immunosuppression is accomplished by monitoring blood concentration levels and other lab values (see Table 15–9). Side effects, including the nutritional-related ones, are generally dose related. Once the dose is adjusted, lab values should return to normal, and symptoms should subside. Blood levels can be affected by the drug dosage, co-administration of multiple drugs or foods with synergistic or antagonistic reactions, noncompliance and organ dysfunction. For example, grapefruit products have been shown to increase blood concentrations of cyclosporine and tacrolimus and it is recommended that transplant recipients who take these medications do not ingest grapefruit products for this reason.[7]

Nutritional Implications of Immunosuppression

Immunosuppressive medications have potential associated gastrointestinal effects that require close assessment, monitoring, and education. Gastrointestinal (GI) side effects, including nausea, vomiting, and diarrhea, are particularly worrisome, as they put the recipient at risk for rejection due to the malabsorption of medications. In addition, prolonged GI side effects can lead to malnutrition and can affect the overall recovery of the patient.[8] Table 15–10 provides a comprehensive review of potential side effects and appropriate nutritional interventions. The home dietitian plays an integral role in assessing for these potential adverse reactions and recommending interventions to alleviate further nutritional harm.

Rejection

Rejection is one of the leading causes of morbidity and mortality in the solid organ transplant recipient. Rejection is a process whereby the body's immune system perceives the transplanted organ as foreign. The immune system's function is to protect the body from infection and other foreign cells. Unfortunately, immune cells cannot differentiate between an invading organism and life-saving transplant tissue. Therefore, the immune system, if not weakened, will attempt to reject the transplant. In general, this response is no different from the body's response to an invading bacteria or virus. Good HLA matching reduces the incidence and severity of rejection; however, the risk of a rejection episode remains because, unless the transplant is from an identical twin, there are still differences between the recipient and the donor.

There are two primary types of rejection that may be seen in the home setting: acute and chronic. Acute rejection describes the clinical situation associated with sudden onset of signs that the immune system is attempting to rid the body of that particular organ. For example, with liver transplantation, the liver will be attacked by lymphocytes, the patient will show clinical signs of liver dysfunction, and unless treated, the patient will lose the liver. See Table 15–11 for a summary of the most common signs and symptoms of acute rejection for each major organ transplant.

TABLE 15–10   Common Gastrointestinal Complications

Complication	Potential Cause	Nutrition Interventions
Alterations in saliva (thick, viscous mucous)	Chemotherapy Radiation therapy Infectious disease Chronic GVHD	• Maintain adequate fluid intake • Clear liquids • Oral hygiene protocol
Anorexia	Altered organ function Chemotherapy Chronic GVHD Disease relapse Radiation therapy Supportive care drugs	• Atmosphere (enhance with smell, variety/texture of foods, attractive physical setting) • Appetite stimulants • Small, frequent meals • Utilize foods high in protein and calorie content
Diarrhea	Altered organ function Chemotherapy Chronic GVHD Radiation therapy Supportive care drugs	• Adequate fluids/electrolytes to prevent dehydration and/or electrolyte imbalance • Avoid caffeine, alcohol, spicy foods • Cool or room temperature foods • Low fat, low fiber • Low lactose intake
Dysgeusia	Chemotherapy Radiation therapy Chronic GVHD Supportive care drugs	• Aromatic foods • Cold, non-odorous foods • Flavor foods (spices, extracts, marinades) • Fruit-flavored beverages • Oral hygiene protocol
Mucositis (oral / esophageal)	Chemotherapy Radiation therapy Chronic GVHD Infectious disease	• Liquid diet • Non-irritating cold foods • Soft or puree textured diet • Soft, bland, moist foods • Oral hygiene protocol • Pain management
Nausea / vomiting	Chemotherapy Radiation therapy Infectious disease Supportive care drugs	• Adequate fluids/electrolytes to prevent dehydration and/or electrolyte imbalance • Antiemetics • Avoid highly sweet or high-fat foods • Cold, clear liquids and solids • High-carbohydrate foods and fluids • Non-acidic juices • Small, frequent feedings
Xerostomia	Chemotherapy Chronic GVHD Dehydration Radiation Therapy	• Add sauces, gravies, broth, etc., and liquids • Artificial saliva (commercial) • Encourage liquids with meals • Moist foods • Oral hygiene protocol • Sugarless candy may stimulate saliva

TABLE 15–11   Signs and Symptoms of Acute Organ Rejection

Organ	Liver	Heart	Lung	Kidney	Pancreas
Signs and symptoms	• Abnormal LFTs • Abdominal tenderness • Dark urine • Light stools • Jaundice • Fatigue • Fever • Biopsy results	• Arrhythmia • Ventricular gallop • Increased CVP • Biopsy results	• SOB • Decreased PFTs • White-out on CXR • Fatigue • Lethargy • Decreased Exercise intolerance	• Elevated BUN & Cr • Decreased u/o • Weight gain • Graft site tenderness • Malaise • Fever • Biopsy results	• Elevated serum glucose • Elevated serum amylase • Decreased urine amylase • Decreased urine pH • Increased Human Anodal Trypsinogen • Fever • Biopsy results

Acute rejection can occur anytime from days to months posttransplant, although it typically occurs in the first three months. In most cases, this form of rejection can be treated successfully with an increase in maintenance immunosuppression and steroid boluses. Additional immunosuppressive medications may be required if the rejection is refractory to this measure.

Chronic rejection is an insidious process that develops over time, usually greater than one year post-transplant. Once initiated, most current immunosuppression is not successful in reversing the effects, and the graft will ultimately be lost and retransplantation will become necessary. Fortunately, this can take years, but graft loss is an eventual reality.

Graft-Versus-Host Disease

Graft-versus-host disease is a complication almost exclusively seen in the allogeneic HSCT patient population and is one of the leading causes of morbidity and mortality, with both an acute and chronic presentation.[9] Historically, acute GVHD (aGVHD) is defined as occurring before day 100, and chronic GVHD (cGVHD) is defined as occurring after day 100. However, more recently, this definition is undergoing revision due to many factors. Chronic GVHD is occasionally diagnosed earlier than 100 days after allogeneic HSCT and is rarely made later than 500 days after HSCT.[10]

Graft-versus-host disease occurs when immunocompetent T-cells from the donor, successfully engrafted and migrating from the patient's marrow into the body, recognize the patient's cells as foreign. The result is varying degrees of damage to target organs. This is in contrast to rejection in solid organ transplantation where the recipient's immunologically competent T-cells recognize the transplanted organ as foreign (host versus graft). Acute GVHD contributes directly and indirectly to death in 15–40% of posttransplant patients who develop the disease. Serious infections are the primary cause of death in these patients.[11]

The probability of GVHD increases with the degree of mismatch between the donor and the recipient. Other risk factors for the development of GVHD include older age (> 18 years), immunosuppressive regimens, female to male donor (especially a female with previous pregnancies), cytomegalovirus infection, and the use of hematopoietic growth factors. Data presented at the International Tandem Blood and Marrow Conference (February, 2005) demonstrated that patients discharged from the hospital during their pancytopenic phase with follow-up care provided in the home environment versus a hospital environment have a lower incidence of GVHD.

Clinical Manifestations and Staging of Acute GVHD

Acute GVHD targets the skin, liver, and gut of the recipient. GVHD of the skin usually begins as a fine, maculopapular rash on the palms of the hands and soles of the feet. If not successfully treated, skin GVHD can progress to total body erythema, bullae formation, de-socking and de-gloving to total desquamation of the skin.

Liver GVHD presents itself as an elevation of the serum alkaline phosphatase and bilirubin levels, jaundice, and hepatomegaly. When unsuccessfully treated, it can evolve into ascites, encephalopathy, and hepatic failure.

Gut GVHD manifests with high-volume diarrhea, pain, nausea, and vomiting and can progress to GI bleeding and denudation of the GI tract lining. In severe cases, patients can have over two liters of diarrhea per day. These GI side effects are particularly worrisome as they put the recipient at risk for further GVHD and other complications due to the malabsorption of medications. In addition, prolonged GI side effects can lead to malnutrition and significantly impact the overall recovery of the patient.[8]

Prevention and Treatment of GVHD

Prevention of aGVHD while allowing the graft-versus-tumor effect is a balancing act. Prevention starts with donor selection. Finding a donor that is as closely HLA matched to the patient as possible will decrease the risk of GVHD. Only 30% of patients will have a matched sibling donor, thus requiring an alternative source of stem cells, such as an unrelated mismatched donor.[5]

Prophylactic immunosuppression is another method used to prevent GVHD. The immunosuppressant medications used in solid organ transplantation to prevent rejection are also effective in GVHD prevention (see Table 15–9). Dual therapy with cyclosporine and methotrexate is the standard for aGVHD prophylaxis. However, newer medications have been developed in recent years and have been shown to be effective. Over time, generally around day 100, HSCT patients will develop tolerance between the host and donor cells. When this occurs, patients can be weaned from their immunosuppressants.

Treatment of GVHD is via administration of many of the same medications as were used for prevention. The medication doses are generally increased, and high-dose steroids are added or increased with a slow taper over several weeks to months. If the GVHD is refractory to these interventions, then other medications may also be added. It is important to remember that treating GVHD increases the patient's net immunosuppression, which can lead to increased infections and medication toxicities.

Nutritional Implications of Acute GVHD

Conventional transplant preparative regimens are the most intensive therapies used in oncology. The dose-limiting toxicity of marrow ablative regimens is almost always associated with effects in the gastrointestinal tract or liver, especially those regimens containing total body irradiation, alkylating agents (cyclophosphamide, busulfan, melphalan, and thiotepa), and etoposide.[12] Metabolic and nutrition management of patients who receive HSCT is dependent on the underlying disease, the conditioning regimen, and pretransplant and posttransplant complications.[13] For example, a regimen that includes cyclophosphamide (Cytoxan) may cause severe stomatitis, leading to the inability to take in oral nutrition and decreasing absorption through the gastrointestinal tract. This drug can also cause acute nausea, vomiting, and diarrhea.

Acute GVHD of the skin is associated with a higher metabolic rate due to the inflammation. Calorie/energy needs should be provided based on measurements of energy expenditure by indirect calorimetry if at all possible.[14] Desquamation leads to fluid and protein deficits similar to those seen in burn patients. These patients require fluids and protein replacement in addition to their general maintenance requirements.

Acute GVHD of the gut is associated with malabsorption of nutrients and large volumes of diarrhea. In the early stages of GVHD, patients may be placed on bland diets and oral nutritional supplements. In severe cases, patients may need to be nil per os (NPO) and placed on PN. Accurate assessment of volume loss due to diarrhea is needed to calculate fluid replacement requirements. Electrolyte levels must also be monitored frequently and treated appropriately. Once diarrhea subsides, a general diet can be slowly resumed. In addition to fluid and volume requirements, patients who have extensive ileal involvement may experience fat intolerance.[14] (See Chapter 14 for information on transitioning to an oral diet.)

Infection

Infection is a leading cause of morbidity and mortality in all types of transplants. Risk factors include the use of immunosuppressive agents, administration of high-dose chemotherapy and radiation therapy in HSCT, diagnosis of immune modulating viruses (e.g., cytomegalovirus [CMV], Epstein-Barr virus [EBV], hepatitis B virus [HBV], and hepatitis C virus [HCV]), and the presence of neutropenia. Additional risks include the use of invasive procedures (e.g., surgery) or devices (e.g., central venous access devices, indwelling catheters) and concurrent metabolic disorders (e.g., malnutrition, uremia, and diabetes).[15] The potential for infection increases with the number of risk factors.

The risk period for the development of an infectious complication is highest at the point of transplant and in the immediate month posttransplant.[16] Patients are at risk for endogenous infections, especially the reactivation of latent infections (e.g., chronic viral infections) as well as infections from normal body flora. For example, post HSCT transplant complications such as vomiting, diarrhea, mucositis, esophageal and stomach ulcerations, or gut acute GVHD may occur, resulting in a disruption of the mucocutaneous barrier, potentially leading to a lethal infection from normal gastrointestinal flora. Patients are also at risk for developing exogenous infections, from the allograft, blood transfusions, and the environment, including both nosocomial and community-acquired pathogens.

Potential infectious etiologies include bacterial, viral, fungal, and parasitic organisms. Common organisms, general development time lines for transplant-related infections, and common pharmacologic measures are depicted in Figure 1.

The use of immunosuppressive agents also contributes significantly to the risk of developing infectious complications. As discussed earlier, medical teams struggle to find the immunosuppression balance between preventing organ rejection in solid organ transplant recipients or GVHD in allogeneic blood and marrow transplant recipients while simultaneously decreasing the risk of life-threatening infectious diseases.

FIGURE 15–1 Infectious Complications Timeline in Transplantation

Signs and Symptoms
Chills, rigors
Cough (wet or dry)
Diarrhea
Dyspnea
Dysuria, hematuria
Fever
Pain (diffuse/localized)
Skin and/or mucous membrane lesions
Rash
Tenderness, erythema, drainage at site of indwelling devices (e.g., CVC) or over surgical incision
New vaginal or penile discharge
Vomiting

Month 1

Gram positive and negative bacteria
Fungus (candida, aspergillus)
Herpes simplex viruses

Bacterial Infections

Gram Positive
Enterococcus
Listeria
Mycobacteria
Norcardia
Staphylococci
Streptococci

Gram Negative
Enterobacter
Escherichia coli
Haemophilus influenzae
Klebsiella
Legionella
Neisseria
Pseudomonas
Salmonella

Months 2–6

Gram positive and negative bacteria
Fungus
CMV, VZV, EBV, other viral infections
PCP

Common Infectious Organisms

Viral Infections
Adenoviruses
Cytomegalovirus (CMV)~
Epstein-Barr virus (EBV)~
Enterovirus
Hepatitis B virus (HBV)~
Hepatitis C virus (HCV)~
Herpes simplex virus (HSV)
Human herpes virus-6 (HHV-6)
Influenza virus
Papovavirus
Respiratory syncytial virus (RSV)
Varicella-zoster virus (VZV

Fungal Infections
Aspergillus
Blastomycosis*
Candida
Cocccidiodomycosis*
Cryptococcosis
Histoplasmosis*

Beyond 6 Months

Pneumococcal organisms
Hemophilus influenza
CMV, EBV, other viral infections
Fungal infections

Parasitic Infections
Cryptosporidium
Pneumocystis carinii (PCP)
Strongyloides stercoralis
Toxoplasma gondii

~ Immune modulating viral infections
* Geographically restricted mycoses (mid-west or southwest United States)
© Coram Healthcare 2005

A key goal in transplantation is the prevention of infection. However, when infectious complications do occur, it is important to recognize how they can contribute to nutritional deficits. This, in part, is because of the antimicrobials used to prevent and treat infectious diseases (see Table 15–12). Also, the clinical manifestations of the pathogens, such as mucositis, esophageal lesions, gastrointestinal ulcerations, and malabsorption, may contribute to further nutritional deficit.

In the 2–6 month posttransplant period, patients continue to be at risk for opportunistic infections and immunomodulating viral infections, especially CMV.[17] These viruses can occur as a primary infection (where the patient has not been previously exposed) or a reactivation (where the latent virus begins to replicate). Additionally, there are three major sources of community-acquired infection: respiratory viruses, geographically restricted mycoses, and exposure to food-borne pathogens.[17]

Nutrition support teams in the hospital, outpatient setting, and home must reinforce general infection-prevention precautions that help patients avoid food-borne illness. These include:

- Maintain effective hand washing
- Avoid raw or partially cooked foods of animal origin
- Avoid cross-contamination between raw and cooked foods
- Avoid unpasteurized products
- Wash raw fruits and vegetables thoroughly before eating
- Avoid herbal and nutrient supplements

Some HSCT centers also implement low bacterial or low microbial diets as an infection-prevention practice. The use of these diets remains controversial and it is recommended that home nutrition support clinicians identify and support center-specific practices to help maintain continuity of care.

Adequate nutrition support is essential in the prevention and management of infectious complications. Nutritional abnormalities can significantly contribute to the infectious complication risk. In turn, the clinical manifestations of infection can contribute equally to further nutritional complications. While the risk for infection in the transplant population is significant, effective prophylactic and treatment measures can minimize the risk for negative outcomes.

TABLE 15-12   Common Antimicrobials and Potential GI Effects

Antimicrobial Therapy Classification	Commonly Prescribed Agents	Potential GI Side Effects
Antibiotics	aminoglycosides (e.g., amikacin, gentamicin, tobramycin)	hepatic toxicity, *nausea, vomiting, anorexia, diarrhea, weight loss,* stomatitis, increased salivation, splenomegaly
	B lactam antibiotics (e.g., aztreonam, imipenem, meropenem)	*nausea, vomiting, diarrhea, colitis*
	cephalosporins (third generation, e.g., cefepime, cefixime, ceftazidime, ceftriaxone)	*nausea, vomiting, diarrhea, anorexia, abdominal pain, flatulence,* pseudomembranous colitis, liver toxicity
	clindamycin	*severe colitis, including pseudomembranous colitis, nausea, vomiting, diarrhea, abdominal pain, esophagitis, anorexia*
	doxycyline	fatty liver, liver failure, *anorexia, nausea, vomiting, diarrhea, glossitis,* dysphagia, enterocolitis, esophageal ulcer
	macrolide antibiotics (e.g., azithromycin, clarithromycin, erythromycin)	*abdominal cramping, anorexia, diarrhea, vomiting,* pseudomembranous colitis, hepatotoxicity
	penicillins (e.g., amoxicillin ampicillin, methicillin, nafcillin, piperacillin, ticarcillin)	*glossitis, stomatitis, gastritis, sore mouth, nausea, vomiting, diarrhea*
	quinolones (e.g., ciprofloxacin, levofloxacin)	*nausea,* vomiting, dry mouth, *diarrhea,* abdominal pain
	rifampin	*heartburn, epigastric distress,* anorexia, nausea, vomiting, gas, cramps, diarrhea, pseudomembranous colitis, *pancreatitis, elevated LFTs, hepatitis*
	trimethoprin-sulfamethoxazole	*nausea, vomiting, anorexia, diarrhea*
	vancomycin	*nausea*

TABLE 15–12 Common Antimicrobials and Potential GI Effects (Continued)

Antimicrobial Therapy Classification	Commonly Prescribed Agents	Potential GI Side Effects
Antifungal agents	amphotericin B (Fungizone, Albecet, AmBisome)	*nausea, vomiting, dyspepsia, diarrhea,* cramping, epigastric pain, anorexia, hypokalemia, hypomagnesemia
	caspofungin	*elevated liver enzymes, nausea, vomiting*
	fluconazole	*nausea, vomiting, diarrhea,* abdominal pain
	itraconazole	*nausea, vomiting, diarrhea, abdominal pain,* anorexia, hypokalemia, hepatic abmormalities
	voriconazole	*nausea, vomiting, diarrhea,* abdominal pain, anorexia, hepatic abnormalities
Antiviral	acyclovir	*nausea, vomiting,* abdominal pain, altered liver enzymes
	cidofovir	*nausea, vomiting, abdominal pain*
	ganciclovir	*altered LFTs,* nausea, vomiting, anorexia, diarrhea, abdominal pain
	famciclovir	abnormal LFTs, nausea, vomiting, anorexia, *diarrhea,* abdominal pain
	foscarnet	*nausea, vomiting, diarrhea,* abdominal pain, dry mouth, pancreatitis, hypocalcemia, hypophsphatemia, hypomagnesemia, hypokalemia
	lamivudine	*nausea, diarrhea, vomiting*
	valacyclovir	*nausea, vomiting,* abdominal pain, altered liver enzymes
	valganciclovir	altered LFTs, *nausea, vomiting,* diarrhea, anorexia, mouth sores

Metabolic Disorders

Metabolic disorders, including and contributing to malnutrition, have been shown to decrease survival in both solid organ and HSCT patient populations.[18,19,20] Many posttransplant patients experience a variety of these metabolic disorders, especially electrolyte imbalances. The HCST recipient may experience electrolyte depletion because of chemotherapeutic agents that are used in the conditioning regimen. All types of transplants are associated with electrolyte imbalances resulting from immunosuppressive and antimicrobial agents (see Table 15–11 and Table 15–12). Close monitoring of electrolytes is critical, and replacement therapy may be given either orally or intravenously.

Depending on the type of transplant and associated complications, an increase or a decrease in various components of nutritional intake may be required. A posttransplant allogeneic HSCT patient may, for example, need an increase in his or her caloric intake because of increased energy expenditure secondary to GVHD.[14] Key parameters for assessment include:

- Calories/Energy
- Protein
- Carbohydrate
- Fat
- Fluids and electrolytes
- Vitamins and minerals

In addition, the method of nutrition support administration may involve the oral, enteral or parenteral route, or a combination. Because transplant patients are immunosuppressed, enteral or parenteral nutrition must be managed with extreme care in the hospital and the home. However, delays in obtaining optimal nutrient intake may further exacerbate nutritional deterioration and increase complications. Exemplary preparation and monitoring of the transplant patient who receives home enteral or parenteral nutrition is essential.

The home nutrition support clinician must closely evaluate the laboratory values as well as the patient's clinical presentation in order to develop an individualized nutrition support care plan. Detailed intervention helps improve clinical outcomes, prevents further complications from metabolic abnormalities, and maximizes the patient's functioning and well-being.

TABLE 15–13   Long-Term Transplant Complications

Potential Long-Term Complications of Transplant

- Acute and chronic rejection
- Infections
- Chronic GVHD
- Osteoporosis, osteopenia
- Hyperlipidemia
- Hypertension
- Diabetes mellitus
- Malignancy
- Sexual dysfunction
- Renal insufficiency

Adapted from Augustine & Flattery (2003)

Long-Term Complications

Because of improved patient and graft survival rates in transplantation, long-term complications such as infection, osteoporosis, and cardiac-related disease have become more common. Patients remain at risk for many long-term complications that require appropriate nutrition intervention to help maximize wellness, physical function, and quality of life. The following is a discussion limited to those complications that will most likely require nutritional intervention, including late onset infections, cGVHD, osteoporosis, hyperlipidemia, hypertension, and diabetes.

Chronic GVHD

Unlike aGVHD, cGVHD is a multisystem, autoimmune-type disease with the date of onset ranging from 2 to 18 months. The incidence of cGHVD is approximately 30% in the HLA-matched related donor and 60–70% in mismatched or unrelated donor transplants.[21] Risk factors include a history of aGVHD, increasing age of the donor, increasing recipient age, poorly controlled aGVHD, female donor to male recipient, and the presence of cytomegalovirus (CMV) infection.[22]

The primary clinical manifestations of cGVHD that impact the nutritional status of the transplant patient are illustrated in Table 15–14. Patients with refractory cGVHD have a poorer prognosis.[11] Other poor prognostic features include progressive presentation, lichenoid changes

TABLE 15–14   Signs and Symptoms of cGVHD That Impact Nutritional Status

Organ	Signs and Symptoms of Chronic GVHD
Mouth	Pain, burning, ulcerations, sensitivity to acidic and spicy foods, loss of taste, xerostomia, sicca syndrome (dry mouth), dental caries, gingivitis
Esophagus	Esophageal web or stricture formation, retrosternal pain, and difficulty swallowing
Gastrointestinal	Anorexia, nausea, vomiting, diarrhea, malabsorption, pain, weight loss, altered linear growth in children
Liver	Cholestasis, malabsorption of fat, steatorrhea

Adapted from Buchsel, Leum & Randolph, 1996

on skin histology, elevated serum bilirubin > 1.2 mg/dL, and thrombocytopenia.[23]

Pharmacologic immunosuppression is used to treat cGVHD. Historically, combination therapy with cyclosporine and corticosteroids has been the most frequently used treatment; however, many cases have proven refractory to this regimen. Extracorporeal photophoresis and other immunosuppression may be considered for salvage therapy.

Patients with cGVHD are also prescribed prophylactic antimicrobial therapies and may potentially receive intravenous immune globulin therapy to support a defective immune system caused by both the clinical manifestations of cGVHD as well as the higher net immunosuppression. Nutritional deficits may be related to cGHVD as well as side effects of these supportive care therapies.

Weight loss is a common phenomenon seen in patients with cGVHD.[24] A body mass index below 21.9 has been demonstrated to be an independent risk factor for mortality.[24] Unfortunately, few studies in the literature have quantified the extent of weight loss in these patients or link weight loss to ongoing clinical symptoms such as dysphagia and oral sensitivities caused by the conditioning regimen. Elevated resting energy expenditure and elevated serum tumor necrosis factor are potential contributors to the weight loss.[24] More research is needed to determine other potential causes. Aggressive treatment of cGVHD with early nutrition intervention is necessary to decrease mortality.

Osteopenia and Osteoporosis

There is a growing awareness among transplant clinicians of the need to assess for, prevent, and treat osteoporosis in the transplant recipient. Many transplant centers obtain a bone density scan during the pretransplant evaluation. This assists in identifying patients with existing disease, those at high risk for the development of bone disease, as well as serves as a baseline for posttransplant comparisons. Other pretransplant risk factors contributing to the development of posttransplant osteopenia or osteoporosis include:

- Calcium-depleting chemotherapy agents
- Utilization of loop diuretics
  (e.g., lasix, bumex)
- Preexisting renal insufficiency

- History of tobacco usage
- Poor dietary calcium intake
- Lack of weight-bearing exercise[25]

Once transplanted, the use of immunosuppressive therapies, most notably steroids, further contributes to the development of osteopenia through both direct and indirect effects on bone and marrow metabolism. Some of the therapy side effects include:[26]

- ↓ intestinal calcium absorption
- ↓ skeletal growth factors
- ↓ bone formation by osteoblasts

- ↑ urinary calcium excretion
- ↑ parathyroid hormone
- ↑ bone resorption

Patients taking either steroids or calcineurin inhibitors (e.g., cyclosporine, tacrolimus) are generally prescribed dietary supplements of calcium (1500 mg) and vitamin D (800–1000 mg).[25] In addition, patients diagnosed with osteoporosis and or bone fractures are usually placed on biphosphonate therapy (e.g., alendronate, etidronate). These agents act as bone resorption inhibitors.

Nutrition support clinicians assist with nutrition supplement and oral intake recommendations that support the daily requirements needed to support bone repair and long-term maintenance. Recommendations for readily available palatable products taking into account patient age, food preferences, and oral intake capabilities will further support the posttransplant management of osteopenia and osteoporosis.

Hyperlipidemia

Hyperlipidemia is another potential long-term complication following all types of transplants. Risk factors include pretransplant hyperlipidemia, obesity, and the use of immunosuppressive therapies. Treatment interventions include nutrition management with a low-fat, low-cholesterol diet as well as the use of statins, which are drugs shown to reduce serum cholesterol.

Hypertension

Hypertension following transplantation has numerous potential etiologies. These include obesity, tobacco and alcohol use, pretransplant hypertension, diabetes, and select immunosuppressive therapies, particularly cyclosporine and steroids.

Hypertensive risk factors unique to the renal transplant population include hypertension in the kidney donor, renal artery stenosis, and uncontrolled renin secretion.[25]

Aggressive management of hypertension is essential. Pharmaceutical interventions include the use of antihypertensive agents, including one or more of the following drug classes: calcium channel blockers, angiotensin-converting enzyme inhibitors, angiotensin II receptor blockers, and vasodilators. Hypertension management includes education and interventions to promote smoking cessation, exercise, and when appropriate, weight loss. A low-sodium diet may also be warranted.

Diabetes

Allogeneic HSCT and solid organ transplant recipients are at an increased risk for the development of diabetes, primarily because of the side effects of immunosuppressive therapies, especially steroids, cyclosporine, and tacrolimus. Posttransplant blood glucose levels must be monitored on a routine basis. Most centers follow the guidelines set by the Diabetes Control and Complications Trial that recommends pharmaceutical and dietary intervention for blood glucose levels > 126 mg/dl on two consecutive tests.[27] This is especially important in transplantation due to the risk of organ damage, most notably renal, resulting from diabetes complications.

The Role of the Dietitian in Transplantation

Nutrition support is integral to the success of transplantation. However, transplant nutrition is a relatively new discipline that has evolved over the past 20 years. The dietitian is involved in all steps of the process from pretransplant through postdischarge, providing nutritional status assessments, recommending nutrition support interventions, and ensuring an appropriate nutrient intake for recovery and maintenance of health.

The goals of support in the transplant patient are to (1) provide substrates that support metabolic function, compensating for drug-nutrient interactions and the patient's medical course; (2) spare lean body mass; and (3) maximize quality of life by reducing the severity of post-transplant complications.[28] Understanding the potential for nutritional disability in transplant patients allows the clinician to be proactive in applying nutrition support principles to accomplish these goals.

A pretransplant nutritional screening and intervention plan is critical to help optimize the transplant candidate's nutritional status prior to transplant as well as the posttransplant outcome. When determining pretransplant nutrient requirements, nutritional status, weight, age, gender, metabolic state, state and type of organ failure, malabsorption, induced losses, goals, and co-morbid conditions must be considered.[2] Assessments should include:

- Weight history, energy level, ability to perform activities of daily living
- Assessment for nausea, vomiting, diarrhea, taste changes, and/or anorexia
- Laboratory baseline studies: protein status (albumin, transferrin), glucose, triglycerides, electrolytes, renal function tests (BUN, creatinine), liver function tests
- Anthropometrics (see Table 15–15)

TABLE 15–15 Components of a Comprehensive Nutritional Assessment for an Adult Organ Transplant Recipient

Component	Purpose	Specific Elements
Physical Assessment	Determine general nutrition condition including fat and muscle store and fluid retention.	Initial interview: • Is the patient of appropriate weight for stature? • Does the patient have noticeable ascities or fluid retention? • Is muscle wasting apparent? • Does the patient require oxygen, wheelchair, or other assistive devices? • Is the patient jaundiced? • Is the patient alert?
	Assess the degree and distribution of deficiencies	Detailed physical examination • Evaluate degree and distribution of fat and/or muscle loss and fluid retention • Examine skin for color, texture, ecchymoses, telangectasias, etc. • Examine the nail beds and hair for symptoms of nutrient deficiencies • Assess the oral cavity for dental problems or signs of vitamin deficiencies History
Anthropometric measurements	Provide objective measurements to evaluate and monitor progress	• Fluid retention may have least effect on upper arm measurements • Anthropometric measurements have limitations in sensitivity and reliability but may be useful if monitored serially over time • Reliability is improved if all serial measurements are made by a single observer • Other functional measurements such as hand grip strength may be helpful as indirect measures of protein

Component	Purpose	Specific Elements
		stores
Laboratory tests	Provide detailed information; must be used selectively to avoid tests using confounded by non-nutritional factors	• Serum protein concentrations are affected by many non-nutritional factors (eg. Fluid status, liver and kidney function, vitamin status) • Urinary tests (eg. Nitrogen balance, creatinine-height index) are also influenced by many non-nutritional factors (eg. Fluid status, liver and kidney function) • Immunocompetence tests (eg. Skin test antigens, total lymphocyte count) are influenced by immunosuppressive drugs

Reprinted with permission from Hasse (2003), *Journal of Parenteral and Enteral Nutrition*, 25(3), pg 120.

This assessment allows for a baseline reference to quickly identify essential nutrition problems and support interventions throughout the transplant continuum.

In the immediate posttransplant period, patients undergo frequent blood tests and evaluations to monitor for infection, rejection, and GVHD. The dietitian monitors the patient's general health issues and co-morbidities such as diabetes and weight loss or gain. Education for long-term health includes preventing excessive weight gain, hyperlipidemia, and hypertension, as well as managing blood sugar. As a result of being immunosuppressed, transplant patients need to know how to avoid food-borne infections. Dietitians in the home can ensure and teach the patient safe food guidelines and handling.

Transplant patients often return to their primary care doctor for routine, long-term follow-up care. The transplant center may or may not be involved with the patient at this time. The home dietitian can oversee, in conjunction with the primary physician, nutrition-related co-morbidities that can occur long term.

Posttransplant nutrition supplementation can be achieved by oral, enteral, or parenteral routes. Oral intake can be significantly impaired at any step of the transplant. When this occurs, enteral or parenteral supplementation may be necessary. The chosen route of nutrition support will depend on the patient's type of transplant, co-morbid states, transplant complications, and tolerance factors. Delivery and monitoring of nutrition supplementation is accomplished according to standard protocols (see Chapters 6 and 8). Adjunctive therapies may be needed to provide improved intake, including antimicrobial therapy, pain management, antiemetics, and electrolyte replacement. These and other potential transplant related therapies that may be seen in the home are listed in Table 15–16.

SUMMARY

In summary, transplantation is an accepted treatment modality for end-stage organ failure and cancers. However, both solid organ and HSCT patients are at risk for complications that may impact survival and present unique nutritional challenges. Rejection, GVHD, and infectious complications continue to be the leading cause of morbidity and mortality in this patient population. As length of hospital stays continue to de-

TABLE 15-16   Potential Transplant Home Intravenous Therapies

Therapy	Pretransplant	Posttransplant
IV antibiotics, antivirals, antifungals	xxx	xxxx
TPN	x (100 % intestinal transplant recipients)	xx
Enteral	xx	xx
Intravenous Immunoglobulins (IVIG)	x (heart, kidney)	xx
Pain Management	x	x
Central Line Catheter Care	xx (100% HSCT)	xxxx
Colony Stimulating Factors (GCSF)	xx (HSCT)	xx
Chemotherapy	x (HSCT)	
Immunosuppressants		xxx
Cardiovascular Agents (inotropes)	xxx (heart only)	

crease and the number of outpatient HSCTs increase, the role of the home dietitian and nutrition team cannot be overemphasized. Nutrition assessment and intervention begin pretransplant and continue throughout the transplant process.

Acknowledgement: The authors of this chapter would like to thank Linda McBride, RN, MSN, for her editing support.

REFERENCES

1. Organ Procurement and Transplant Network. Available at: http://www.optn. org. Accessed May 14, 2006.
2. Allard J. The role of nutrition before and after transplantation. *Curr Opin Clin Nutr Metab Care.* 1999;2(4):313–314.
3. Hasse J. Nutrition assessment and support of organ transplant recipients. *J Parenter Enteral Nutr.* 2001;25(3):120–131.
4. Intestinal Transplant Registry. Available at: http://www.intestinaltransplant. org. Accessed May 14, 2006.

5. Muscaritoli M, Grieco G, Capria S, et al. Nutritional and metabolic support in patients undergoing bone marrow transplantation. *Am J Clin Nutr.* 2002; 75(2):183–190.

6. O'Connell S, Schmit-Pokorny K. Blood and marrow stem cell transplantation: indications, procedure, process. In: Bakitas-Whedon M, Wujcik D, eds. *Blood and Marrow Stem Cell Transplantation: Principles, Practice, and Nursing Insights*, 2nd ed. Sudbury, MA: Jones and Bartlett Publishers;1997:66–99.

7. Dumas-Hicks D. Immunosuppression. In: Cupples, Ohler, eds. *Transplantation Nursing Secrets.* Philadelphia, PA: Hanley & Belfus;2003:67–74.

8. DiCecco S, Francisco-Ziller N, & Moore D. Overview and immunosuppression. In: Hasse, Blue, eds. *Comprehensive Guide to Transplant Nutrition.* Chicago, Ill: American Dietetic Association;2002:1–30.

9. Ringden O. Introduction to graft-versus-host disease. *Biology of Blood and Marrrow Transplantation.* 2005;11(2 suppl 2):17–20.

10. Vogelsang G. How I treat chronic graft-versus-host disease. *Blood.* 2001; 97(5):1196–1201.

11. Anasetti C. Advances in the prevention of graft-versus-host disease after hematopoietic cell transplantation. *Transplantation.* 2004;77(suppl 9):S79–S83.

12. Lenssen P, Bruemmer B, Aker S, McDonald G. Nutrient support in hematopoietic cell transplantation. *JPEN.* 2001;25(4):219–228.

13. Mattox T. Specialized nutrition management of patients receiving hematopoietic stem cell transplantation. *Nut Clin Prac.* 1999;14(1):5–15.

14. Lenssen P, Aker S. Adult hematopoietic stem cell transplantation. In: Hasse, Blue, eds. *Comprehensive Guide to Transplant Nutrition.* Chicago: American Dietetic Association;2002:123–152.

15. Fishman JA, Rubin RH. Infection in organ-transplant recipients. *N Engl J Med.* 1998;338(24):1741–1751.

16. Cupples S. Infectious disease. In: Cupples, Ohler, eds. *Transplantation Nursing Secrets.* Philadelphia, PA: Hanley & Belfus;2003:247–270.

17. Chiu L, Domagala B, Park J. Management of opportunistic infections in solid-organ transplantation. *Prog Transplant.* 2004;14(2):114–129.

18. Selberg O, Bottcher J, Tusch G, Pichlmayr R, Henkel E, Muller M. Identification of high- and low-risk patients before liver transplantation: a prospective cohort study of nutritional and metabolic parameters in 150 patients. *Hepatology.* 1997;25(3):652–657.

19. Deeg H, Seidel K, Bruemmer B, Pepe M, Appelbaum F. Impact of patient weight on non-relapse mortality after marrow transplantation. *Bone Marrow Transplant.* 1995;15(3):461–468.

20. Fleming D, Rayens M, Garrison J. Impact of obesity on allogeneic stem cell transplant patients: a matched case-controlled study. *Am J Med.* 1997;102(3): 265–268.

21. Antin JH. Clinical practice. Long-term care after hematopoietic cell transplantation in adults. *N Eng J Med.* 2002;347(1):36–42.

22. Remberger M, Kumlien G, Aschan J, Barkholt L, Hentschke P, Ljungman P, Mattsson, J, Svennilson, J, Ringden, O. *Biology of Blood and Marrow Transplantation.* 2002;8:674–682.
23. Buchsel P, Leum E, Randolph S. Delayed complications of bone marrow transplantation: an update. *Oncol Nurs Forum.* 1996;23(8):1267–1291.
24. Jacobsohn D, Marolis J, Doherty J, Anders V, Vogelsang G. Weight loss and malnutrition in patients with chronic graft-versus-host disease. *Bone Marrow Transplantation.* 2002;29(3):231–236.
25. Augustine S, Flattery M. Long-term complications of solid organ transplantation. In: Cupples, Ohler, eds. *Transplantation Nursing Secrets.* Philadelphia, PA: Hanley & Belfus;2003:271–278.
26. Rodino MA, Shane E. Osteoporosis after organ transplantation. *Am J Med.* 1998;104(5):459–469.
27. Diabetes Control and Complications Trial Research Group. The effect of intensive treatment of diabetes on the development and progression of long-term complications in insulin-dependent diabetes mellitus. *N Engl J Med.* 1993;329(14):977–986.
28. Fredstrom S. (1998). © Coram Healthcare.

CHAPTER 16

Reimbursement for Home Nutrition Support

Frank R. Wojtylak, RD/CDN
Karen Hamilton, MS, RD, LD, CNSD

INTRODUCTION

Health care reimbursement is affected by insurer and employer mandates for cost containment, quality monitoring, and provision of basic services. Many insurance products are available to the consumer, with an increasing number of insurance plans developing defined standards of care. Insurance coverage for home nutrition support may be from governmental, commercial, and/or private insurance plans. With each insurance plan, specific guidelines exist. In the case of governmental insurance plans, for example, the Centers for Medicare and Medicaid Services (CMS) outline specific medical condition requirements that must be present to qualify for benefit coverage for either enteral or parenteral nutrition therapy. These guidelines must be followed to ensure payment. This chapter outlines the requirements for successful reimbursement for nutritional therapy along with the documentation most often required.

When advocating for their patients' insurance coverage, many practitioners verbalize frustration regarding the guidelines set forth by insurers for coverage of enteral and parenteral therapies. One must remember, however, that cost containment and consistency are the key concerns related to many insurance decisions. In general, the decision-making follows established coverage rules, and most personnel from insurance companies who implement and monitor the initial medical claims and approval process are not clinicians. They are simply responding to directives and policies that define a limited scope of coverage rules established by their company. Thus, if a case is not presented per the specific payor guidelines, coverage may be denied simply because of miscommunication or misunderstanding of the case. Accordingly, it is incumbent upon clinicians and institutions to familiarize themselves with insurance products, provisions, and limitations to provide patients the most appropriate and thorough care.

CATEGORIES OF INSURANCE COVERAGE

Overall, it is the population of the United States that dictates insurance needs and requirements. An aging population and its many needs drive new insurance/coverage products. Generally, there are four basic categories of insurance and various components of these:

Four Basic Categories of US Insurance Coverage			
Commercial	**Governmental**	**Disability**	**Uninsured**
—Umbrella Coverage	—Medicare:	—Short Term	—Patient Assistance Programs (PAP):
	Part A	—Long Term	
or	↓		
	Part D		
—Full Benefit Plans			Private Local Government Institutional
—Capitated	—Medicaid		
	—Federal Benefits Program		
	—TRICARE for		
—Supplemental	Life		
	—Railroad Benefits		
	—Social Security		
	—Disability		
	—Veterans/ Indian Affairs		

In addition, patients may pay out of pocket or "private pay" for services that are not covered or when they do not have insurance coverage of any kind. Insurance contracts delineate the services covered. Some plans have limits, also known as lifetime maximums or deductibles. A review of a recipient's insurance product and associated benefit allows clinicians and recipients to make an informed and intelligent choice about available options that can direct and determine the course of therapy offered. Although, generally speaking, inpatient or hospital insurance benefits largely cover the cost of care, patients who are discharged to home and receive outpatient or alternate site services may find significant differences in insurance coverage and their ability to receive their provision (i.e., nursing, infusion, rehabilitation, long-term care, hospice, and extended care therapies). It is important never to assume that coverage is adequate to meet all the needs required by any individual, especially in the home setting. Many people have a combination of insurance plans that may or may not provide coverage benefits for alternate site or home care services. An example of this would be a patient who has Medicare Part B as a primary insurer and a supplemental commercial product as a secondary insurer and who requires parenteral nutrition (PN) therapy. If the patient's medical condition does not meet the pre-set Medicare criteria, then the supplemental policy will also deny coverage, and the patient will be left to pay the entire bill out of pocket.

There has been a move to ensure that patients are aware of what they can expect financially. A guarantee or informed consent of financial responsibility is a right afforded to patients prior to the acceptance of any service provided. The Patient Bill of Rights universally guarantees that every patient will be a participant in his or her care and that an itemization of costs be provided to them, as well as what prescribed services are not covered. Current laws firmly uphold the disclosure of patient rights and prior consent.

In reviewing the available insurance coverage and needed services, it is important to determine the following:

- What is the primary insurance?
- What are the dictates of the policy?
- Who may provide the service desired?
- Are there one or more insurance plans available?
- Are there limits/deductibles/maximum coverage limits?
- Are time limits associated with this particular policy?
- Is there any coverage from a spouse/partner?

- Will insurance be maintained or changed during the course of the current treatment?
- What are the limits of any supplemental plans?
- Has the patient applied for any insurance that is currently not in effect?
- Is prior approval or authorization required for coverage?
- Are parameters/qualifications met to provide coverage?
- Is the patient aware of his or her insurance coverage, what it means, and what services will be provided?
- Has a delineation of costs associated with the therapy been reviewed with the patient?
- Is the patient aware of what will be provided and by whom?
- Is the patient/recipient able to afford any non-covered costs associated with the therapy?

COMMERCIAL INSURANCE

Commercial insurance can vary from state to state and from person to person. Commercial insurers dictate the parameters of the policies they develop. Some corporations work directly with commercial carriers to provide employees with specific levels of service, service providers, and coverage. The size of the corporation, the premiums paid, and the mix of the personnel in the insured group all determine the product available to members. Although there is a desire to provide high-quality care with a degree of cost containment, maintaining the balance between need and cost is an ongoing process.

Before a service agency, care provider, or supplier provides any non-emergent services, the patient's policy must be examined to determine what coverage limits are afforded. This information should then be communicated to the patient so that he or she can make an informed decision regarding his or her care. This should be done in concert with the patient's medical team so that the most cost effective and best medical treatment can be determined. Coverage can vary according to the types of services approved. Admissions departments and insurance representatives can specifically outline the requirements and coverage provisions related to any patient or recipient.

When clinicians anticipate required services, particularly outpatient services, they need to ascertain the following:

- What is the exact scope of the services required?
- What is the duration of the expected service?
- Is the patient a willing participant in the care being given?
- Is the patient safe in an outpatient setting?
- Is there a dedicated support mechanism in the home?
- Are prior approvals needed for services provided?

A coordinated effort needs to match the services required with the coverage available. Case managers, social workers, and other personnel who understand insurance coverage should work with clinicians involved in the care of the patient. The patients' diagnosis and medical condition necessitating the specific therapy needs to be expertly conveyed by the managing clinician to those coordinating the actual care and interpreting insurance regulation and coverage. It is essential to review the overall case, coverage requirements, diagnosis, and anticipated needs in order to ensure a complete picture of what tests and documentation may be needed for coverage and goal attainment. Once a patient is being managed in the alternate site, it is important to establish a monitoring process for patient safety and compliance with therapies. Many insurers expect periodic updates as to the patient's progress toward goals for continuation of payment. As a result, a greater emphasis is being placed on outcomes monitoring as it relates to therapies provided for individuals.

PRIVATE PAY

When services are not covered by a given insurance policy, a patient may opt to pay privately or "out of pocket" for services. The private pay option is generally reserved for those who have the financial means to pay for highly-defined and costly services and for those who desire to receive these services at home in lieu of hospitalization. Despite the fact that the patient is not using a commercial or government policy, it remains important to establish a clearly defined policy that includes total disclosure of services and their costs to the patient. Private payment is often the choice of last resort for an individual who requires outpatient therapy. It is important to note that in some cases, such as Medicare, even if there is a desire to have private payment services provided, any existing primary insurance must be billed first.

MEDICAID

Medicaid is health care coverage for certain groups of low-income people who do not have any medical insurance or do not have enough medical insurance. Qualifications and eligibility for Medicaid differ from state to state because each state sets its own guidelines for eligibility and services. These eligibility groups are either categorically financially needy, medically needy, or special groups. In general, Medicaid may provide coverage to people receiving Aid to Families with Dependent Children, pregnant women, and persons younger than age 21 and if they receive or are eligible for Supplemental Security Income (SSI). It also offers coverage to the blind and disabled and income-qualifying people age 65 years and older. This list is not inclusive and is subject to change. For more information go to http://www.cms.hhs.gov/MedicaidEligibility or http://www.cms.hhs.gov/MedicaidEligibility/02_AreYouEligible_.asp Payments are not made to the patient, but rather, are made to the provider of services.

When reviewing the scope of Medicaid services, it is important to ascertain the following:

- Has the patient/recipient been "qualified" for services under his or her state Medicaid program?
- What is the state of primary residence of the recipient?
- Is there a prior approval process mandated by state statute for services provided?
- What is the relative reimbursement provided to purveyors, suppliers, and health care providers?
- Are specific certified agencies and service providers required?
- What is the duration of the services provided? Do they need to be recertified on a timely basis?
- What paperwork and forms are required for services and recertification?

The federal government regulates Medicaid services through the Centers for Medicare and Medicaid Services. An excellent resource for specific Medicaid questions can be found on the government website: http://www.cms.hhs.gov/medicaid/asp.

MEDICARE

Medicare is a federal program enacted by Congress as part of Title 18 of the Social Security Act of 1965. It is the largest insurance program in the United States. Information related to current coverage can be found at: http://www.medicare.gov.

Medicare is available to select recipients. To qualify for Medicare coverage, an individual must be:

- 65+ years of age
- Entitled to Social Security benefits and/or Railroad Retirement
- Younger than age 65 years, but disabled for > 2 years
- Younger than age 65 years, with end-stage renal disease

Medicare coverage is divided into Parts A, B, C, and D, each of which provides different covered benefits (Table 16–1). Home parenteral and enteral nutrition (HPEN) services are covered under Medicare Part B. Enrolling in Part B Medicare is the choice of the recipient/beneficiary. Those who already receive Social Security or Railroad Retirement benefits are automatically enrolled in Part B starting the first day of the month that they turn age 65. Those who are younger than age 65 and disabled are automatically enrolled in Part B after receiving Social Security or Railroad Benefits for 24 months. Those who opt not to take Part B at the first time of eligibility are penalized at a rate of 10% premium increase per year, for each year they opt not to subscribe. Individuals who are receiving military benefits or who are governed under the provisions of TriCare/VA have different enrollment periods and eligibility criteria.

For purposes of management, Medicare beneficiaries are assigned to one of four Durable Medical Equipment Regional Carrier (DME MAC) regions; assignment is based on the beneficiary's permanent address. The four formerly known DMERCs were realigned beginning in 2006, and with the advent of DME MACs, there are new areas of responsibilities and jurisdictions. For a comprehensive listing of areas of jurisdiction, see the CMS map link and state listings, which can be found at: http://www.cms.hhs.gov/MedicareContractingReform/Downloads/Primary_AB_MAC_Jurisdiction_MAP.pdf.

The DME MAC contract for Jurisdiction A (Connecticut, Delaware, District of Columbia, Maine, Maryland, Massachusetts, New Hamp-

TABLE 16–1   Medicare Covered Benefits

Medicare Part A
- Inpatient health coverage
- Intermittent skilled care
- Rehabilitation treatment
- Short-term skilled nursing therapy
- Hospice care
- Some medical equipment/supplies
- Blood/blood products

Medicare Part B
- Outpatient hospital services
- Physician services and advanced practice nurse services
- Emergency department visits and services
- Laboratory services and diagnostic tests
- Home health services not covered under Part A
- Durable medical equipment and supplies
- Medical nutrition therapy
- Prosthetic devices

Medicare Part C
- Programs that might help an individual to pay health care costs that Medicare does not cover*

Medicare Part D
- Prescription drug program—effective January 1, 2006

*More details can be found at www.medicare.gov in the Personal Plan Finder section.

shire, New Jersey, New York, Pennsylvania, Rhode Island, and Vermont) was awarded to National Heritage Insurance Company (NHIC). Effective date of implementation: July 1, 2006.

The DME MAC contract for Jurisdiction B (Illinois, Indiana, Kentucky, Michigan, Minnesota, Ohio, and Wisconsin) was awarded to AdminaStar Federal, Inc.

The DME MAC contract for Jurisdiction C (Alabama, Arkansas, Colorado, Florida, Georgia, Louisiana, Mississippi, New Mexico, North Carolina, Oklahoma, Puerto Rico, South Carolina, Tennessee, Texas, and the U.S. Virgin Islands) was awarded to Palmetto GBA, LLC.

The DME MAC contract for Jurisdiction D (Alaska, American Samoa, Arizona, California, Guam, Hawaii, Idaho, Iowa, Kansas, Missouri, Montana, Nebraska, Nevada, North Dakota, Northern Mariana Islands, Oregon, South Dakota, Utah, Washington, and Wyoming) was awarded to Noridian Administrative Services. Effective date of implementation: End of calendar year 2006.

TABLE 16–2   DME MAC Providers and Websites

DME MAC: Jurisdiction A — National Heritage Insurance Company
  www.medicarenhic.com/dme/index.shtml

DMERC B: Jurisdiction B — AdminaStar Federal
  www.adminastar.com/Providers/DMERC/ContractorReform/ContractorReform.html

DME MAC: Jurisdiction C — Palmetto GBA
  http://www.palmettogba.com/palmetto/palmetto.nsf/template/Palmetto/Home?
  Opendocument

DMERC D: Jurisdiction D — Noridian
  https://www.noridianmedicare.com/bene/

Provider's Handbook:
http://www.cms.hhs.gov/MedicareContractingReform/Downloads/DME%20MAC_
DME_MAC_Implementation_Handbook.pdf

The DME MACs are the governing and coordinating entities that will administer federally mandated Medicare policies (see Table 16–2).

PROVIDING HOME NUTRITION SUPPORT FOR THE MEDICARE PATIENT

To ensure the most accurate, complete, and updated Medicare coverage information for home nutrition services, go to www.cms.hhs.gov/ MedicareContractingReform. It is important to note that changes may be enacted at any time and can affect coverage for Medicare recipients. Payments are not made to the patient, but rather, are made to the provider of services. It is important to note that there will also be significant changes to the CMN (certificate of medical necessity) process that will include reporting, completion, and documentation. To keep current with the changes occurring, refer to the CMS website.

QUALIFICATION FOR HOME NUTRITION THERAPY

In order for patients to qualify for HPEN coverage under Medicare Part B, the following must be ascertained:

- Has the patient/beneficiary been "qualified" for services under Part B Medicare?

- When does the patient turn age 65?
- What is the state of primary residence of the recipient?
- Is the patient or spouse the primary holder of the insurance?
- Are there other supplemental insurances that may affect overall coverage?
- What is the duration of the services provided?
- Are specific criteria obtained for provision of services under Medicare policy?
- Are the patient, health care practitioner, and health care providers in agreement with sound, long-term plans of care?
- Is the ordering physician willing to complete and sign a CMN and/or is there a completed DME MAC Information Form (DIF) demonstrating the need and justification for the nutrition therapy?
- Is the patient fully informed of services provided and costs associated with the therapy he or she is receiving?
- Is there anatomic impairment to the gastrointestinal tract and a need for "permanent" or ongoing long-term therapy?

Certificate of Medical Necessity/ DME MAC Information Form

The Certificate of Medical Necessity (CMN) has been replaced by a DME Information Form—[CMS 10126]—Enteral and Parental Nutrition Form. This provides a mechanism for suppliers of durable medical equipment and medical equipment and supplies to demonstrate that the item they provide meets the minimal criteria for Medicare coverage. A DME MAC Information Form (DIF) is the supplier form as of October, 2006 and it is to be completed and signed by the supplier. It does not require a narrative description of equipment and cost or a physician signature. Contractors review the documentation provided on this new form and determine if the medical necessity and applicable coverage criteria for DMEPOS have been met. As of October 2006, the following forms will no longer be accepted: external infusion pump CMS form 851, Parenteral Nutrition CMS form 852 and Enteral Nutrition CMS form 853. These forms are replaced with the following forms: external infusion pump (CMS-10125), Parenteral and Enteral Nutrition (CMS-10126) and can be found at http://www.cms.hhs.gov/CMSForms/CMSForms.

It will be important for the supplier to maintain appropriate documentation according to the requirements outlined by Medicare. This

---

TABLE 16–3   Requirements for CMNs for Home Enteral Nutrition

Initial Enteral CMNs
- All new patients
- All patient changes in B-code formulas when the patient had not previously been on that formula
- All patients resuming therapy after a 60-day break in need
- Any patient beginning pump therapy (i.e., from bolus, syringe feedings)
- Any patient who becomes Medicare-eligible

Revised Enteral CMNs
- To show a route of administration change from syringe to gravity
- With changes in calories per day, number of days of administration, route of administration (tube to oral when billing for denial), supplier, or physician
- For a change in supplier address or location from which services are provided
- For B4154 and B4155 formula changes

Recertification of Enteral CMNs
- By the DMERC at any point during the therapy provided
- When a physician indicates on the CMN less than lifetime therapy and changes the CMN at a later date to show an extension of overall therapy provided

---

documentation may be required for auditing and payment purposes. This documentation must be kept on record and updated according to all governing Medicare policies.

Home Enteral Nutrition

A number of parameters must be documented when providing enteral therapy for patients/beneficiaries with Medicare benefits (see Table 16–3). Governing rules for coverage may be found at: http://www.cignamedicare.com/articles/Jan05/Cope1879.html.

Among the information that must be fully documented are the following questions:

- Does the patient/beneficiary meet the need for permanence of enteral therapy? (i.e., is enteral therapy required for > 90 days)
- Is there documentation that the patient is receiving enteral therapy by means other than orally?
- Is there an identified diagnosis of impaired gastrointestinal dysmotility or inability to swallow, as evidenced by objective testing and ICD-9 code?
- Is there documented evidence of disease that prevents food or nutrition from reaching the bowel and being absorbed?

- Is there a documented trial of a standardized enteral formula or "lower B-code" before utilization of a specialty enteral formula when a specialty product is required?
- Is there an ongoing program of monitoring patient/beneficiary compliance with the therapy established?
- Is there a completed CMN/DIF showing the need and justification for the enteral therapy?
- Is there documentation showing that the patient requires tube feedings to maintain weight and strength commensurate with overall health status?
- Is it not possible to provide adequate nutrition by dietary adjustment and/or oral supplements?

If a patient requires an enteral pump for the therapy, then justification of the need and rationale for providing this device is required, which can be provided through objective medical documentation or through an ICD-9 code. Commonly documented reasons for needing a pump include failure to tolerate gravity feedings due to:

- Reflux with potential for aspiration
- Severe diarrhea
- Dumping syndrome
- Required administration of feeding at a rate of less than 100 cc/hour
- Utilization of a jejunostomy tube for feedings
- Blood glucose fluctuations

When developing and maintaining the CMN/DIF, the clinician should be aware of the requirements of the initial, revised, and recertified processes (see Table 16–4).

To assist with overall documentation needs and qualification, Medicare has outlined the requirements/documentation required for enteral coverage. A documentation checklist can be downloaded from: http://www.cignamedicare.com/dmerc/mr/CERT/Pdf/Enteral.pdf.

When assembling and maintaining documentation on a patient who is receiving enteral therapy, a properly documented patient chart should include:

- Physician orders (updated accordingly)

TABLE 16–4   Requirements for CMNs for Home Parenteral Nutrition

Initial Parenteral CMNs

- Any new patient on parenteral nutrition therapy
- A patient who is resuming parenteral therapy after a 60-day break in need
- Any patient becoming Medicare-eligible

Revised Parenteral CMNs

- A change in pump
- An HCPCS code change for lipids and/or amino acids
- A change in days per week infused for amino acids that necessitates an HCPS code change
- A change in lipid volume (increase)
- Physician indicates a less than lifetime need and subsequently orders a greater length of need
- Change in physician or supplier
- Change in supplier address

Recertification of Parenteral CMNs

- Six months from the date of initial date of service (all recertification requires appropriate documentation and certifying need for continued therapy)
- By the DMERC on a requested basis

- Objective laboratory and diagnostic tests that support the reason for enteral therapy
- ICD-9/diagnostic codes that support the need for enteral therapy
- Evidence of tube placement
- Calories, type of feeding, administration instructions
- Method of administration (e.g., pump, syringe)
- Ongoing proof of delivery
- Ongoing proof of patient compliance
- Copy of CMN/DIF on file
- Reasons for the need/use of any specialty enteral formulas

Home Parenteral Nutrition

To qualify for reimbursement, patients receiving parenteral nutrition must meet the explicit criteria according to Medicare policy. The following information provided is taken directly from the Medicare policy and is noted as such. AdminaStar Federal defines the qualifications in the policy as the following:

"The patient must have a permanent impairment. Permanence does not require a determination that there is no possibility that the patient's condition may improve sometime in the future. If the judgment of the attending physician, substantiated in the medical record, is that the condition is of long and indefinite duration (ordinarily at least 3 months), the test of permanence is considered met. Parenteral nutrition will be denied as noncovered in situations involving temporary impairments.

The patient must have (a) a condition involving the small intestine and/or its exocrine glands which significantly impairs the absorption of nutrients or (b) disease of the stomach and/or intestine which is a motility disorder and impairs the ability of nutrients to be transported through the GI system. There must be objective evidence supporting the clinical diagnosis.

Parenteral nutrition is noncovered for the patient with a functioning gastrointestinal tract whose need for parenteral nutrition is only due to:

a) a swallowing disorder,

b) a temporary defect in gastric emptying such as a metabolic or electrolyte disorder,

c) a psychological disorder impairing food intake such as depression,

d) a metabolic disorder inducing anorexia such as cancer,

e) a physical disorder impairing food intake such as the dyspnea of severe pulmonary or cardiac disease,

f) a side effect of a medication,

g) renal failure and/or dialysis."

Medicare delineates the services provided under medical policy if one of the following criteria are met and substantiated. AdminaStar Federal outlines the following criteria according to Medicare policy.

Parenteral nutrition is covered in any of the following situations:

Criteria A:

A patient has undergone recent (within the past 3 months) massive small-bowel resection leaving < 5 feet of small bowel beyond the ligament of Treitz.

Criteria B:

The patient has a short-bowel syndrome that is severe enough that the patient has net gastrointestinal fluid and electrolyte malabsorption such that on an oral intake of 2.5–3 liters/day the enteral losses exceed 50% of the oral/enteral intake and the urine output is < 1 liter/day.

Criteria C:

The patient requires bowel rest for at least 3 months and is receiving intravenously 20–35 cal/kg/day for treatment of symptomatic pancreatitis with/without pancreatic pseudocyst, severe exacerbation of regional enteritis, or a proximal enterocutaneous fistula where tube feeding distal to the fistula is not possible.

Criteria D:

The patient has complete mechanical small-bowel obstruction where surgery is not an option.

Criteria E:

The patient is significantly malnourished (10% weight loss over 3 months or less and serum albumin < 3.4 gm/dL) and has very severe fat malabsorption (fecal fat exceeds 50% of oral/enteral intake on a diet of at least 50 gm of fat/day as measured by a standard 72-hour fecal fat test).

Criteria F:

The patient is significantly malnourished (10% weight loss over 3 months or less and serum albumin < 3.4 gm/dL) and has a severe motility disturbance of the small intestine and/or stomach, which is unresponsive to prokinetic medication and is demonstrated either:

(1) scintigraphically (solid meal gastric emptying study demonstrates that the isotope fails to reach the right colon by 6 hours following ingestion), or
(2) radiographically (barium or radiopaque pellets fail to reach the right colon by 6 hours following administration).

These studies must be performed when the patient is not acutely ill and is not on any medication, which would decrease bowel motility. Unresponsiveness to prokinetic medication is defined as the presence of daily symptoms of nausea and vomiting while taking maximal doses. For criteria A–F above, the conditions are deemed to be severe enough that the patient would not be able to maintain weight and strength on only oral intake or tube enteral nutrition.

Criteria G/H:

Patients who do not meet criteria A–F above must have a documented trial and failure of diet modification and/or tube feeding trial and pharmacologic intervention to manage malabsorption, plus criteria G and H below:

G) The patient is malnourished (10% weight loss over 3 months or less and serum albumin < 3.4 gm/dL), and

H) A disease and clinical condition has been documented as being present and it has not responded to altering the manner of delivery of appropriate nutrients (e.g., slow infusion of nutrients through a tube with the tip located in the stomach or jejunum).

The following are some examples of moderate abnormalities which would require a failed trial of tube enteral nutrition before parenteral nutrition would be covered:

- Moderate fat malabsorption fecal fat exceeds 25% of oral/enteral intake on a diet of at least 50 gm of fat/day as measured by a standard 72 hour fecal fat test)
- Diagnosis of malabsorption with objective confirmation by methods other than 72 hour fecal fat test (e.g., Sudan stain of stool, d-xylose test, etc.)
- Gastroparesis, which has been demonstrated (a) radiographically or scintigraphically as described in F above with the isotope or pellets failing to reach the jejunum in 3–6 hours, or (b) by manometric motility studies with results consistent with an abnormal gastric emptying, and which is unresponsive to prokinetic medication
- A small-bowel motility disturbance that is unresponsive to prokinetic medication, demonstrated with a gastric emptying to right colon transit time between 3–6 hours
- Small-bowel resection leaving >5 feet of small bowel beyond the ligament of Treitz
- Short-bowel syndrome that is not severe (as defined in B)
- Mild to moderate exacerbation of regional enteritis or an enterocutaneous fistula
- Partial mechanical small-bowel obstruction where surgery is not an option

DEFINITION OF A TUBE TRIAL

A concerted effort must be made to place a tube. For gastroparesis, tube placement must be postpylorus, preferably in the jejunum. Use of a double lumen tube should be considered. The Centers for Medicare & Medicaid Services recommend:

"Placement of the tube in the jejunum must be objectively verified by radiographic studies or fluoroscopy. Placement via endoscopy or open surgical procedure would also verify location of the tube, however they are not required.

"A trial with enteral nutrition must be made, with appropriate attention to dilution, rate, and alternative formulas to address side effects of diarrhea."

Examples of a failed tube trial would be:

- A person who has had documented placement of a tube in the post-pyloric area continues to have problems with vomiting and on radiographic recheck the tube has returned to the stomach.
- After an attempt of sufficient time (5–6 hours) to get a tube into the jejunum, the tube does not progress and remains in the stomach or duodenum. An attempt of enteral tube feeding with a very slow drip was made. It was initially tolerated well, but vomiting occurred when the rate was increased.
- After placement of the tube in the jejunum and 1–2 days of enteral tube feeding, the person has vomiting and distension.
- A tube is placed appropriately and remains in place. Enteral nutrition is initiated and the concentration and rate are increased gradually. Over the course of 3–4 weeks, attempts to increase the rate and/or concentration and/or to alter the formula to reach the targeted intake are unsuccessful, with increase in diarrhea, bloating, or other limiting symptoms, and the person is unable to meet the needed nutritional goals (stabilize at desired weight or gain weight as needed).

Parenteral nutrition can be covered in a patient with the ability to obtain partial nutrition from oral intake or a combination of oral/enteral (or even oral/enteral/parenteral) intake as long as the following criteria are met:

1a) a permanent condition of the alimentary tract is present, which has been deemed to require parenteral therapy because of its severity (criteria A–F), or 1b) a permanent condition of the alimentary tract is present which is unresponsive to standard medical management (criterion H); and the person is unable to maintain weight and strength (criterion G).

"Parenteral nutrition would usually be noncovered for patients who do not meet these criteria but will be considered on an individual case basis if detailed documentation is submitted."

DOCUMENTATION REQUIRED FOR QUALIFICATION

According to the AdminaStar Federal Web Site, the following documentation is required for the Medicare patient to qualify for home parenteral nutrition:

1. DME Information Form—CMS—10126—(DIF) Enteral and Parenteral Nutrition Form. This form (see Table 16–5) is to be completed by the supplier. The form must be completed in full and contain the signature of the supplier (*note—this is subject to civil and legal penalty when signed.) The DIF Form must be reviewed for the accuracy of the information and signed by the supplier who is providing the services.
2. As of October, 2006 a DIF is required to be completed by the supplier instead of the CMN. This form does not require physician signature.
3. *Medical Justification*: The type of documentation relates to which situation (A–H) in Coverage and Payment Rules, General serves as the basis for coverage. For situations A–D, the documentation should include:
   a. copies of the operative report and/or
   b. hospital discharge summary and/or
   c. x-ray reports and/or physician letter that documents the condition and the necessity for parenteral therapy.

For situations E and H (when appropriate), include:

   a. results of the fecal fat test and dates of the test.

For situations F and H (when appropriate), include:

   a. copy of the report of the small-bowel motility study
   b. list of medications that the patient was on at the time of the test.

For situations E–H, include:

a. results of serum albumin and date of test (within 1 week prior to initiation of parenteral nutrition)
b. copy of a nutritional assessment by a physician, dietitian, or other qualified professional within 1 week prior to initiation of parenteral nutrition, to include the following information:
1) current weight, with date and weight 1–3 months prior to initiation of parenteral nutrition
2) estimated daily calorie intake during the prior month and by what route (e.g., oral, tube)
3) statement of whether there were caloric losses from vomiting or diarrhea and whether these estimated losses are reflected in the calorie count
4) description of any dietary modifications made or supplements tried during the prior month (e.g., low fat, extra medium-chain triglycerides)

For situations described in H, include:

a. statement from the physician
b. copies of objective studies
c. excerpts of the medical record giving the following information:
1) specific etiology for the gastroparesis, small-bowel dysmotility, or malabsorption
2) a detailed description of the trial of tube enteral nutrition, including the beginning and ending dates of the trial; duration of time that the tube was in place; the type and size of tube; the location of tip of the tube; the name of the enteral nutrient; the quantity, concentration, and rate of administration; and the results
3) a copy of the x-ray report or procedure report documenting placement of the tube in the jejunum
4) prokinetic medications used, dosage, and dates of use
5) nondietary treatment given during prior month, directed at etiology of malabsorption (e.g., antibiotic for bacterial overgrowth)
6) any medications used that might impair GI tolerance to enteral feedings (e.g., anticholinergics, opiates, tricyclics, pheno-

TABLE 16–5 Sample DME Information Form

INSTRUCTIONS FOR COMPLETING DME INFORMATION FORM
FOR ENTERAL AND PARENTERAL NUTRITION (CMS-10126)

CERTIFICATION TYPE/DATE:	If this is an initial certification for this patient, indicate this by placing date (MM/DD/YY) needed initially in the space marked "INITIAL." If this is a revised certification (to be completed when the physician changes the order, based on the patient's changing clinical needs), indicate the initial date needed in the space marked "INITIAL," and also indicate the revision date in the space marked "REVISED." If this is a recertification, indicate the initial date needed in the space marked "INITIAL," and also indicate the recertification date in the space marked "RECERTIFICATION." Whether submitting a REVISED or a RECERTIFICATION DIF, be sure to always furnish the INITIAL date as well as the REVISED or RECERTIFICATION date.
PATIENT INFORMATION:	Indicate the patient's name, permanent legal address, telephone number and his/her health insurance claim number (HICN) as it appears on his/her Medicare card and on the claim form.
SUPPLIER INFORMATION:	Indicate the name of your company (supplier name), address and telephone number along with the Medicare Supplier Number assigned to you by the National Supplier Clearinghouse (NSC) or applicable National Provider Identifier (NPI). If using the NPI Number, indicate this by using the qualifier XX followed by the 10-digit number. If using a legacy number, e.g. NSC number, use the qualifier 1C followed by the 10-digit number. (For example. 1Cxxxxxxxxxx)
PLACE OF SERVICE:	Indicate the place in which the item is being used, i.e., patient's home is 12, skilled nursing facility (SNF) is 31, End Stage Renal Disease (ESRD) facility is 65, etc. Refer to the DMERC supplier manual for a complete list.
FACILITY NAME:	If the place of service is a facility, indicate the name and complete address of the facility.
HCPCS CODES:	List all HCPCS procedure codes for items ordered that require a DIF. Procedure codes that do not require certification should not be listed in this section of the DIF.
PATIENT DOB, HEIGHT, WEIGHT AND SEX:	Indicate patient's date of birth (MM/DD/YY) and sex (male or female); height in inches and weight in pounds, if required.
PHYSICIAN NAME, ADDRESS:	Indicate the physician's name and complete mailing address.
PHYSICIAN INFORMATION:	Accurately indicate the treating physician's Unique Physician Identification Number (UPIN) or applicable National Provider Identifier (NPI). If using the NPI Number, indicate this by using the qualifier XX followed by the 10-digit number. If using UPIN number, use the qualifier 1G followed by the 6-digit number. (For example. 1Gxxxxxx)
PHYSICIAN'S TELEPHONE NO.:	Indicate the telephone number where the physician can be contacted (preferably where records would be accessible pertaining to this patient) if more information is needed.
QUESTION SECTION:	This section is used to gather clinical information about the item or service billed. Answer each question which applies to the items ordered, circling "Y" for yes, "N" for no, a number if this is offered as an answer option, or fill in the blank if other information is requested.
SUPPLIER ATTESTATION:	The supplier's signature certifies that the information on the form is an accurate representation of the situation(s) under which the item or service is billed.
SUPPLIER SIGNATURE AND DATE:	After completion, supplier must sign and date the DME Information Form, verifying the Attestation.

According to the Paperwork Reduction Act of 1995, no persons are required to respond to a collection of information unless it displays a valid OMB control number. The valid OMB control number for this information collection is 0938-0679. The time required to complete this information collection is estimated to average 12 minutes per response, including the time to review instructions, search existing resources, gather the data needed, and complete and review the information collection. If you have any comments concerning the accuracy of the time estimate or suggestions for improving this form, please write to: CMS, Attn: PRA Reports Clearance Officer, 7500 Security Blvd. Baltimore, Maryland 21244.

DO NOT SUBMIT CLAIMS TO THIS ADDRESS. Please see *http://www.medicare.gov/* **for information on claim filing.**

Form CMS-10126 (09/05) INSTRUCTIONS EF 08/2006

TABLE 16–5   Sample DME Information Form—*(cont'd)*

DEPARTMENT OF HEALTH AND HUMAN SERVICES
CENTERS FOR MEDICARE & MEDICAID SERVICES

Form Approved
OMB No. 0938-0679

DME INFORMATION FORM
CMS-10126 — ENTERAL AND PARENTERAL NUTRITION

DME 10.03

All INFORMATION ON THIS FORM MAY BE COMPLETED BY THE SUPPLIER

Certification Type/Date: INITIAL ___/___/___   REVISED ___/___/___   RECERTIFICATION ___/___/___

PATIENT NAME, ADDRESS, TELEPHONE and HIC NUMBER		SUPPLIER NAME, ADDRESS, TELEPHONE and NSC or applicable NPI NUMBER/LEGACY NUMBER
(__ __) __ __ __ - __ __ __ __ HICN _____		(__ __) __ __ __ - __ __ __ __ NSC or NPI #_____
PLACE OF SERVICE_____	HCPCS CODE	PT DOB ___/___/___ Sex ___ (M/F) Ht. ___(in) Wt ___(lbs.)
NAME and ADDRESS of FACILITY *if applicable (see reverse)*	_____ _____ _____ _____	PHYSICIAN NAME, ADDRESS, TELEPHONE and applicable NPI NUMBER or UPIN
		(__ __) __ __ __ - __ __ __ __ UPIN or NPI #_____
EST. LENGTH OF NEED (# OF MONTHS): _____ 1-99 *(99=LIFETIME)*		DIAGNOSIS CODES (ICD-9): _____ _____ _____ _____

ANSWERS	ANSWER QUESTIONS 1–6 FOR ENTERAL NUTRITION, AND 6 - 9 FOR PARENTERAL NUTRITION (Circle Y for Yes, N for No, Unless Otherwise Noted)
Y N	1. Is there documentation in the medical record that supports the patient having a permanent non-function or disease of the structures that normally permit food to reach or be absorbed from the small bowel?
Y N	2. Is the enteral nutrition being provided for administration via tube? (i.e., gastrostomy tube, jejunostomy tube, nasogastric tube)
A)_____ B)_____	3. Print HCPCS code(s) of product.
A)_____ B)_____	4. Calories per day for each corresponding HCPCS code(s).
1 2 3 4	5. Circle the number for method of administration? 1 – Syringe 2 – Gravity 3 – Pump 4 – Oral (i.e. drinking)
_____	6. Days per week administered or infused (Enter 1 – 7)
Y N	7. Is there documentation in the medical record that supports the patient having permanent disease of the gastrointestinal tract causing malabsorption severe enough to prevent maintenance of weight and strength commensurate with the patient's overall health status?
	8. Formula components: Amino Acid _____(ml/day) _____concentration % _____gms protein/day Dextrose _____(ml/day) _____concentration % Lipids _____(ml/day) _____days/week _____concentration %
1 2 3	9. Circle the number for the route of administration. 1 – Central Line (Including PICC) 2 – Hemodialysis Access Line 3 – Peritoneal Catheter

Supplier Attestation and Signature/Date

I certify that I am the supplier identified on this DME Information Form and that the information provided is true, accurate and complete, to the best of my knowledge. I understand that any falsification, omission, or concealment of material fact associated with billing this service may subject me to civil or criminal liability.

SUPPLIER SIGNATURE_____ DATE _____/_____/_____

thiazines) or that might interfere with test results (e.g., mineral oil) and a statement explaining the need for these medications

Any other information that supports the medical necessity for parenteral nutrition may also be included.

INITIAL MEDICARE CERTIFICATION, REVISIONS, AND RECERTIFICATION

(Note: requirements stated below are as of October, 2006 and are subject to ongoing change and revision. Check the following web site for alterations in CMN/DIF policy http://www.cms.hhs.gov/MLNMatters Articles/downloads/MM4296.pdf.

"For the Initial Certification and for Revised Certifications or Recertification involving a change in the order, there must be additional documentation to support the medical necessity of the following orders, if applicable.

1) the need for special nutrients (B5000-B5200)
2) the need for dextrose concentration less than 10%
3) the need for lipids more than 15 units of a 20% solution or 30 units of a 10% solution per month."

An excellent source provided by Cigna outlines the necessary documentation required: http://www.cignamedicare.com.

When developing and maintaining the CMN, specific requirements apply to initial, revised, and recertified CMNs (see Table 16–4).

REQUIRED DOCUMENTATION FOR ANY PAYMENT SUBMISSION

When submitting a claim for payment, there are specific pieces of documentation required to be on file. When initial/subsequent claims are submitted, the following documentation may be required for auditing purposes:

- Completed/Signed DIF Information Form
- Signed and dated physician orders

- Letter of Medical Necessity outlining/summarizing the criteria and reasons for total parenteral nutrition and any need for specialized formulations.
- Appropriate documentation as required—laboratory tests, diagnostic tests, intake and output, history and physical, documented weight history, progress notes, etc.
- Consultant/Operative Reports
- Objective tests and notations as related to the patient's case

(It should be noted that Medicare will *not* accept unsigned notations, reviews of verbal conversations, and generalized statements.)

CONCLUSION

Home parenteral or enteral nutrition support can restore or maintain nutrition status in a patient who is unable consume adequate nutrients orally. Working with the patient to assist with his or her ability to receive reimbursement for these services at home is a valuable and important component of overall care of patients at home. Clinicians as well as administrative staff should be aware of the qualifications for coverage, whether these are from commercial or governmental sources, as they plan the home nutrition support regimen to best meet the needs of individual patients. As reimbursement qualification requirements and coverage changes often, it is important to ensure there is a process of ongoing reauthorization of benefits in place to maintain payment for services provided.

READINGS

The policies governing the use and requirements of Applicable Certificates of Medical Necessity are subject to change. Please refer to the following Web sites for updates.

Enteral CMN: http://www.cms.hhs.gov/forms/cms853.pdf.

Parenteral CMN: http://www.cms.hhs.gov/forms/cms852.pdf.

Determination of Individual Medicare Coverage: http://www.medicare.gov/Coverage/Home.asp.

Listservs—E-mail of updates: http://www.cms.hhs.gov/mailinglists/default.asp?audience=3.

CHAPTER 17

Home Nutrition Support from the Patient's Perspective

Robbyn S. Kindle, RD, LD
Rick Davis
Linda Gravenstein
Carol S. Ireton-Jones, PhD, RD, LD, CNSD, FACN

INTRODUCTION

There are a wide variety of disease processes that can occur that may require the initiation of parenteral or enteral nutrition. With long-term home parenteral nutrition (HPN) or home enteral nutrition (HEN) therapy, it is necessary to keep in mind the person as a whole, both physiologically and psychologically, in addition to any and all other medical issues that may be present. Every patient is unique.

The other chapters in this book are focused on caring for the clinical needs of the person receiving home nutrition support. Several chapters mentioned the need for psychosocial support and have provided some patient resources as well. However, none of these authors have lived life on HPN or HEN. The following three sections are from real people who know what it is really like to depend on HPN or HEN. When reading this, it is important to note that these people are no longer "patients"—they are HPN or HEN "consumers." They consume HPN or HEN to live, but that is not the center of their lives—they are actively living life, and nutrition support is just a part of their lives. That is why they do not want to be called "patients." As one long-term consumer said, "HPN is my lifeline—why should I complain about it? I just go on with what I need to do." That is not always the case, but hopefully the information presented here, in the consumers' own voices, will help clinicians and other consumers alike.

Robbyn depended on HPN for 12 years before she had a multivisceral organ transplant. She then received HEN and HPN for some time after her transplant until she was able to eat adequately again. She is also a dietitian, choosing to become a dietitian following her hospitalization and subsequent time on HPN. She has an interesting insight that is both personal and clinical.

Rick suffered a stroke and lost his ability to swallow. He was a successful businessman and his story is a journey of challenge, learning about his feeding modality, and finally accepting and, in fact, making the best of his need for HEN.

Linda is caregiver and mother of a long-term HPN consumer. Her daughter started on HPN as an infant and has grown up into a beautiful, independent, and successful young woman who depends on HPN. Linda has helped numerous consumers by sharing her experiences.

—CIJ

ROBBYN

My expertise is based on my personal journey into the world of HPN that began in early 1991 due to a malrotation of my gut, resulting in a volvulous and subsequent resection of the majority of my small bowel and right half of my colon. Until that time I lived the average life of a college student with no extraordinary health issues. After that tragic day I quit school and prepared myself for what I thought was my imminent death. Fortunately that did not occur, and so I eventually returned to school to pursue a new path as a dietitian. Then, ten years after the original bowel resection, I developed liver cholestasis and could no longer tolerate HPN therapy; therefore, I needed a liver/small-bowel transplant. In May 2000, 5 months later, I received a liver, kidney, pancreas, and small intestine transplant. Much of what I have included in my section of this chapter is from personal experience, with the addition of various facts that have been concluded scientifically.

The Development of HPN Therapy

In the early years of parenteral nutrition (PN), there was no consideration given to sending the person home while on therapy. The choice was to either stay in the hospital indefinitely, or go home to die. Eventually physicians began to realize that neither scenario was sufficient and therefore began to devise a way to allow these patients to go home with their PN therapy.[1]

For those first few pioneering consumers in the 1970s, HPN was very complicated and required multiple bottles of HPN components, intravenous (IV) lines, bulky mechanical pumps, and hours spent mixing and hanging bottle after bottle of PN solutions. Complications were frequent, as were hospitalizations, but at least the consumer had the opportunity to be in the comfort of his or her own home. We should admire the tenacity of these individuals, both consumers and physicians, because if it were not for their desire for a better quality of life for PN consumers, we would not be where we are today.

Today's HPN Therapy

The world of HPN today is much different and significantly easier for both the consumer and the physician. Each year, more changes and improvements are made that enhance the quality of life for HPN consumers. Instead of multiple bottles of HPN solutions to infuse daily with bulky mechanical pumps, we now have the opportunity to have one HPN bag infused per day with the majority of the necessary components pre-mixed (with the exception of multivitamins and some medications that cause HPN stability problems). The need to "piggyback" lipids into the HPN solution is not required, thanks to development of the dual chamber bag that keeps the lipids separated from the dextrose and amino acid solution until just prior to hanging and infusing. Infusion pumps have become much smaller and smarter. They can be preprogrammed for each individual consumer, including his or her specific HPN delivery rate, ramp up rate, and ramp down rate. Mechanical pumps have progressed from the size of a mailbox to the size of a small hand. These pumps are almost noise free, as opposed to the older models that could be heard from several feet away.

Today, manufacturers are making products specifically for HPN consumers such as prefilled syringes for flushes, and needle-less positive-pressure caps that keep HPN lines free from blood back-up. This helps to reduce central venous catheter occlusion and infection rates. Backpacks are available that are designed specifically to hold the infusion pump and HPN bag, allowing the consumer more mobility and independence. These advancements have allowed HPN-dependent children to participate in regular school classes rather than being home schooled, HPN students to be in college rather than in self-study programs, and other HPN consumers the ability to work full-time.

Improved HPN formula stability has allowed HPN deliveries to be made weekly, or even monthly. There is a greater understanding of how to adjust HPN macronutrients or micronutrients, allowing each individual consumer to remain physiologically stable, thus reducing their hospitalizations and complications from long-term HPN. Home care dietitians who are certified in nutrition support can calculate the proper fluid and nutritional requirements of an HPN consumer. Pharmacists who are certified in nutrition support can supervise HPN compounding, ensuring that the many HPN components are stable in solution. Nurses provide education and re-education to consumers to help keep them well. These clinician caregivers maximize the safety of each individual patient. All of these advancements have led to a better quality of life and longer estimated life spans for the HPN consumer.

The Patient and HPN Therapy

Transitioning PN therapy to the home setting can be a very frightening experience for the consumer. Most consumers have little medical experience or education. Their knowledge of human anatomy is also very limited. Every physician who starts a patient on PN therapy should make a strong effort to explain HPN therapy in simple terms, including showing the consumer and caregivers diagrams so that they can better understand the physical reason for HPN and what will happen in the future. This may require multiple education sessions for a more complete understanding depending on each consumer's previous medical knowledge and level of education.

Taking nutrition orally is the first instinct for every living mammal, so NPO (nil per os or "nothing by mouth") orders are difficult to comply with. It seems impossible to comply with being placed on indefinite restrictions of no, or severely limited, food or liquid intake orally. Take, for example, in psychology, Maslow's hierarchy of needs. At the base of his pyramid are the basic physiologic needs that every person must fulfill before progressing up to the next level. In humans, as in all animals, we are born with the instinct to first find nourishment. From birth we accept that whatever nourishment is needed is generally taken orally.

Although it can be reasonably explained that HPN is now the patient's primary source of calories and nutrients, it can be difficult for someone who does not have the medical knowledge to make this connection. As a result, some patients may become noncompliant to the order of NPO. Also understand that the patient may still feel the sensation of hunger, which further accentuates the perception of the need for oral nourishment. Although the patient may have the knowledge that HPN is now their sole source of calories and nutrients, the instinct is still there to eat by oral means, particularly when they experience hunger. Overcoming this instinct requires that major consequences to oral nutrition be in place. A simple physician order of NPO is not enough to ensure patient compliance. Repeated education and encouragement is required.

With this feeling of unbalance with the generally accepted norms of sustenance, some patients may be noncompliant because they feel that they are being starved. Denial or even refusal of HPN will occur with some patients. Even those who initially accept the diagnosis while in the hospital might discontinue therapy for a short time because of their desire to be normal again, and also in an attempt to eliminate the pangs of hunger. But eventually, most of the patients in this group will start back on their therapy once they discover the negative side effects of not consuming HPN. Personally, I made the choice to discontinue HPN, and after realizing the effects of not consuming my HPN, I no longer denied my need for the HPN and even began to accept that this was now a new way of life for me.[2] Eventually, just the thought of being without my HPN for a short time was very frightening because I knew how much my life depended on my nightly feedings.

Another consideration is the need for the patient to grieve the loss of their own expectations of how their life should be. Depression and anger can be a part of the grieving process. Unfortunately, because the patient cannot be angry with himself or herself or the HPN, his or her anger could be directed at members of the hospital staff. They may feel the need to blame someone, and often that someone is their physician. Just remember that the patient may need an outlet in order to deal with their new reality, a reality that they did not want. At times, when my own life was assuming its new norm, any reminder of my dependence on HPN would be an irritation or a point of anger because it pointed out my difference to the accepted norm, or my inadequacies.

Points to Keep in Mind

When dealing with patients who will need HPN for any length of time, there are a few things to remember that can make the process easier for both the clinician and consumer.

1. Be polite and respectful. The consumer is likely already confused and hurting, so being brash and disrespectful only furthers the fear of what is happening.
2. Ask the consumer if it is okay to discuss his or her condition while there are other people in the room.
3. Remember that although the person is a patient in the hospital, he or she is a *consumer* of HPN. The difference being that while in the hospital there may be other conditions that have brought them there, but once that person leaves the hospital, he or she is a consumer and no longer a patient.
4. Never forget that the consumer is a person with feelings and is most likely scared and confused about his or her condition.
5. Talk directly to the consumer, not to the others in the room. Although the consumer may be under the influence of medications, he or she is still the one who is being treated and therefore needs to know what is happening.
6. When dealing with HPN consumers, always try to keep in mind that each person and situation is unique, and that different people react differently to each situation.
7. Remember that the HPN consumer may not understand what is happening; therefore, you may need to explain things again, or put them into a way that the consumer can begin to grasp.
8. Be considerate of the person's faith. For some HPN consumers, their faith is a form of personal strength that they may need in order to deal with this medical crisis.
9. Allow the consumer to maintain dignity when you are examining him or her. Explain what you are doing, and try to reveal as little

of his or her body as necessary. Do not randomly expose the consumer, thereby invading his or her personal space.

10. Make eye contact. This way you can tell if the consumer understands what you are saying.

11. If possible, try to make level eye contact. Do not hover over consumers; rather make them feel comfortable by speaking with them at their level. Hovering can be intimidating to the consumer.

12. Do not be afraid of touching the HPN consumer. Greet him or her with a handshake if possible. The touch of another person can be soothing, even just a pat on the shoulder can create a sense of ease for the consumer.

13. If possible, find a way to make the consumer smile when you leave. Even a stupid joke can lighten an otherwise tense situation.

14. Finally, and most importantly, have patience with us as consumers. We are doing our best to understand the situation and deal with life the best way we can.

Life Continues

Now, 16 years after my initial bowel resection, I find that life and my health continue to change. My "adventures" with short-bowel syndrome have slowed me down some, but I deal with it, as it is just a natural part of who I am. I am able to work, go out with friends, actively participate in church, and am now even planning to return to school with the hopes of applying to medical school next year. I have big plans for my life, something I would not have had it not been for HPN. Home parenteral nutrition changed my life and helped me keep living, and it by no means has stopped my life.

RICK DAVIS

In the Beginning

It was 6:00 AM, Friday, December 22, 2000. When I woke up, I felt terrible. Something was stuck in my throat. It felt raw and irritated. Something was taped over my nose. Something was stuck in my arm. Some things were taped to my chest. Where was I? What was happening? Why did I feel so weak? It seemed like all the energy had been drained out of me.

The doctors and nurses said I had a stroke. That morning, I woke up in the intensive care unit. Electrodes were taped to my chest. My blood pressure and heart rate were visible on a small machine beside my bed that made a regular "beeping" sound. I had an IV line dripping fluid into my arm. And, I had a tube stuck down my nose. I learned later that it is called an NG tube, and it was being used to feed me.

HEN Patient Perspective

This is the perspective of a patient who has been 100% dependent on home enteral nutrition (HEN) for 5 years. It will compare an initial period of distress, depression, frustration, and physical challenge with a successful transition to a normal lifestyle. No, better than a "normal" lifestyle; my current lifestyle is one of thriving, in large part because of, and in spite of, receiving my nutrition by enteral therapy. The personal anecdotes included in this chapter are supplemented by experiences of other enteral nutrition patients who have shared their stories with me in my role as a "counselor" for the Oley Foundation, a support group for Home Enteral and Parenteral Nutrition patients. Comments from other persons are included in *italics*. Much of the information shared with the reader is based upon personal experience and additional information is available through the Oley Foundation.

The first 18 months of enteral therapy were very difficult for me. Some patients resolve their challenges more quickly. A description of the difficulties I faced early in my therapy, compared to my success with enteral therapy more recently, will illustrate some of the problems clinicians encounter with their patients and provide examples of successful outcomes. Topics will include a comparison of my activity level and socialization, emotional and psychological challenges, discovering resources and finding support, feeding tube management, and the evolution of my daily nutrition support routine.

Life Before Home Enteral Nutrition

Before it became a part of my life, I knew nothing about enteral nutrition. I was reasonably well educated (with a couple of college degrees), I was a successful businessman, the president and CEO of a small company, and I was very involved with other leaders in my community. Despite this, I felt overwhelmed by the complexity of medical technology and medical terms used to describe my new way of life. I had been active, athletic, and outgoing. I traveled frequently, often to Europe and Asia. I was recognized as a leader in my industry. I had a good life. Suddenly, it was all lost.

Underlying Illness or Incident

Difficulty swallowing (dysphagia) can result from several different causes: cancer, stroke, digestive diseases, trauma, and so on. For some patients, the need for enteral therapy develops slowly, and the decision to place a feeding tube is arrived at slowly and thoughtfully. For others, like me, there is no time to think about it. It is done because you need it done. A nasogastric (NG) tube is an immediate solution. Some patients begin to adapt to their feeding tube right away, and they can focus on learning self-management of their feeding tube and coping with their new way of getting nutrition. For other patients, the underlying illness or incident is their primary focus. For me, the feeding tube was of no more consequence than the electrodes taped to my chest, although the NG tube was considerably more uncomfortable. My focus was on recovering from my stroke; learning to walk again; learning to talk again, learning to think logically; and trying to regain my energy, my muscle tone, and my strength.

Stroke

There are 500,000 strokes a year in the United States. Of those, 170,000 are fatal. Stroke is the third leading cause of death in the United States, and stroke is the number one cause of disability. I had a stroke in my brain stem. A small blood vessel carrying nutrients and oxygen to a few million of my several billion brain cells failed. It may have been clogged up by a blood clot, it may have ruptured, or it may have just worn out and collapsed. Whatever the cause, the result was dead brain cells. Deprived of nutrition and oxygen, the brain cells died. The ones that died controlled the muscles that opened and closed my cricopharyngeal sphincter (the valve between my esophagus and the back of my throat) and the muscles of my esophagus that caused peristaltic motion, moving food down my esophagus to my stomach. The stroke also affected the muscles and nerves on my right side. My right leg was too weak to support me. I had difficulty raising my right arm and had almost no grip strength in my right hand. I had no sensation of pain or temperature on my right side. Proprioceptor nerves on my right side were impaired, causing apparent balance problems. Additional brain stem stroke syndromes of vomiting, nausea, vertigo, and hiccups complicated my nutrition and feeding tube therapy.

Enteral Feeding Tube

A day or two after being admitted to the hospital, my NG tube was replaced with a percutaneous, endoscopically placed gastro-jejunostomy (PEG-J) tube by an interventional radiologist (see Chapter 5). The tube and the placement were decided by my doctor—I was not consulted although I would not have been able to ask questions about other tubes, anyway.

Priorities of the Patient

Learning about how to recover from my stroke delayed my learning about how to manage my enteral therapy. More important to me, the day after my stroke, a physical therapist asked me to stand up beside my bed. I put my feet on the floor and would have fallen on my face if he had not caught me. Physical therapy and learning to walk again started right away. It was a challenge.

I was told that swallowing disorders were not uncommon following a stroke and that most stroke survivors would recover their ability to swallow within 6 months. My feeding tube was only a temporary inconvenience. I may have received excellent training from the hospital's nutrition support staff while I was in the rehab ward, but I probably did not pay much attention because it was not something I had to worry about for very long, and I had much more important issues to deal with. My priorities did not include my feeding tube. The extent of the patient's focus on his or her underlying illness will affect the patient's ability to learn about his or her feeding tube.

Experience with Health Care Providers

The clinician's ability to help the patient will also be affected by the patient's experience with other health care providers. A positive experience will create a positive expectation by the patient for the help provided by the nutrition support clinician. The doctor of rehabilitative medicine assigned to my case could not answer any of my questions about the cause of my stroke or the gastric distress I was having, or give me any hope for continued recovery. Many medical doctors are very good. Some could use additional training. A gastroenterologist called the Oley Foundation and asked, *"Do tube feeders have bowel movements?"* A retired doctor who learned I had a feeding tube said, *"I don't think I would want to go on living if I could not enjoy a good meal."* Another HEN patient said, *"I am frustrated with the lack of information from my doctor. He doesn't communicate very well, even when I ask direct questions."* When I was discharged from rehab, I stayed in a hotel for two more weeks because I was not strong enough to climb the stairs to our bedroom at home. The first weekend at the hotel, the enteral feeding pump stopped working. We called the home care company and asked for someone to bring us an instruction book for the pump. Instead, they sent a home care nurse who had no clue about how an enteral pump worked. She suggested that I try to swallow something. I thought it was obvious that if I could swallow, then I would not need an enteral pump, and I told her so. We called the hospital's nutrition support number and got a recording giving us a pager number. We called the pager number and entered the hotel phone number at the prompt. No one called back. We finally went to an emergency room, where they hooked me up to a pump and fed me. We learned that it is important to have a home care company with experienced clinicians with specific experience with enteral feeding, because providing supplies and formula is not enough. Having someone to call who is familiar with enteral feeding is essential. If this is not available through the home care company, then the hospital dietitian may be able to help.

Slow Recovery, Activity Level, and Socialization

Stroke recovery was slow. In the hospital, I gradually pushed my walker a little bit farther each day. At the hotel, I could slowly shuffle down the hall without my walker if I supported myself against the wall. At home, I walked with my wife every day. At first, I held on to her for support and walked only a short distance. Eventually, I could walk the length of a block. Two months after my stroke, I could walk several blocks.

In the months following my stroke, there was very little time for activities or socialization. I spent 10 hours a day sitting under an IV pole. I was fed four times a day, for two and one-half hours each time. Sometimes, I was fed up to seven times a day if a feeding needed to be discontinued because of nausea, reflux, bloating, cramps, or vomiting. In spite of the time needed for feeding, I forced myself to get out. Every day, my wife took me for a walk. Every day, we walked a little farther, measuring our progress by the number of houses we walked past, and, later, by the number of blocks we could walk. After 3 months, I tried to ski. Skiing was my passion. After 4 months, I tried to work, going to my office for a few hours once or twice a week. I took my IV pole, my pump, my gravity bags, formula, tubes, syringes, and other paraphernalia to the office with me. Hooked up to my feeding tube, spitting into a cup every few minutes (because I could not even swallow my own saliva), making rude sounds to clear mucous from the back of my throat, and looking as bad as I felt, I was not the image of a strong, successful CEO. Obviously, I could not "wine and dine" clients. Obviously, I could not travel. After trying to work, I was exhausted and realized I was ineffective. I could not work and, consequently, I retired on disability. Except for daily walks and doctor visits, I spent most of my time at home. I did not share meals with my family. I did not go out to dinner with friends. I did not go skiing. I did not go shopping or to movies. I could not travel. I was isolated.

I was laid low by a stroke. Being unable to swallow and unable to enjoy all the pleasures of eating added insult to my injury. It was devastating emotionally and psychologically. I felt overwhelmed. I was depressed. The sister of a new HEN patient sent me an email that said, *"My brother got a feeding tube last week. He is struggling with putting eight cans of formula into his system every day. I am more concerned about his mental state. This seems to have thrown him into a life-isn't-worth-living tailspin and I feel powerless to know what to say or do to help."* Another HEN patient said, *"Sometimes I feel like, why did this happen to me? Is God testing me?"* Sitting under an IV pole ten hours a day, I watched a lot of television. Do you know how many TV commercials are about food or restaurants? Too many! Enteral therapy provides the basic requirements for nourishment, but patients must still cope with being unable to enjoy the social, cultural, religious, and sensory pleasures of eating. It is a challenge for enteral nutrition patients to enjoy Thanksgiving, Rosh Hashanah, Easter, birthdays, weddings, anniversaries, reunions, or picnics. I could not work. Much of "who I was" was "what I did." I had been "somebody" before my stroke. Now, I was "nobody" and I felt alone. Another HEN patient said, *"I felt like I was the only one this way."*

However, I had a desire to get better, or maybe even get to my best—and I did!

Current Level of Activity and Socialization

Now, I am as active, or more active, as I ever was. During the past ski season, I skied three to four days a week. During the summer, I hiked and rode my bike. Even though I cannot eat or drink, I go to restaurants with my friends and family. I just do not order. I realized how many social activities involve food. If I did not go out to eat with friends and family, I would miss their company and conversation. Now, we have friends to our home for dinner and I cook and serve. We go to movies, concerts, the theatre, football games, gymnastic meets, and play cards in several bridge clubs. I consult in my former business. I teach skiing to persons with disabilities. I serve as president of our condominium development homeowner's association, write articles for magazines, and speak to civic clubs and at clinical meetings. In the past few years, my wife and I have traveled to New Zealand, England, Denmark, Germany, Norway, Russia, Hawaii, Alaska, and dozens of other states. From isolation and minimal activity, I have progressed to a full, active life with friends and family. The progression occurred over time, in purposeful, gradual increments.

My life is good! I do the things I want to do whenever I want to do them. Every day is like a vacation day. I can play hard. Volunteer work is very satisfying and emotionally rewarding. Comments from other HEN patients I have talked with include, *"You helped me realize that I should be happy for all the good things I still have in my life."* There is almost no stress in my life. I have no major worries. I cannot recall when I felt more emotionally and psychologically healthy. From depression and anger, I have progressed to genuine happiness and great satisfaction with my life. It did not change for the better overnight but, rather, it was a slow and gradual process. But, in one regard, positive change occurred relatively quickly. Five months after my stroke, I still felt extreme fatigue and exhaustion. I wanted to know if this would be a permanent consequence of my stroke and made an appointment with the neurologist who was on call when I came into the emergency room and who told me about the effects of my stroke the following day. From our first visit, he knew that I liked to ski and he asked if I had been skiing yet. I told him that I had tried, but I could not do it. He said he would be very depressed if he could not ski and prescribed an antidepressant, which came in a liquid form and was easy to infuse through my tube. Apparently, I was as much physically depressed as I was mentally depressed. Within a month, I felt less fatigued and more optimistic about my recovery. I became mellow and less irritable. The antidepressant made me easier to live with. My wife said it was the best thing to happen to her!

Resources and Support for Successful HEN

From the first day, my wife has been the strongest source of my support. Our son, who had lived out of state for 10 years, returned to the city we lived in only a few months before my stroke. As much as my wife was my strongest support as my caregiver, he was her strongest support. A supportive family has been very important to my recovery. The Oley Foundation was the other major area of support. The support from my wife has been a constant factor, but the support and resources of the Oley Foundation have had an increasingly positive effect over time.

Current Daily Routine for Tube and Formula Management

I have a low-profile gastrostomy tube that is very easy to care for. Each morning, I infuse ~600 mL, my morning meds and a cup of coffee, and I fill two thermos bottles, each with 400 mL of formula. I put the remaining 600 mL in the fridge. I take the thermos bottles in a backpack when I go skiing and take breaks for feeding in the late morning and the late afternoon. I infuse the remaining 600 mL (warmed up in the microwave) with my evening meds and six ounces of red wine. It is a good reminder that I need to hydrate after I feed (because I never get thirsty, I sometimes forget to hydrate). From ten hours a day and a preoccupation with the management of my tube and formula, I have progressed to less than two hours a day, and my tube and formula are only incidental parts of my life.

Strategies and Techniques for Coping and Resilience

The ability to cope emotionally and psychologically develops concurrently with the ability to manage your feeding tube, other supplies, and your formula. An attitude of personal responsibility is most important to successful coping and will empower the patient to manage the challenges of enteral therapy. A study describes five internal and external resources that compliment and derive from the attitude of personal responsibility:[3]

- accepting the need for enteral nutrition and the associated therapy

- seeking and accepting support from family, friends, health care professionals, the Oley Foundation and similar organizations, and from spiritual sources
- taking charge of your personal well being
- maximizing independence and achieving "normality"
- maintain a positive focus

The concept of "personal responsibility" is an underlying factor in all the strategies and techniques used to make progress from the initial difficulties associated with enteral therapy to efficient management of the therapy and achievement of a high quality of life.

Setting Goals and Measuring Progress

Goal setting can be used for many challenges. Goals should be achievable and progress toward the goal should be measurable. Initially, I recovered my ability to walk by setting a goal of pushing my walker from my bed to the door in my hospital room—only a few steps. My first goal, the day after my stroke, was not to hike across the Grand Canyon!

My next goal was to walk a short distance down the hospital hallway. At home, I measured my progress by the number of blocks I could walk. My tube-feeding goal was to reduce the time I spent under an IV pole. Gradually, I increased the volume of formula I infused during the first and last feedings of the day. I reduced the volume of formula infused for the middle two feedings during the day. At the same time, I gradually increased the flow rate of the pump. I made the changes as quickly as my gut would tolerate. When too much formula was being infused too quickly, causing bloating, cramps, vomiting, or diarrhea, I cut back for awhile until my gut would settle down. Then I would start the process again. It was several months of gradual change. I thought of this period as "Boot Camp for My Gut." A similar approach helped me regain my strength and endurance. Resistance training (lifting weights) at the gym began with very small weights and very few repetitions. Weight and repetitions increased in small, gradual increments each time I went to the gym. Eating with family and friends also followed a gradual process. At first, I only watched while my family ate during their meals. Gradually, I sat down with them and entered the mealtime conversations. Eventually, I began cooking again on our grill. To become "acclimatized" to restaurants, I went with family to fast food restaurants with no table service. From there, I progressed to casual family restaurants. And, finally, I went to nice restaurants with friends who knew of my condition and my desire to "normalize" my life. In most other ways, I progressed from difficulty to competency in gradual and incremental steps.

The Oley Foundation

After 18 months of focusing my efforts on walking and regaining strength after my stroke, and of searching for a swallowing solution from experts around the country, I turned my attention to my enteral nutrition opportunity. Since first going home, a dietitian from the Nutrition Support Department at my hospital followed my case. She called regularly to ask how much I weighed and how well I was tolerating my feedings. When I asked her about traveling, she sent me a photocopy of an article about traveling, which had been printed in the newsletter of the Oley Foundation. That was when I first realized that I did not need to feel isolated. That was when I realized there were other people like me. I called the Oley Foundation and learned more. A few weeks later, I attended their annual conference. It was a life-changing event. I met people who had gotten on with their lives in spite of having a tube in their tummies. From the patient-oriented clinical conferences presented by experienced clinicians, I learned all about enteral nutrition because they really cared about people who depended on enteral therapy. I used the Oley website and read past issues of their newsletter. I ordered copies of their videotapes. I corresponded by email and telephone with several of the people I met at the Oley conference. I learned that for most patients who become involved with Oley (membership is free) the annual conference is their most valuable resource. A patient I recently talked with said, *"I'm going to try to come to an Oley conference because I would like to meet other people like you and me."* Another patient said, *"You are the only person that has a feeding tube that I have been in contact with."* The Oley Foundation has done so much for me that I am glad to volunteer as a regional coordinator and board member so that I can help other home enteral nutrition patients cope with their therapy as well as they possibly can. Another patient said, *"I am hopeful that with the information from you and the Oley Foundation, that I can regain and maintain my independence."*

Conclusion

I am very fortunate. My diet is as healthy as it can be. I can adjust my calorie intake to match my calorie output and maintain an ideal weight. I have high energy. I can ski, hike, travel, and enjoy being with friends and family. I do volunteer work that is rewarding and satisfying. I have no worries and no stress. Five years ago, I was miserable, frustrated, angered, and overwhelmed by the sudden change in my life and an unpleasant means of receiving nutrition. Today, I am thriving on home enteral nutrition support.

LINDA

Introduction

From the moment we discover we are going to become a parent, the topic of conversation seems to center around breast milk versus formula, when to start solids, and what foods to avoid. Whether through an anomaly at birth or an injury, the issue of feeding becomes all encompassing for the parent of a child whose life depends on home parenteral or enteral nutrition (HPEN).

My darling daughter is now 25 years old. She has been on either enteral or parenteral nutrition most of her life due to a surgical complication at 2 months of age. She now lives independently in her own apartment at college. She dates, travels, gets speeding tickets, and is an all-around "normal" person. She is a successful woman with a bright future ahead of her. Hers is not always an ideal life, but I have never met anyone whose life is picture perfect all of the time. We all must face the challenges of life, and with a child whose existence is dependent on HPEN, we as parents have an extraordinary role in their development. What I relay in this chapter is solely based on my experience as a parent and what I found to be successful.

Accepting the Diagnosis

As strange as it might seem, it was easier to accept the implementation of HPN than HEN. When my daughter was put on enteral nutrition, I received less than 1 hour of instruction and then I was sent home. I was nervous and felt alone. I educated myself and talked with other parents. I knew that she needed help with her nutrition and did feel relived when she started to get her energy and stamina back.

When it became obvious that she would need HPN, she was an inpatient and the support and education I received has been life sustaining for many years. I did feel threatened as a parent that I could not furnish this naturally to my child. Through the education I was given I learned to accept the need for HPN and how to avoid complications. One physician even arranged for me to visit a parent and child in his home. There is no substitute for education.

Growing Up with HPN

When we agreed to HPN, we developed a motto that is still with us today. Having this condition is a reason but never an excuse to short-change your life. We would not place her on this life-sustaining therapy with its potential for life-threatening complications if it were not for her will to live her life all-embracing. It is essential that the child on HPEN be given support to live the childhood experience to his or her capability. Sleepovers, field trips, school trips, dating, and hobbies are all feasible. Timing of appointments needs to honor the lifestyle of the child when possible. School nurses can be trained to help with infusions. Letters with details to the appropriate school departments can ease many fears and help the parents advocate for their child to arrange for help and guidance.

Hospitalizations

Hospitalization is a scary time for anyone. You find yourself among strangers and your privacy is compromised in the best of circumstances. Children find themselves thrust into a world of unknown people, procedures, and possibly pain. Sadly, sometimes they know what will be happening. The parents are sleep deprived from sleeping in a chair and they now find their role in caring for their child is altered.

The one most fearful issue is hand washing. To a parent of a HPN child, protecting the central venous line from infection is as important as protecting your child from running in front of a car. I realized that most clinicians washed their hands before entering the room, but that was not enough. I would only feel safe when I saw them wash their hands. I developed a handout to make this request. It was a hot pink business card that said, "Thank you for taking care of our daughter. If you feel that we are overprotective, it is because we are. We will never wash our hands of her. **PLEASE WASH YOURS.**"

When the time to discuss treatment, further testing, or possible surgery comes, it is usually better to wait until the parent is alone. Young children tend to get scared. But when the child becomes a teenager, they need to know what is going on. Parents will have to agree to give this right to the clinician but once it is obtained, the clinician can talk directly to the child and in terms they can understand. I think you will be amazed at their level of understanding. Most young people become more compliant when they are involved in the decisions.

Developing Relationships

When it is first evident that a child needs to be on HPEN, developing a trust between so many people can be difficult. The child's physical, social, and mental well-being is primary. Developing a relationship with parents can smooth a sometimes rocky road. Realize that they are sharing one of the most primary roles they have with you—nourishing their child, and you, in return, are asking parents to take on the role of medical caregiver and sometimes being responsible for treatments that only a few are allowed to administer in an inpatient setting. With these extremes it is vital that everyone involved be trusting, respectful, and cooperative.

Preparing for the Future

The one thing that I have found to be true is that people can live a lifetime on HPEN. Given this, it is important to prepare the pediatric patient to be independent. I feel very proud that my daughter has realized her independence and is out there experiencing all that life has to offer. She has her issues to deal with, and I am proud that she has developed skills that help her cope. She still can get acutely ill and need my help, and I step into the role of caregiver when asked and quietly step down when she is back on her feet. The fact that she can take care of herself and plan for her future is a testimonial to each and every person who helped take care of her while she grew up.

REFERENCES

1. Dudrick SJ. History of vascular access. *J Parenter Enteral Nutr.* 2006; 30(suppl 1):S47–56.
2. Kindle R. Life with Fred. *Nutr Clin Prac.* 2003;18:235–237.

3. Cheryl W. Thompson. PhD Dissertation. *Fostering coping skills and resilience in home enteral nutrition consumers.* Department of Health Promotion and Education: 12/2005.

Additional Credits

CHAPTER 3
Table 3-5 Morrison SG. Clinical nutrition physical examination. *Support Line*. 1997;19(2):16-18.

CHAPTER 4
Table 4-1 Reprinted with permission from Fuhrman MP, Newton A. Transitioning the Patient from Acute Care to Home Care, DNS Home & Alternate Site Home Page, http://www.dnsdpg.org.

CHAPTER 8
Figure 8-1 Adapted with permission from L.E. Matarese, E. Steiger, D.L. Seidner (eds.), Intestinal Failure and Rehabilitation, A Clinical Guide, p. 238, Copyright, 2005, CRC Press LLC.

Table 8-3 Reprinted with permission from L.E. Matarese, E. Steiger, D.L. Seidner (eds.), Intestinal Failure and Rehabilitation, A Clinical Guide, p. 237 Copyright, 2005, CRC Press LLC.

Table 8-16 Reprinted with permission from L.E. Matarese, E. Steiger, D.L. Seidner (eds.), Intestinal Failure and Rehabilitation, A Clinical Guide, p. 240 Copyright, 2005, CRC Press LLC.

Table 8-18 Reprinted with permission from Hamilton C, Parenteral nutrition-associated metabolic bone disease. Support Line 2003; 25(5): 12.

Subject Index

A

Abbot, W. O., 61

Abdominal distention, complicating enteral nutrition, 98

Accreditation Commission for Health Care, Inc. (ACHC), home infusion providers accredited by, 225

Activities of Daily Living (ADLs), in nutrition assessment, 45

Actual, measured body weight (ABW), 35, 38

Acute care patients, energy requirements of, 49

Acyclovir, potential GI effects of, 376

Additives
administration of, 215
in pediatric PN, 238

Adiposity, 39. *See also* Fat

AdminaStar Federal, Inc., 396

Advocate, nurse as patient's, 276

Aid to Families with Dependent Children, 394

Air embolism, as potential complication, 270

Albumin, 45, 48

Alpha 1-antitrypsin deficiency, 280

American Academy of Pediatrics (AAP), on infant formulas, 165

American Diabetes Association
disease classification of, 291
guidelines of, 292

American Dietetic Association (ADA), nutrition care process of, 30, 32

American Medical Association (AMA), Nutrition Advisory Group of, 52

American Society for Parenteral and Enteral Nutrition (A.S.P.E.N.), 215–216
Clinical Evidence Rating System of, 13
Clinical Guidelines, 29
HPN standards of, 134
mission of, 12
on nutrition assessment, 30–31, 33
practice guidelines of, 17, 20, 21, 83–84, 116
'Safe Practices for Parenteral Nutrition Formulations' of, 128

American Society of Gastrointestinal Endoscopy, 61

Amino acids. *See also* Protein